To Rob P Allen —
Something to fill those
empty bookshelves

with love
and in friendship,

Ruth

PIOUS TRADERS IN
Medicine

PIOUS TRADERS IN

Medicine

A German
Pharmaceutical
Network in
Eighteenth-Century
North America

Renate Wilson

The Pennsylvania State University Press
University Park, Pennsylvania

Library of Congress Cataloging-in-Publication Data

Wilson, Renate, 1930–
    Pious traders in medicine : a German pharmaceutical
network in eighteenth-century North America /
 Renate Wilson.
        p.   cm.
    Includes bibliographical references and index.
    ISBN 0-271-02052-0
    1. Medicine—United States—History—18th century.
    2. Medicine—Germany—History—18th century.
    3. Pietists—United States—History—18th century.
    4. Pietists—German—History—18th century.
    5. Pharmacy—United States—History—18th century.
    6. Missionaries, Medical—United States—History—
    18th century.   I. Title.

R151.W54 2000
610'.973'09033—dc21   99-086276

Copyright © 2000 The Pennsylvania State University
All rights reserved
Printed in the United States of America
Published by The Pennsylvania State University Press,
University Park, PA 16802-1003

It is the policy of The Pennsylvania State University Press
to use acid-free paper for the first printing of all cloth-
bound books. Publications on uncoated stock satisfy the
minimum requirements of American National Standard
for Information Sciences—Permanence of Paper for
Printed Library Materials, ANSI Z39.48–1992.

Contents

Figures

Tables

I first encountered a German Pietist physician practicing in colonial North America in the detailed reports home by his superior in the colony of Georgia. Ernst Thilo had studied medicine at the Friedrich University in Halle in Brandenburg-Prussia and had come over in 1737 as *medicus* for a settlement of Salzburger refugees, among whom he practiced until his death in 1765. Despite his superior's generally disapproving accounts of his medical practice and practices, which extended over thirty years, he died leaving behind considerable property. I was intrigued by several aspects of this practice, which included large orders of drugs and materia medica from his Halle motherhouse, the Francke Orphanage Foundations. His generally expectationist attitude toward aggressive medical treatment evoked the principles of his German mentors, who had been students of the vitalist and chemical philosopher Georg Ernst Stahl, and suggested that vitalist medicine was not entirely unknown on these shores.

Thilo's orders from Germany threw light on the extent of the large-scale manufacture and trade in carefully labeled proprietary medicines under the Halle Orphanage label. These proprietaries—intended both for professional use and for the self-medicating public—had been developed by the brothers Richter, pious entrepreneurs and themselves students of Georg Ernst Stahl. The trade was well known, mainly in terms of its *arcana*, in German accounts of eighteenth-century pharmacy. But the notion of a continuous trade into the British colonies is not to be found in either the German or the North American literature, although the dispensing of Halle Orphanage medications by Lutheran clerics had been noted by Whitefield Bell Jr., Rosalind Wolman, and other careful readers of the diaries of Heinrich Melchior Mühlenberg in Pennsylvania.

Mühlenberg, a pastor trained at the Halle Orphanage, came to North America to take over a number of German Lutheran parishes in the early 1740s, and, like other Halle missionaries to the East and West Indies prepared for their mission in this extraordinary institution, he had been given a measure of medical instruction in a large dispensary that used the Orphanage medications for charity and commercial purposes. As the patriarch of Pietist pastors in this country, Mühlenberg was at the center of the network of information and influence that stretched between Halle, the Pietist establishment in London, and the North American British colonies. His example is the best known, but his vicars and catechists and eventually his sons and sons-in-law all were engaged in the occasional practice of medicine, a route well known to the clergy of the time who needed to augment their stipends.

When I worked my way back to the origin of these medications—their composition, their place in a changing European system of therapeutics, their shipment through London as charitable and untaxed goods—I found in the copious and well-preserved Halle archives of the Francke Foundations a treasure trove of sources unknown to English-language historians of medicine. The sources documented a pious trade in medicines, not only within Germany, but across Europe and the oceans, to Tranquebar in East India and to North America. The trade was driven largely by the need of the Foundations to invest and leverage their capital from charitable bequests and legacies, which they used to fund a large printing press and the manufacture of medications.

In the pharmaceutical trade, the Foundations were indeed extraordinary. Like Halle and the pious Bible societies in England before them, eighteenth-century evangelicals like George Whitefield and John Wesley tapped into the extraordinary, and extraordinarily profitable, demand for the written Christian word both in England and on these shores. But in terms of medical supplies, Halle could command the medical resources and reputation of a famous medical school and, in this country, a network of clergy, their spouses, and their commercial associates in the clusters of German-speaking congregations and settlements that were willing to increase their stipends and their influence by dispensing these medications on the charity and for profit.

So much for the closely and well-documented supply side. On this side of the Atlantic, it was far more difficult and in many cases impossible to trace this modest but continuous trade under favored philanthropic auspices into the German communities and beyond. Although large volumes of the Orphanage medications are known to have been dispensed throughout Europe and into Russia, at considerable profit by mid-century, their North American presence other than through the channels described in this book can be glimpsed only through a variety of indirect sources. There are occasional advertisements in colonial journals, references to the disapproval of English-language physicians in correspondence home, and hints that travelers brought these and other medicinals in their luggage as part of a modest but steady shipboard trade over the decades from 1730 to 1815.

One explanation for this little-noted persistence of a German medical niche in a well if spottily supplied colonial market in materia medica is language and brand recognition. The medications from Halle, although expensive and scarce, were well known, above all for their safety and constant composition. In other words, they had predictable effects. Moreover, their nomenclature was familiar to persons of German-language background; they were accompanied by German-language product sheets and manuals; and they were distributed, among others, by reputable German clergy. This assumption of language driving medical preference in a multilingual and open community of medical providers and patients made sense of the broader but still little-known community of German medical men and women, many but not all of sectarian religious backgrounds, some well trained, some not, who practiced in German ways in German congregations from New York to South Carolina and Georgia.

Like other recent scholars of Halle Pietism in North America, I have concentrated in this book on the well-documented exchanges between Halle and its clergy, using the widely dispersed literature on other German medical practitioners, lay and clerical, to show that the men from Halle did not practice their charitable brand of medicine in a vacuum. By setting out, in some detail, the background of the trade from Halle and its medical and philanthropic underpinnings, I hope to show that traditions and therapeutic approaches of mainstream German medicine were well established on these shores by the middle of the eighteenth century. Additional work on the academics trained in this Central European tradition and its therapeutic preferences—Adam Kuhn and Casper Wistar come most readily to mind—will be needed to show how these traditions fed into the botanic and eclectic medicine of the early American republic.

To readers interested in the mechanisms of eighteenth-century transatlantic trade, the German sources also offer some extraordinary insights into the transfer of philanthropic capital and interest through both London and Amsterdam. Heading a voluntary organization located in the backwaters of eighteenth-century colonial enterprise, the founders of the Francke Foundations and their successors used established banking connections in Hamburg, Frankfurt, and the Netherlands as well as the Protestant colonial networks to the East and West Indies with an extraordinary and aggressive skill that belies the notion of a quietist and unenterprising civil society. And despite the perils of religious stewardship during a period of growing state control and secularization, the charitable capital invested into the Foundations by German benefactors over the course of the century found its way into the new United States, where it could be safely invested—or so it was hoped—at better rates of interest. That pharmaceuticals, Bibles, and books were the means of transferring these funds throws some light on the perceived opportunities, however short-lived, of trade with the United States under a new polity.

In piecing together this story of a pious trade in medicine, I have incurred many debts of gratitude to archivists, colleagues, and organizations on both sides of the Atlantic. My early work at the Halle archives in the 1980s fell in a period of difficult access. Once inside the magic castle of the Francke archives, however, those privileged to work there were taken in hand by the then archivist, Jürgen Storz, and given glimpses of untold archival riches. The hours spent in a tiny upstairs office of the still-extant if crumbling Orphanage buildings with materials nobody had seen since the 1950s or earlier are part of the magic of archival research. My entry into the complexities of Halle pharmaceutical manufacture was eased by the challenging collaboration with Pharmazierat Hans Joachim Pöckern, who generously shared with me the inside story of these medications and their development. For much valuable advice and tolerance of my lack of theological training and innocence of doctrine, I owe a special debt of gratitude to Professors Friedrich de Boor and Udo Sträter, both renowned Pietist historians from both sides of the former German divide. And I wish to take this opportunity to recall the gracious advice to students and scholars offered by the late Georg Harig, of the Department of the History of Medicine at the Charité, who although certainly no admirer of Pietism and its medicine, shared with me and many foreign visitors the riches of an astute, learned, and critical mind.

The Francke Foundations have weathered the transition to a new world, to computers and new buildings, and my thanks for many acts of kindness and research support go to their archivist, Thomas Müller-Bahlke, and his staff, the head librarian of the gloriously reconstituted library, Britta Klosterberg, and of course to Professor Paul Raabe, to whom the Foundations owe, literally, the roof over their head and much else. The Center for the Study of Pietism, under the knowledgeable and deft leadership of Udo Sträter, was throughout supportive of my work. I thank as well Professors Richard Töllner and Christa Habrich for advice and shared knowledge in the history and implications of Pietist medicine and ethics. Professor Fritz Krafft gave me the opportunity to discuss my work with colleagues during a month at the Marburg Institute for the History of Pharmacy, and Robert Jütte of the Robert Bosch Institute extended the same welcome courtesy at his dynamic center in Stuttgart.

For the core problems in the history of pharmacy addressed in this book, my work would not have been possible, in the fullest sense of the word, without the support, advice, and astute criticism of David L. Cowen, John Worth Estes, and

John K. Crellin. I thank the members of the National Library of Medicine study panel who considered the questions in the history of medicine and pharmacy raised in my various proposals not unworthy of some support. That I have been unable to answer all of them in a definitive fashion they probably foresaw, and I appreciate their forbearance. Gregory Higby and Glenn Sonnedecker of the Institute for the History of Pharmacy at the University of Wisconsin gave generously of their advice and support. I owe them and the then chair of the History of Medicine Department, Harold Cook, and Phyllis Kaufmann, the curator of books, for a rewarding month in the Wisconsin Medical School Library, which I used mainly for a rare in-depth reading of all 1,200 pages of the Richter tract that figures so prominently in these pages. In the 1980s, when I started my work on Pietist medicine, Gert Brieger, chair of the Institute for the History of Medicine, encouraged me to delve into the history of therapeutics of the eighteenth century, and Jerome Bylebyl shared generously his historical knowledge. Edward Morman, Christine Ruggere, former and present rare book curators at the Institute, and Linda Bright were helpful and resourceful, as were Donald Peterson of the Lutheran Theological Seminary at Germantown, Pennsylvania, Adele A. Lerner, archivist of the New York Hospital and Cornell Medical Center, and the staff of the archives of the New York Public Library. Pastor Frederick S. Weiser of Oxford, Pennsylvania, the keeper of the Mühlenberg flame and himself no mean historian of American religion, was both helpful and generous in his practical support and in his advice. I have enjoyed many and fruitful exchanges on Pietist history in eighteenth-century North America with A. G. Roeber, professor of History and of Religious Studies at The Pennsylvania State University; this book would be much poorer without his multifaceted and innovative work on the German element.

Institutional financial support for this study was provided, in chronological order, by the Taylor Foundation in Atlanta, Georgia, the New Jersey Historical Commission, and a National Library of Medicine Publications Grant (R01 LM 05470). The National Library of Medicine grant made it possible, with the kind help of Professor Richard Töllner, to obtain additional funding from the Alexander von Humboldt Foundation in Bonn under a TransCoop collaborative grant. This additional financial support made it possible to secure the necessary technical help for documenting and summarizing overlapping orders and bills of lading; I thank in particular Jeannette Staudte, Antje Matthäus, and Shahana Sakar for their skill, their patience, and their willingness to tackle the mysteries of eighteenth-century ledger entries. A senior fellowship of the Fulbright

Commission afforded time and opportunity in 1996–97 for final source work on the mechanisms of the pharmaceutical trade.

Some of the material in this book has appeared in preliminary or partial form in German and American journals in the field, in particular a special issue on eighteenth-century German medicine in the British North American colonies, which appeared in volume thirteen of *Caduceus, A Journal for the Medical Humanities*. I thank the journal editors, John S. Haller and Mary Ellen McElligott, for the opportunity to test the ground and, with the help of my co-authors for the guest issue, to revise some historical opinions. The College of Physicians in Philadelphia and the American Philosophical Society and their curators and staff, in particular Thomas Horrocks and Mary Beth Horrocks, generously permitted extensive and repeated access for J. Woodrow Savacool and myself to the deBenneville manuscript and the diaries of Gotthilf Heinrich Ernst Mühlenberg, respectively.

Throughout, Professor Hartmut Lehmann, first at the German Historical Institute in Washington, D.C., and then as director of the Max Planck Institute in Göttingen, followed with interest tempered by his natural skepticism my attempts to make German philanthropy and Pietist medicine part and parcel of a revised history of mutual acculturation and persistence of Central European scholarly traditions in North American society. He may disagree with the implications of some of my findings, but I am most grateful for the encouragement and friendship he and Silke Lehmann have given me over these last ten years.

This book describes medical practices, transatlantic pharmaceutical commerce, and the evolution of a distinct medical market and medical culture in the German Lutheran and Reformed communities of eighteenth-century North America. The story centers on several generations of Pietist ministers who in conjunction with their clerical office provided medical services and imported pharmaceuticals and medical literature during the period from 1740 to 1810. They were supported by the religious, political, and financial network of the Francke Orphanage, their German motherhouse and a famous religious and philanthropic foundation. The pharmaceuticals were manufactured and sold throughout Europe as part of a commercial enterprise founded in support of the Francke Foundations' charitable goals.

The Protestant alliances that had been fostered by the Foundations since the end of the seventeenth century, especially in London, provided favored access to the Lutheran and Reformed congregations of the British North American colonies. The demographic and economic growth of these congregations in both urban and rural areas in turn offered a contiguous field of influence from the 1750s onward for the Pietist ministers and a potential market for the medications manufactured and sold by their motherhouse. In addition to being used in congregational charity practice supported by donations from Germany, the medications and the German self-help texts explaining their indications and appropriate uses attracted the more prosperous segments of the German-language population until the early nineteenth century.

The American medical practice by the men and women of this German network has remained largely unexamined beyond local and anecdotal accounts. This book brings together the findings from a large array of primary sources in European and American archives to provide a full chronological narrative from 1700, when the Foundations started their missions and their manufacture, to 1810, when their North American clergy had become independent from their motherhouse and American medical practice and education had begun to follow its own course.

Scope and Context

One purpose of this study is to describe the genesis of this German Pietist network and its interaction with an American medical environment that during the eighteenth and early nineteenth centuries gave equal place to medical practitioners of varying degrees of training, orthodoxy, and therapeutic orientation. Another purpose is to investigate how and why German patients might have been drawn to these medical ministers and the medications they offered.

The continued ability of the Francke Foundations in establishing and maintaining this link to North America was made possible by a constellation of political and religious trends. Originating in the Protestant territories of Southwest Germany in the 1670s, German Pietism was an evangelical movement of social and religious reform with roots in the mysticism of Johann Arndt.[1] Its followers were found in all social classes and alike among men and women. The right of Pietist laypersons and clergy to preach, teach, and provide charity was contested by orthodox Lutheranism, first in the South German duchy of Württemberg and several of the large Protestant trading cities and subsequently in Saxony and Prussia. In Prussia, the founder, A. H. Francke, and his mentor, Philipp Jakob Spener, eventually managed to turn the tables on their opponents because of the protection extended by the first two Prussian kings, Frederick I (III) and Frederick William I. The latter in particular used the advocates of independent religious and educational reform in his fight against the privileges of the Prussian nobility, which he turned into a class oriented to military and civil service and which had to yield to the crown clerical preferments and local teaching positions.

In seeking a profitable and independent economic base for domestic reform and colonial missions, the Francke Foundations entered into the production and sale of Bibles and edification tracts and of pharmaceutical products early in the eighteenth century. In this commerce, the Halle Orphanage enjoyed some unique advantages deriving from the juncture of religion and medicine. Its medical associates, in particular the brothers Richter, developed and exported a well-defined set of proprietary remedies, including the *essentia dulcis,* a tincture of gold. Some of the success of this trade over the course of the century was based on the consistent quality and reputation of these medications, which providers and patients repaid by brand recognition and loyalty.

Even after the pharmaceutical business became an independent enterprise in the 1740s, its profits continued to accrue to a charitable enterprise that took

---

1. Wallmann, *Philipp Jakob Spener;* Brecht, *Geschichte des Pietismus,* vol. 1, sections III–VIII, H. Lehmann, "Pietismus und weltliche Ordnung"; idem, "Pietismus und soziale Reform"; Hinrichs, *Preussentum und Pietismus.*

great care to preserve its philanthropic status and reputation. Gifts and bequests on behalf of Pietist missions were often channeled wholly or in part to pay for the products of the pharmacy and the printing houses, which then sent their products abroad for charity distribution and sale. In their financial transactions in a period of underdeveloped financial markets, the Foundations relied on many of the stratagems noted by English historians of medicine and pharmacy, including a trade in discounted drafts and letters of credit.[2] The medicines became part of the trade in military physic chests used in the many wars of the eighteenth century, and Pietist officers and merchants promoted them in numerous campaigns. Although the developers and proponents of the medications would have rejected any claims that they practiced sectarian medicine, it can be argued that the mechanisms of this trade prefigured the later development and marketing practices of closed sectarian therapeutic systems, particularly in North America, such as Thomsonianism, eclectic pharmacy, and homeopathy.[3]

An advocate of social and charity reform, Halle Pietism also acted as an aggressive missionary movement in the eighteenth-century colonial context, providing clergy to Danish and English stations in India and the Near East and the settlements of North America. Its German antecedents of social and evangelical reform largely defined and may eventually have restricted the place of Pietist medicine in the development of a distinct and competitive American medical culture. Until the early nineteenth century, however, Pietist pharmaceuticals retained a market niche in German communities and profited from the persistent ties of the German population to medical instruction and self-help texts provided in the German vernacular.

Throughout, the Pietist community in the colonies was not sectarian and isolated. Cotton Mather, himself a major contributor to early American medicine,[4] had been drawn by the growing reputation of the Francke Orphanage to start in 1714 a lengthy correspondence with August Hermann Francke that included book lists and similar items. The Great Awakening of the 1730s in New England and the middle colonies had provided an enthusiastic audience for the social and religious reforms of the Halle Pietists. A Latin biography of Francke

---

2. See in particular Porter and Porter, "Rise of English Drugs Industry." See also Steele, *Atlantic Merchant Apothecary*.

3. Beyerlein, *Die Entwicklung der Pharmazie zur Hochschuldisziplin (1750–1875)*, 72; Haller, *Kindly Medicines*; Berman, "Neo-Thomsonianism"; idem, "Thomsonian Movement." For Hahnemann, see the recent collection of essays published by Dinges, *History of Homeopathy*.

4. Duffy, *Healers*, 96; Mather, *Angel of Bethesda*.

was published by Samuel Mather in Boston in 1733.[5] In the 1740s, the Pietists were well received by Swedish Lutherans and by many of the Reformed German clergy, although their long-standing ties with supporters of the Anglican establishment tested the diplomatic mettle even of Heinrich Melchior Mühlenberg, the main placeholder of Halle Pietism in the colonies. But in terms of therapy and medical concepts, denominational differences and affinities proved less important than the incentives to trade in the Halle medications and a joint European medical tradition. This tradition, and to some extent the trade, was shared with clergy from other denominations and with secular practitioners from Central Europe.

In providing medical care both as charity and on a fee basis, several generations of Pietist ministers and their wives and widows followed the colonial and missionary tradition of joining medicine and religious practice, a phenomenon also observed for Anglican and congregational ministers in New England. In both cases, the augmentation of ministerial stipends was clearly a major motive. However, the first generation of Pietist ministers from the Francke Orphanage could not rely only on the famous medications produced by the motherhouse but had received clinical training in a large dispensary associated with a famous university and medical school in Halle in Brandenburg-Prussia. Several of the second, American-born generation of these clerical and other German practitioners trained in Germany and on their return became part of the clerical and academic American establishment.

The 1760s saw the transition from colonial practice to the self-definition of American physicians. John Morgan and other proponents of the tighter, more professional, and academically oriented medicine they had observed in their student days in Europe, particularly in Scotland and England, frowned on the crossing of professional boundaries between clerics and physicians.[6] But in rural areas and towns of the backcountry, clerics of many denominations persisted in their joint practice of religion and medicine. Although the commercial element that the sale of pharmaceuticals introduced into relationships with parishioners may have confirmed academic prejudice in many cases, others could combine their practice with major contributions to the sciences of the young republic. The case of the minister, botanist, and educator Gotthilf Heinrich Ernst Mühlenberg,

5. The best account of the relationship between Cotton Mather and G. A. Francke is still Lovelace, *American Pietism*.

6. Duffy, *Healers*; Bell, *John Morgan*; Gevitz, *Other Healers*.

the youngest son of Heinrich Melchior Mühlenberg, is one example that this study investigates in some detail.

The religious rivalries of the colonial period have obscured much of the academic path of this clergy. Although we know from board minutes and agendas that the major members of the Lutheran clergy were trustees and professors at the College of Pennsylvania, King's College, and the Society of New York Hospital, to name just a few, Lutheran Pietists and their German Reformed colleagues were barred by political considerations from openly choosing sides between the Presbyterian and Anglican establishments before the Revolution. After the Revolutionary War, many of these Germans were, or were accused of being, loyalists. Among these were Adam Kuhn and Casper Wistar, prominent sons of prominent German settlers and professors of medicine and botany at the forerunner of the University of Pennsylvania. John Housiel, who cofounded New York Hospital but remained loyal to England, went to Nova Scotia. The influence of their European training on medical teaching remains an important area of critical investigation beyond the Pietist clergy that is the core of this book.[7]

Medical providers—both secular and clergy, German and English—eventually adjusted their practice to the challenges of competition and a multicultural society. The reactions of patients and their families—the consumers of medical care—are of equal interest in this study. The general assumption has been that German colonial settlers were isolated from contemporary and professional medical care and quickly lost touch with European trends. But here again, there is evidence to the contrary. The Halle motherhouse was famous for its Bible press and edification tracts, which it produced and shipped to colonial North America in competition with both the Anglican establishment and the Herrnhuters or Moravians during the colonial period.[8] When imports opened up again in the 1790s, a whole new German print market sprang to life, which, together with renewed imports from the Halle motherhouse, covered the entire social spectrum of the German-language communities in the middle colonies.

This new market reflected considerable social stratification in both urban and rural German communities. A diverse German public could and did accommodate traditional folk medicine as well as a more sophisticated therapeutic

---

7. Adam Kuhn's medical views are of particular interest but generally receive only passing mention (see Duffy, *The Healers*, 96; Bell, "A Portrait of the Colonial Physician," 23).

8. Butler, *Awash in a Sea of Faith*; Roeber, "German and Dutch Books and Printing."

armamentarium.[9] A financially well-off section of this public agreed with the social and congregational policies of the Pietist ministers and through them maintained its link to the eighteenth-century European mainstream and even attempted to use it for commercial ends. In both its medical and literary choices, this public insisted on a godly and Christian tradition of medicine and on the active use of the means of healing.[10]

The argument in this book for a specifically German medical culture and market in eighteenth-century North America derives in large part from a large reservoir of materials printed in Gothic type in the High German vernacular, from the mid-century almanacs of the Saur Press to later American imprints of traditional German medical and self-help texts of all descriptions to sophisticated imports from Europe.[11] For it was in good part through the language of transmission and recording of medical knowledge and advice that this culture perpetuated itself and permitted the growth of a market in printed matter and pharmaceuticals that was independent of English intermediaries.

The Pietist and other clergy practicing medicine and dispensing the Halle Orphanage medications in rural areas had at their disposal two Pietist vernacular medical treatises originating at the Halle motherhouse. The more weighty text—the *Höchst-nöthige Erkenntnis des Menschen sonderlich nach dem Leibe* (A most necessary understanding of the body and its natural life)—was followed, in the 1740s, by an abbreviated version—*Kurtze Nachricht* or *A Short Account*—prepared by David Samuel von Madai, a Viennese-trained physician who headed the pharmaceutical commerce of the Orphanage from 1740 to 1777. During the eighteenth century, the text gained a considerable international reputation and was carried by Pietist missions and trade interests across Europe into Dutch, Danish, and English possessions in the East and West Indies.[12] In North America, the Richter text was used by medical providers in the German-language settlements of the southern colonies beginning in 1733 and in the middle colonies shortly thereafter.[13] The mission accounts for Pennsylvania alone show imports of roughly 200 of the 1,200-page volumes by the 1750s, not counting those brought along in the baggage of medical practitioners,

9. Cowen and Wilson, "Traffic in Medical Ideas: Popular Medical Texts as German Imports and American Imprints."

10. Dehmel, *Arzneimittel in der Physikotheologie*.

11. Cowen and Wilson, "Traffic in Medical Ideas."

12. See also Chapter 3 below.

13. Wilson, "Waisenhausmedikamente."

clergy, and laymen. The work thus became part of the medical discourse of North America at least in clerical and medical settings related to German congregations. The Richter *Erkenntnis* and Madai's *Kurzer Bericht* were ordered both in German and in Latin and French translations, indicating their acceptance beyond the German communities. Benjamin Franklin's 1749 translation into German of John Tennent's *Every Man His Own Doctor* during a surge of German immigration thus competed with an imported and a local German print culture.

This is not to imply that there was competition between different national systems of medicine and medical understanding. European medicine of the seventeenth and eighteenth centuries drew on and perpetuated similar traditions of knowledge regardless of country, and any differences between systems of medical thought were a matter not of national but of medical culture. Academic travelers could have picked up the same disputes at Paris as at Copenhagen and Leiden.[14] At the level of vernacular medical literature, the same lack of national boundaries prevailed. Self-help texts, midwife manuals, herbals, and similar material in particular had been printed in the vernacular since the late Middle Ages and translated across Europe without much in the way of reliable attribution, following the unrestrained translation practices of the early modern period.[15] A good portion of these imprints were in the tradition of astrological and even magical medicine, but they also supplied useful information on dyes and veterinary medicine and female complaints. Much of the new German-American print market of the 1790s was thus neither specifically German nor imported to fit a specific therapeutic community. The crucial distinction in our context was that its products were in German, set in German type, and thus both familiar and accessible.[16]

Finally, in the transition from the colonial period to the slow and tortuous socialization of academic and practical medicine over the early part of the nineteenth century, this study seeks a broader understanding of how the American social polity alternately integrated and rejected transatlantic traditions from different cultural and social frameworks. In many ways, early Pietist reforms of charity and charity medical care were closely linked to the state-centered and

14. French and Wear, *Medical Revolution of the 17th Century*; Shackelford, "Rosicrucianism"; Debus, *English Paracelsians*; Cook, "Henry Stubbe."
15. Eamon, *Secrets of Nature*; Getz, *Charity, Translation, and the Language of Medical Learning*; Leibrock-Plehn, *Hexenkräuter oder Arznei*.
16. Butler, *Awash in a Sea of Faith*, chap. 3; Cowen and Wilson, "Traffic in Medical Ideas."

pragmatic medical and public health reforms in the German territories and Vienna. But Pietism was distinguished from the secularist and Enlightenment approach by the juncture of religious and social reform in the lives and duties of evangelical Christians. In Europe, until the French Revolution and even beyond the Napoleonic Wars, this element constituted a socially conservative rather than reactionary force in the polity of what remained of the German nation. In the American environment, this Christian tradition defined the social, economic, and political space that Pietist missionaries from Halle and kindred German elements occupied in the German immigrant community of the colonial and early republican periods.

This transatlantic perspective invites readers to examine more closely the historical origins of American medical practice outside state control, regulation, and support and nourished by voluntarism and philanthropy. Despite their Central European origins and thus their proximity to an increasingly regulated model of medical care,[17] the transatlantic emissaries of the Francke Foundations appear to have fit well into the social dynamics of the emerging American republic. The young polity lacked the traditional European mechanisms that linked welfare policy to an established church. Committed to interdenominational tolerance and civic activism, medical charity not only offered opportunity for but relied almost entirely on the Protestant philanthropy that had developed in Northern Germany and England a century earlier among the evangelical movements of the eighteenth century.

The Cast of Characters—Men and Women in Europe and North America

This study uses a number of concepts and constructs borrowed from social medicine, in particular the notion of a medical market in which medical providers— physicians, apothecaries, midwives, and other trained and untrained men and women—offer their services to patients and their families in times of sickness and other medical need. This market is influenced by the social conditions of the environment in terms of the regulation and hierarchy of medical providers, of patients' expectations and their ability to pay, and of the disease environment. Such market and social and cultural factors are aggregates that permit us to reconstruct the social field in which therapeutic decisions are made. They

---

17. For this background, see the classic works by Rosen (*History of Public Health*) and Lesky (*Österreichisches Gesundheitswesen*).

cannot, however, reflect the individual therapeutic decisions and choices made from the large medical armamentarium that was available to eighteenth-century patients and practitioners even on the fringes of the European medical world.

In our narrative, we can additionally rely on a good amount of personal information about the people who made these choices and about the principals who initiated and pursued the transatlantic traffic in medicines and medical ideas. For reasons of economy, we must rely on the secondary literature for brief accounts of the founders of the Halle enterprise, their competitors, and their religious and medical circle: August Hermann Francke and his son Gotthilf August, and Court Chaplain Friedrich Michael Ziegenhagen in London; Count Nicholas Zinzendorf and other members of the Pietist nobility; the physicians Georg Ernst Stahl, Friedrich Hoffmann, Johann Juncker, and Johann Samuel Carl; and the manufacturers of the pharmaceuticals, the brothers Richter and their successor, David Samuel von Madai.[18] But there is also a rich personal and business correspondence, both published and in manuscript, which is the backbone of this study and which brings to life many of the Halle men and women in America. These people are headed by such familiar names as Heinrich Melchior Mühlenberg, the first ordained minister sent by Halle in 1741 to head an American congregation, and, somewhat less familiar, Johann Martin Boltzius and his successors, who headed the Salzburger congregation in Georgia from its founding in 1733. There are the three Mühlenberg sons—Peter, Friedrich August, and Gotthilf Heinrich Ernst—the first known for his role in the War of Independence; the second Postmaster General of the new republic; and the youngest a minister, founder of Franklin College, and an early and famous American botanist. We also know the paths of several Halle ministers who came in the decade before the Revolution, above all Justus Heinrich Helmuth and Johann Christoph Kunze, who were sent by the Halle Orphanage and were to play major roles among the German clergy and the educational establishment of the late colonial period. There were some trained physicians from Europe, such as Ernst Thilo, George de Benneville,

---

18. For the Halle Pietists and the Moravians, see the wide range of essays in Brecht et al., eds., *Geschichte des Pietismus*, vols. 1 and 2. For the Halle physicians, see the work by Geyer-Kordesch, Konert, and Habrich discussed in greater detail in Chapter 2 of this volume. For the brothers Richter and David Samuel von Madai, see Wilson, "Traffic in Medicines," and the German literature cited in Chapter 3 of this volume.

and Abraham Wagner, and, less accessible through our sources, several dozen German medical providers active in the colonies.[19]

The business ledgers at Halle documenting the pharmaceutical trade also offer a new perspective on a whole range of German merchants in North America, from Heinrich Keppele and the sugar factor Heinrich Schleydorn to the various merchants in Lancaster ordering books, medications, and German lace at the end of the eighteenth century. The Halle archives also offer a rare glimpse of Pietist women, as philanthropic benefactresses in Europe and as patients and pharmaceutical agents in North America. Just as important, we can gain some insight into the demands and opportunities for medical providers and the pharmaceutical trade posed by pregnancy, birth, and female complaints. These offer an additional dimension within the framework of Halle medical practice at the end of the early modern period and for North America before the turn to the nineteenth century.

Presentation and Sources

This account is based on a wide range of primary sources, which in part have only recently come to the attention of scholars engaged in German-American studies.[20] The diaries of Heinrich Melchior Mühlenberg, for instance, are familiar to most historians of the period, as are the journals from Georgia. They have been used to demonstrate the congregational history of the German Lutheran communities and, on an anecdotal basis, the practice of medicine by Mühlenberg in Pennsylvania and by Ernst Thilo in Georgia.[21] The present study in addition

19. For summary descriptions of the German clergy, see Glatfelter, *Pastors and People*, vol. 1. Specific studies of a few of these men are cited in context in Chapters 4 and 5. For the Georgia clergy, see Jones, *The Georgia Dutch*, and for German physicians in North America, see the studies cited in Chapters 4 and 7.

20. An overview of primary sources is provided in a source note preceding the composite bibliography.

21. The corpus of Mühlenberg writings is a well-known and major source for the history of Lutheran and Reformed congregations and German communities in the colonies (Tappert and Doberstein, *Journals of Henry Melchior Mühlenberg*). This study has above all drawn on the more recent and invaluable edition of his unemended letters (Aland et al., eds., *Die Korrespondenz Heinrich Melchior Mühlenbergs*, hereafter referred to as KM) and, for medical practice in the Georgia settlement, on the correspondence and diaries of the Salzburger ministers and their physicians in Missionsarchiv Franckesche Stiftungen [MAFSt] 5 (for Georgia). The diaries are accessible in English as Jones et al., eds., *Detailed Reports of the Salzburger Emigrants Who Settled in Georgia*. For the biographies and work of the corpus of the Halle ministers in the middle colonies, see the comprehensive work by Glatfelter, *Pastors and People*.

draws on the full range of administrative, congregational, and missionary correspondence in the archives of the Francke Foundations, which continue to provide a rich and new source for colonial and early republican studies within the transatlantic context. This applies in particular to the mission ledgers for Pennsylvania and Georgia and to the financial archives, which give a detailed record of a century of commercial and charitable transactions under philanthropic and missionary auspices. The ledgers and attached correspondence include as well the transactions with England, in particular with the court chaplain in London, Friedrich Michael Ziegenhagen, which were crucial for the success of the Pietist missions.[22]

Oriented to both social history and the history of medical practice, this study of religion and medical commerce uses both a narrative account and a topical approach supported by some descriptive statistics. Findings from German archives are integrated with material from American depositories, including some contemporary journals[23] and newspaper accounts. A chronological account of clerical practitioners, their wives, associates, and competitors is developed, as is a record of the geographical dispersal of their practice. Numerical data supported by correspondence and related accounts summarize the trade. The secondary literature, in a composite bibliography at the end of this volume, is drawn from German, English, and American studies on Pietism and its American missions, on the German Lutheran element in North America, and on eighteenth-century medical care and therapy in both Europe and the colonies. For reasons of space, it was necessary to make choices in citing the wide range of German and English works on the topics discussed.

Detailed listings in German and English of the medications used in the charitable commerce from Halle, provided in Chapter 3, guide readers through the welter of eighteenth-century indications for use. To the extent possible, botanical and mineral ingredients are shown, as are prices, unit sizes, and doses suggested by the manufacturer for the more elusive chemiatric preparations. In Chapters 6 and 7, a small set of tables gives an overview of a group of orders

22. This study uses the rarely accessed business archives of the Franckesche Stiftungen at Halle (Wirtschafts und Verwaltungsarchiv, Repertorium ii) and the individual business ledgers for the Georgia (MAFSt Section 5, Series c–e) and Pennsylvania (MAFSt Section 4, Series c–g) missions.

23. Major American primary sources used are the little-known journals of Gotthilf Heinrich Ernst Mühlenberg at the American Philosophical Society in Philadelphia and the de Benneville formulary at the College of Physicians. I thank the present and former curators of manuscripts of the American Philosophical Society and the College of Physicians for their help and generosity in providing access to this complex and little-used material.

placed from North America during the 1770s and 1790s, permitting a modest degree of standardization of quantities ordered and their monetary values. As historians of pharmacy and science know, for the eighteenth century, such standardization may be subject to considerable and multiple errors; I have preferred not to err on the side of caution. However imperfect, these data might be of value in view of the renewed interest in the materia medica of the period.

A final note concerns the treatments of currency equivalents. The transatlantic trade described in this study covers close to nine decades; clearly currency conversion rates and even the currencies involved changed continually against one another and against the pound sterling, both in Europe and in North America during this period. Although the ratio of the pound sterling to the Reichthaler stood at approximately one to five until roughly 1785, using a fixed equivalency rate would introduce numerous and confounding errors and deprive readers and scholars of the opportunity to verify other data sets or transactions against this study. Adjusting each amount to the time series available from McCusker would be both clumsy and of marginal value. Readers interested in approximate valuations of this trade are referred to McCusker's times series for currency equivalents across Europe to the period to 1775 and the more recent work of Markus Denzel for the period to 1815.[24]

24. McCusker, *Money and Exchange in Europe and North America,* chap. 2, esp. tables 2.11–2.17, chap. 3, table 3.7; Denzel, "Die Einbauung der Vereinigten Staaten."

PART one

European Philanthropy,

Pietist Medicine, and the

Pharmaceutical Trade

The Fruit

of Religious

Reform

The first three decades of the eighteenth century saw the rise to prominence of the Francke Foundations in Halle in Brandenburg-Prussia as the major voluntary charitable institution of Protestant Germany. The choice of Halle as home to the Foundations, far from the origins of German Pietism in the German Southwest and its large urban centers like the imperial cities of Frankfurt and Augsburg, was due more to dynastic coincidence than to deliberate preference. The city of Halle and its environs had recently been ceded by the King of Saxony to the Elector of Brandenburg. A medieval town on the river Saale that had lost its status in manufacture and salt extraction during the seventeenth century, Halle lay on the road between the old Magdeburg bishopric and the commercially vibrant city of Leipzig with its fairs and its printing industry. Halle both needed and offered potential for new manufactures and communal reforms. It had a tradition of religious plurality if not tolerance and shared in the rich cultural and musical heritage of Protestant Thuringia and Saxony.

Under the guidance of Ludwig von Seckendorff, author of a famous seventeenth-century treatise on how to reform the estates and centralize administration and tax policy in the German territories,

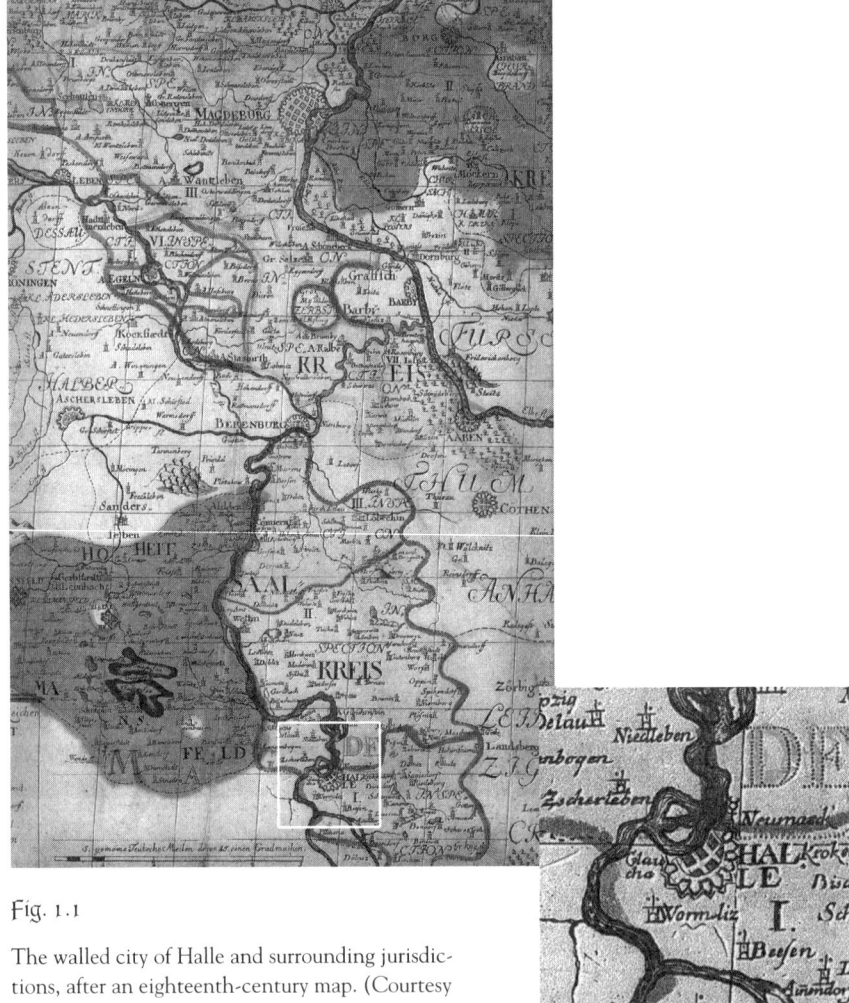

Fig. 1.1

The walled city of Halle and surrounding jurisdictions, after an eighteenth-century map. (Courtesy Franckesche Stiftugen.)

reformers at the Hohenzollern court in Berlin sought to create a new and forward-looking academy emphasizing political economy and natural philosophy.[1] A new and pragmatic academy, which offered its faculty a place of opportunity and European influence, was indeed founded as the *Friedrichs Universität* in 1694, named after its patron, the elector Frederick III, later to be crowned first King of Prussia. His pious but progressive advisers also, if tentatively, encouraged the new charity proposed by evangelical groups outside the Lutheran Church.

The Foundations and their best-known institutional component, the Halle Orphanage, bore the name of their founder, August Hermann Francke (1663–1727), a professor of theology. Francke was a major and combative proponent of the Pietist movement of the latter third of the seventeenth century, which demanded and practiced reform of personal Christian belief and lifestyle and attacked the orthodoxy and the hierarchical institutions of the Lutheran Church as inimical to personal piety, conversion, and revival. In 1692, having been driven from a chair at Leipzig University and a vicarate at Erfurt for his reforming zeal and contentious proposals to reorganize public and private worship, A. H. Francke found refuge, a congregation, and a position of influence at the new university in Halle.[2] He used his influence with pious circles at the Hohenzollern court in Berlin and with Queen Amalia Sophia to set up a large and influential department of theology, placing many of his academic supporters on the faculty.

The philosophical breadth and intellectual excellence of the Halle faculty from the time of its founding to the 1720s were extraordinary for a new university: Among its founding members were Christian Thomasius, the famous legal scholar, humanist, and proponent of the German vernacular in academic teaching, and Friedrich Hoffmann and Georg Ernst Stahl, the two great German contributors to eighteenth-century medical philosophy and practice. Christian Wolff, a famous rationalist philosopher, joined the faculty; other prominent professors included Simon Gasser, who occupied the first Cameralist chair in

1. Written in the aftermath of the Thirty Years' War and the Treaty of Westphalia, volume 1 of the *Teutsche Fürstenstaat* was first published in 1655. Volume 3, the *Christenstaat,* was published in 1685. See Stolleis, "Veit Ludwig von Seckendorff," in *Staatsdenker im 17. und 18. Jahrhundert, Reichspublizistik, Politik, Naturrecht,* 148–73. Seckendorff died in 1692, before the official inauguration of the university. For Prussian administrative reforms during the period 1690–1730, see Hinrichs, *Preussentum und Pietismus: Der Pietismus in Brandenburg-Preussen als religiös-soziale Reformbewegung,* and Deppermann, *Der preussische Staat unter Friedrich III (1).*

2. Brecht, *Geschichte des Pietismus,* vol. 1, Sections VI and VIII.

Germany in 1727, and Michael Alberti, considered by many the founder of forensic pathology. Unfortunately, Francke and his Pietist associates did not repay the tolerance shown to them when they joined the faculty. In the 1720s, at the height of their influence under the pious Frederick William I, they forced out Christian Wolff, who returned in 1740 only at the behest of Frederick II.[3]

But A. H. Francke himself was a pragmatist above all, and he and his larger circle of supporters did not rely on academe alone. They established a firm and lasting base of power and influence in the new philanthropy of the eighteenth century, both at home and abroad. As pastor of a poor and derelict congregation in Glaucha,[4] an impoverished town outside the city walls of Halle, he took up the cause of voluntary charity on behalf of poor children and widows and of discharged and unemployed soldiers left without sustenance after the end-of-century wars with Sweden and France. He urged a program of moral reform—advocating the closing of taverns, education for poor children, and domestic and institutional care for widows and orphans. Starting with a legendary anonymous gift of modest proportions, he placed his confidence first in God and then in the thirst for direct religious experience and for social and educational reform among large sectors of the public—from court nobility to country gentry, influential urban interests, and last but not least common men and women. Their support secured him a famous court privilege or charter in 1698, which exempted him from numerous corporate strictures and municipal supervision and taxes. By the time of his death in 1727, his educational and charity institutions were known all over Europe and were described as a "city of schools" in their own right, and as a place dedicated to instilling new principles of hard work and Christian seriousness in pupils from all ranks of society, including girls and foreigners.[5]

3. See Hinrichs, *Preussentum und Pietismus*.

4. Strictly speaking, the Francke Foundations and their Orphanage were located just outside the city walls in the suburb of Glaucha. The *Churfürstlich brandenburgische Privilegium* to the Orphanage is entitled *zu Glaucha an Halle*. But the city of Halle increasingly and by 1720 almost exclusively served as the geographical point of reference for the Foundations. For a history of the city of Halle, see the classic *Ausführlich diplomatisch historische Beschreibung* by Dreyhaupt.

5. There is now much recent European work on the genesis and structure of early modern Pietism. The classic work in the theological domain remains Ritschl, ed., *Geschichte des Pietismus*, 3 vols. (1880–86), although newer research has taken a more sympathetic approach. For the beginnings of seventeenth-century German Pietism as an identifiable movement of religious reform, see Wallmann, *Philipp Jacob Spener und die Anfänge des Pietismus*, 2d ed. There is no modern full biography of A. H. Francke, but Peschke (*August Hermann Francke, Werke in Auswahl*) has provided a critical selection and discussion of some of A. H. Francke's voluminous work. In addition to a continually updated biography in the journal *Pietismus und Neuzeit*, a multivolume series synthesizing current

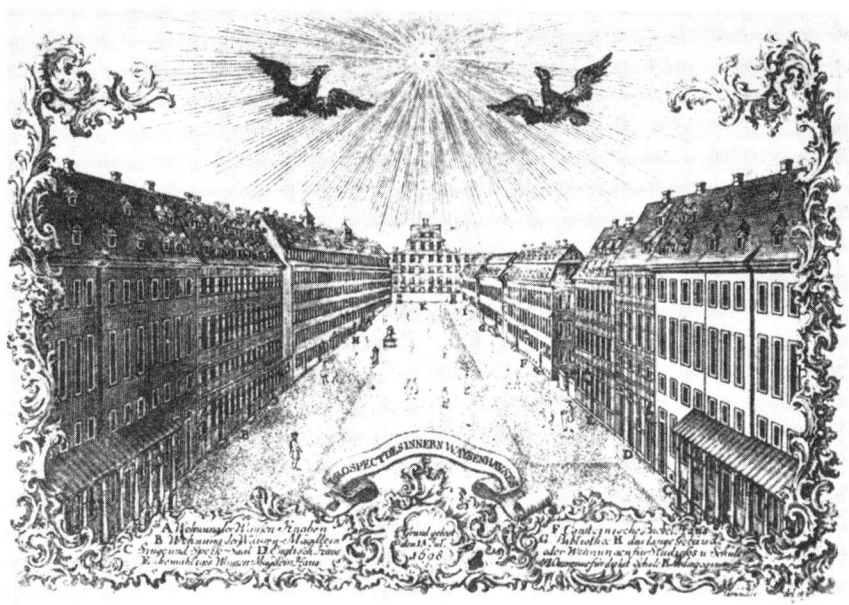

Fig. 1.2

The Francke Orphanage in Halle.

After Francke's death in 1727, his son Gotthilf August and a circle of associates continued the founder's work, but with the ascent to power of Frederick II to the Hohenzollern throne in 1740, the Foundations no longer enjoyed the full support of a pious ruler in Berlin. Apart from Frederick's distaste for religion, the accelerating centralization of control by the Prussian state over universities, commerce, and social services, including medical care, forced the Foundations to abandon the goal of universal Christian reform they had shared with their earlier English and Dutch allies. However, they could and did concentrate their

research is in progress as *Geschichte des Pietismus*, ed. Martin Brecht, K. Deppermann (dec.), Ulrich Gäbler, and Hartmut Lehmann, 2 vols. to date. The major American sources remain Stoeffler, *The Rise of Evangelical Pietism*; idem, *German Pietism During the 18th Century*; idem, *Continental Pietism and Early American Christianity*; Lovelace, *The American Pietism of Cotton Mather: Origins of American Evangelicalism*. Major studies linking Pietism to the political and social domains of the early modern period are Hinrichs, *Preussentum und Pietismus*; Lehmann, *Das Zeitalter des Absolutismus*; idem, "Zur Erforschung der Religiosität im 17. Jahrhundert."

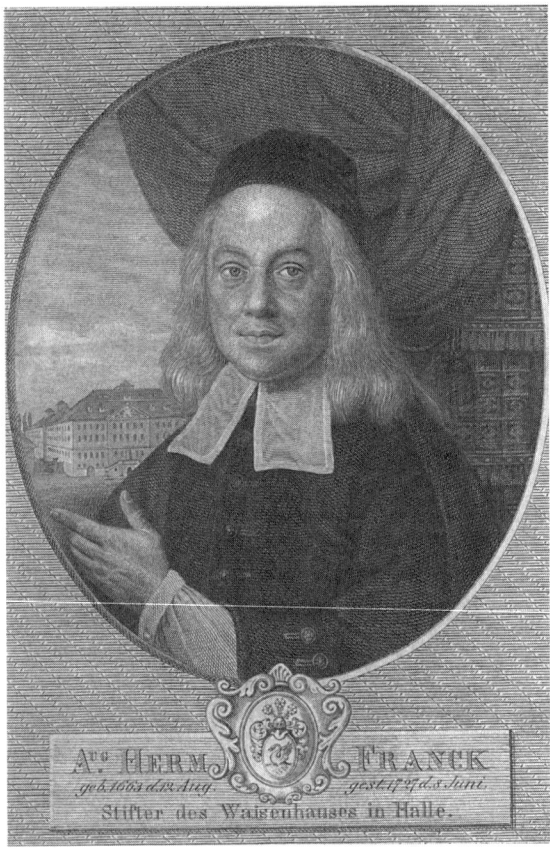

Fig. 1.3

The founder, August Hermann Francke (b. 1663 Lübeck, d. 1727 Halle). (This portrait is reproduced from the holdings of the Francke Foundations in Halle, Germany, with their kind permission.)

resources on the narrower legacy of colonial mission and education bequeathed by the founder. This legacy they were able to continue even beyond the death of Gotthilf August Francke in 1769.[6] The educational institutions and legacy of the Foundations continued well into the nineteenth century, although they had to withstand much competition and implicit and explicit criticism by

6. Gotthilf August Francke is a much-neglected person in the annals of Halle Pietism, and most scholars either ignore him completely or speak of him with reservation as the weak son of a strong father or a mere administrator. (See Brecht, *Der Hallische Pietismus in der Mitte des 18. Jahrhunderts, seine Austrahlung und sein Niedergang.*) This judgment is the result of a serious *Forschungslücke* and is urgently in need of revision, although this study is not the place to attempt it. It is obvious from the primary sources and recent work centered on North America, however, that without G. A. Francke's tireless and autocratic supervision of the American missions and Halle Pietist emissaries, reflected in many volumes of correspondence with Pennsylvania and Georgia (MAFSt Series 4–5; *Detailed Reports*

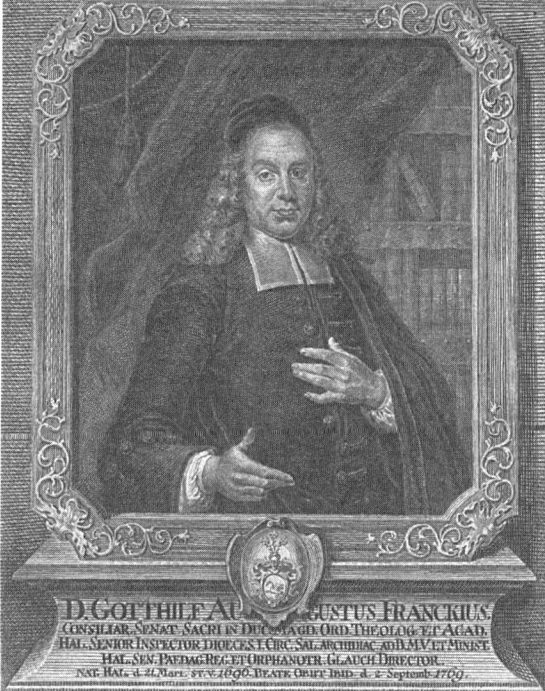

Fig. 1.4

The founder's son and the "Father" of Halle's emissaries to North America, Gotthilf August Francke (b. 1696 Halle, d. 1769 Halle). (This portrait is reproduced from the holdings of the Francke Foundations in Halle, Germany, with their kind permission.)

supporters of the educational enlightenment promoted by men like Wilhelm Basedow and Jean Jacques Rousseau.[7]

Support of and interaction with foreign missions in Tranquebar and Madras in East India and German Lutheran congregations in North America continued until the first decades of the nineteenth century. By that time, the Foundations and many of their German aristocratic patrons had been reduced to a state of genteel poverty. The second generation of Halle emissaries, now well entrenched in the American social and clerical establishment, offered help and support, mainly in the form of purchases of books and medications, but also through commercial contacts. Many of these exchanges remained tied

---

of the Salzburgers; Korrespondenz Mühlenberg; Roeber, *Palatines;* Wilson, "Public Works and Piety") this and many other studies of Pietism in North America would have been moot.

7. For eighteenth-century educational reform in a variety of settings, see Lempa, *Bildung der Triebe: Der deutsche Philanthropismus, 1768–1788,* in particular chap. 3.

to the generous legacies for the American missions that had been made by noble benefactors and benefactresses earlier during the century.[8]

Protestant Evangelical Reform and the New Philanthropy

"'Charity,' as observed by Henry Fielding as chief magistrate for Westminster to a grand jury in 1749, 'is the very characteristic virtue at this time. I believe we may challenge the whole world to parallel the examples which we have of late given of this sensible, this noble, this Christian virtue.'"[9]

The educational, social, and economic institutions that had grown up between 1696 and 1720 were indeed impressive in scope and depth.[10] The orphanage school had been only the first small step in the far-reaching plans of Pietist reform of all estates, particularly the young, through educational reform at each level of society and the introduction of Christian principles of frugality and social concern in economic life. The provision of social services to the deserving poor was to ensure their eventual conversion to Christ through improving their material circumstances.[11]

A. H. Francke had advocated the establishment of social and religious institutions and their replication for the purpose of universal Christian reform in several major treatises, among them the 1701 *Projekt: Zu einem Seminario*

8. The Degendorf legacy is a good example. It was in American hands until the end of the nineteenth century (see also Chapter 5, below). See also Roeber, " J. H. C. Helmuth, Evangelical Charity, and the Public Sphere in Pennsylvania, 1793–1800," and Wilson, "The Development of Eighteenth-Century Voluntary Institutions: Medical Care and Social Reform."

9. The quotation is from Owen's classic study, *English Philanthropy, 1660–1960*, and illustrates contemporary perception.

10. There is little literature in English on the planning and implementation of the charity and medical structure of these institutions in the scheme of Pietist reform. See however Ward, *The Protestant Evangelical Awakening*; Wilson, "Development of Eighteenth-Century Voluntary Institutions"; and idem, "Pietist Universal Reform and Care of the Sick and the Poor: The Medical Institutions of the Francke Foundations and Their Social Context."

11. The term *deserving poor* is not in fact one used by Francke, for whom Christian repentance and conversion were the major criteria for acceptance and for soliciting outside support. I use it here to indicate the generic similarities in the rise of the voluntary institutions of the new philanthropy. Among others, Pelling, "Healing the Sick Poor: Social Policy and Disability in Norwich, 1550–1640"; Cavallo, "The Motivations of Benefactors: An Overview of Approaches to the Study of Charity"; and Porter, "The Gift Relation: Philanthropy and Provincial Hospitals in Eighteenth-Century England," point out the fluidity of this term, which may well have been introduced by historians of charity to set off modern Protestant philanthropy from medieval charity that embraced all poor as children in the image of Christ. In his *Grosse Aufsatz*, Francke did make distinctions in eligibility, although these were probably utilitarian.

Universali oder Anlegung eines Pflantz-Gartens . . . and *Der Grosse Aufsatz.*[12] In building his orphanage in particular, Francke relied on a number of features of the leading Dutch charity facilities of the period. The inquiries of his close associate and emissary, Georg Neubauer, in the 1690s extended from personal and environmental hygiene, including the cleanliness of latrines and diet, to the rigid structure of staffing and financial and personnel supervision.[13] In Halle, however, inmate labor had neither an explicit punitive nor a financial objective, as was true for many contemporary Dutch and later English charitable institutions,[14] but was closely joined to the improvement and salvation of orphans and widows through religious conversion and education. Although manual tasks such as spinning, knitting, and carding were as elsewhere a major educational tool to orient the young to work, the expectation of major monetary gain from inmate labor was more of a rhetorical exercise in line with the tenets of the period. Also, the educational offering was purposely rich and vertically open, again in some contrast to the often strictly mercantilist efforts in England.[15]

By 1710, the Orphanage proper had expanded into a large and famous complex of day and boarding schools for the different estates: an establishment for the nobility and the gentry, a Latin school for future teachers and missionaries, a short-lived gynecaeum for ladies, and a so-called German school for the lower orders (sons of artisans and the lower commercial classes). The Orphanage school for the poor, which performed social functions of education and reform while accustoming its inmates to useful work, was only a small part of this large educational edifice.[16] In addition, the founder continued to pay close attention to the academic sector, where the new and dynamic Friedrich University gave

12. Peschke, *Francke Werke in Auswahl,* 108–15; Podczeck, ed., *Grosse Aufsatz.* The *Grosse Aufsatz* originally dated to 1704 but was revised in 1709, 1711, and 1716 during a period when the author and his collaborators slowly expanded their base of operations and sought means of securing economic independence.

13. Staatsbibliothek Berlin, Francke Nachlass Kapsel 28, fasc. 1–5, instructions to Georg Neubauer, 1697.

14. Spierenburg, *The Prison Experience, Disciplinary Institutions, and Their Inmates in Early Modern Europe;* Hitchcock, *The English Workhouse: A Study in Institutional Poor Relief in Selected Counties, 1696–1750.*

15. Hitchcock, "Paupers and Preachers: The SPCK and the Parochial Workhouse Movement." For vertical open access at Halle, see LaVopa, *Grace, Talent, and Merit: Poor Students, Clerical Careers, and Professional Ideology in Eighteenth-Century Germany.*

16. For the educational scheme of Francke and his associates, see Oschlies, *Die Arbeits-und Berufspädagogik A. H. Franckes.* For the gynecaeum and its female director, see Witt, *Bekehrung, Bildung, und Biographie.* For a chronological overview of the growth of the institutions of education,

him access to an academic reservoir of teachers, instructors, and even medical staff for the Orphanage institutions.

Replication of the Orphanage was attempted on several occasions and in several locations, such as in Augsburg and, most directly and successfully, at the new university of Göttingen, and in some of the Russian areas of Pietist influence. In general, these institutions had varying success and were not necessarily permanent.[17] Within Brandenburg-Prussia, concern with improving the lot and the skills of the poor and the disabled and of those dislocated by a century of dynastic and confessional strife continued to render the Halle institutional experiment attractive to the Hohenzollern monarchy, which by the turn of the seventeenth century was launched on a course of political and economic reform and in need of administrative cadres and skilled labor.[18] Religious accommodation was rendered both more urgent and feasible by the coexistence of the Reformed and Lutheran denominations since Prince Elector Johann Sigismund of Hohenzollern had converted to the Reformed faith in the early seventeenth century, and by the continuing accession to the Hohenzollern crown of territories with large Reformed populations. The Reformed element was also continually replenished by the import of skilled labor from Holland and France.[19] This had required much in the way of official religious toleration, which despite the ongoing battles between the Protestant and Catholic powers was a not uncommon phenomenon in mercantilist societies.

For the Halle Pietists, this royally sanctioned toleration brought a good amount of operational freedom. But it was bought at the price of close collaboration with the crown, which enlisted the Pietist clergy in its struggle for control over glebes and preferments with the Lutheran orthodox establishment and its patrons in the country gentry. In contrast to the Pietist stronghold of Württemberg,[20] Philipp Spener as well as Francke, both newcomers to the Hohenzollern territory, had no natural alliance with the landed estates against

---

see Kramer, *August H. Franckes pädagogische Schriften*. Sträter, "Pietismus und Sozialtätigkeit," 220, pointed out that the ratio of students, largely although not exclusively orphans, to student instructors was eleven to one early in the century; by the late 1720s, students of all kinds outnumbered true orphans at the rate of twenty to one.

17. Sträter, "Pietismus und Sozialtätigkeit"; de Boor, "Franckesche Stiftungen als Fundament"; Winter, *Halle als Ausgangspunkt*.

18. Hinrichs, *Preussentum und Pietismus*.

19. See, for example, Klingebiehl, "Huguenot Settlements in Central Europe," in Lehmann et al., eds., *In Search of Peace and Prosperity*; Hinrichs, *Preussentum und Pietismus*; idem, *Friedrich Wilhelm I*.

20. Lehmann, *Pietismus und weltliche Ordnung in Württemberg*.

the growth of absolutist central power. Thus, despite original and continuing suspicion of the crown's intentions, which the Hohenzollern court often reciprocated, Spener and Francke joined the Prussian monarchy in its efforts to reform schools and social institutions and to break the monopoly of the landed estates over clerical and educational patronage.[21]

After the accession of Frederick William I in 1713, clergy trained at the Halle Orphanage headed the crown's own orphanages for the children of deceased or impoverished soldiers, provided ministers to its troops, and carried educational reform into backward rural communities.[22] What has been less observed by German authors but noted by an astute English observer[23] is that despite outward subservience to the temporal power, not much in the way of dynastic loyalty was apparent in those disciples of Halle Pietism who managed to escape this new union between faith and state. There was little affection for or even mention of Prussia or its monarchs (whether Frederick William I or his son, Frederick II) in the correspondence between Halle and its dependencies in India and North America. The son of the founder, Gotthilf August Francke, commented on the coronation of Frederick II in 1740 with much and justified suspicion, because the new king promptly forbade the Francke enterprises to expand their by then very substantial real estate holdings.[24]

The Protestant Network

In his pursuit of a godly society similar to that proposed by the English Puritan reformers around Samuel Hartlib and Johann Comenius, the elder Francke had from the outset sought independence from both the established Church and the power of the state.[25] To this end, he sought his allies across territorial and national boundaries. Born in Lübeck as the son of a jurist who had been an administrator at the court of Ernest the Pious of Saxe-Gotha, he was the brother of a merchant situated in Venice and a member of the commercially active and enterprising section of the German *Bürgertum* at the threshold of the eighteenth

---

21. The best accounts of this history of mutual accommodation and occasional breaks in relationships between Halle and the Hohenzollern dynasty until 1727 remain the classic studies of Hinrichs and Deppermann. For a brief account to mid-century, see Brecht, *Geschichte des Pietismus*, vol. 1, Section IV.

22. Hubatsch, *Geschichte der evangelischen Kirche in Ostpreussen*.

23. Ward, *Protestant Evangelical Awakening*, 63.

24. Wirtschafts-und Verwaltungsarchiv Franckesche Stiftungen, Repertorium II.

25. Webster, *Great Instauration*; Lehmann, *Das Zeitalter des Absolutismus*.

century. Both the merchants and a large and highly educated clerical and administrative diaspora at the numerous territorial courts of the German Empire and
Northern Europe attempted to establish new links with the outside world and
to maintain old ones. Francke and his mentors, who included famous and well-
connected diplomats and linguists like Hiob and Heinrich Wilhelm Ludolf, were
well aware of the limitations by which territorial systems of traditional privileges
and economic controls hampered Germans in their encounters with the aggressive mercantilism of Holland and England. They were also aware of the need to
remain united with their Protestant brethren across Europe in the face of continuing Catholic attempts to retake territories and reconvert populations that
had come under Protestant control, as in Silesia. From the beginning of his Halle
ministry, A. H. Francke therefore expended his forces and his faith on securing
a strong base for his goal of universal Christian reform.

Among his supporters in this task was the reform-minded aristocracy
throughout the Holy Roman Empire. Until the end of the Seven Years' War
(1763), this aristocracy's interests often and openly ran counter to those of the
Prussian kings. From the Protestant nobility in Austria who employed theology
students from Halle as house chaplains[26] to the Counts Stolberg at Wernigerode
who used a remaining episcopal privilege to have Halle theologians properly
ordained on their way into the colonies, these pious nobles—both reigning aris-
tocrats and country gentry—remained a central pillar of the Halle institutions.
Francke's larger German network was strengthened and rendered partly independent by this camara of familial and dynastic ties, which included many pious
Lutheran counts and countesses at the midsize and small courts of Central and
Southwest Germany, from Saxe-Gotha and Waldeck to Sayn-Wittgenstein and
Ysenburg-Büdingen. Many, like the numerous Imperial Counts Reuss, still
answered directly to the Emperor in Vienna and to the Diet at Regensburg, and
most had played an independent role in turning the tide of the Counter-
Reformation in the seventeenth century. They reformed education and charity
in their territories and participated actively in the rise of the new philanthropy
of the eighteenth century.[27]

26. I owe this information to Hungarian colleagues from the Jozsef Attila University at Szeged.
I thank in particular Dr. Csepregis and Dr. Suzanna Font. There is little useful and almost no recent
work on this subject, despite its importance for the history of Southeast European Protestants.

27. For this network, see most recently the important contributions to vol. 2 of Brecht et al.,
eds., *Geschichte des Pietismus*, in particular by Schneider ("Der radikale Pietismus," 107–97) and Meyer
("Zinzendorf und Herrnhut," 5–106).

In looking beyond Prussian borders, the Francke enterprise also shared mutual interests with a large network of imperial officers who had fought under Eugene of Savoy in Holland and the Balkans since the end of the seventeenth century. These men had maintained connections to the Hapsburg court in Vienna and knew many bankers and merchants in the large Imperial cities like Frankfurt, Augsburg, and Nuremberg. Their association with the Halle Orphanage is reflected in the support by noble benefactors and their little-known attempts at North American colony building, in particular in Georgia. Immigrant groups to the Salzburger settlement at Ebenezer, for instance, were led by a nobleman in Hanoverian services, the Baron Georg Philip von Reck, in 1733 and 1742, and in 1751 by Gerard William de Brahm, a former artillery officer of the Empress Maria Theresa. One Georgia sponsor was the Imperial Field Marshall Friedrich Wilhelm von Seckendorff, a nephew of the founder of Friedrich University. As Imperial Ambassador at the court in Berlin in the 1720s and 1730s, he had been intimately involved in the negotiations over the fate of the Salzburger refugees from Catholic oppression. He remained loyal to the Empress Maria Theresa during the Silesian Wars of the 1740s, and Frederick II promptly had him imprisoned. There is good evidence that he and his circle remained interested in settling in the Georgia colony until the 1760s.[28]

From the start, Francke had joined the larger European and Protestant network of philanthropy and foreign mission. His Orphanage soon became famous among the early charity movements on the continent and in the England of Queen Anne, where a group of Anglican promoters of the Halle cause in the Society for Promoting Christian Knowledge (SPCK) translated Francke's *Fusstapfen* and other tracts beginning in 1708.[29] Since its founding in 1699, the SPCK had entertained close and continuing relationships with A. H. Francke and his circle, first through Heinrich Wilhelm Ludolf, secretary and agent of George of Denmark, Queen Anne's consort, and then through Francke's pupils Anton Wilhelm Böhme and Friedrich Michael Ziegenhagen (Fig. 1.5), successively

28. Jones et al., eds., *Detailed Reports of the Salzburger Emigrants*, vols. 1, 9, 10, 15; G. F. Jones, "Commissary van Reck's Report"; De Vorsey, ed., *De Brahm's Report*. For Count Seckendorff, see Walker, *Salzburg Transaction*. His correspondence in the Halle archives, mainly through one of his aides, shows him in retirement on an estate close to Halle, from where he advised the younger Francke on a number of issues. His name is prominently featured in the introduction to several volumes of Urlsperger's *Ausführliche Nachricht* (Archiv Franckesche Stiftungen, Series F, and biography by his nephew). See also Wilson, "Land, Population, and Labor."

29. Woodward, ed., *Francke's Pietas Halensis, Short Instruction, Nicodemus, or On the Fear of Man* (London, 1708).

the Lutheran court chaplains in London during the reigns of the first Hanoverian kings, George I and II. As Francke's placeholders in London, they cemented both ecumenical and missionary partnerships between the Anglican Church and the Halle Pietists. Ludolf in particular had opened access to the English and Danish merchant companies operating in the colonial territories, first in the Levant and East India, and then in British North America. By the 1730s, a good number of the Anglican clergy on the Common Council and the general board of the Georgia Trust were close associates of Halle Pietism. Most were members of the Associates of Dr. Thomas Bray, founder of both the SPCK in 1699 and the Society for Promoting the Gospel in Foreign Parts in 1701. In the 1690s, Bray had been a missionary to North America and the British West Indies; by the 1720s, he had become one of the persistent advocates of English social reform that brought the members of the Georgia Trust together before his death in 1730. The Trust made up the core of the Tory–High Church missionary and philanthropic establishment and included, in addition to the Earl of Egmont and James Oglethorpe, (Captain) Thomas Coram, also an associate of Dr. Bray, the famous Welsh philanthropist Sir John Philips, and the brothers Robert and Stephen Hales. Thomas Coram, an early advocate of the settlement of foreign Protestants in the American plantations, first in Nova Scotia in 1719 and subsequently in Georgia, was a prominent member of the British philanthropic establishment and founder of the London Foundling Hospital.[30] In English-speaking North America, Francke's work was enthusiastically received by the First Great Awakening of the 1740s, and the Orphanage served as the model of George Whitefield's Savannah institution built in 1740.[31]

Philanthropy and charity, then, were obvious and accepted common concerns among the SPCK and the Halle Pietists. According to the Society for Promoting Christian Knowledge, charity was "a dividend in the improved happiness and morality of the poor" or, as put more pragmatically by Francke, in

30. In Great Britain under William of Orange and Queen Mary and later under Anne and her Danish consort, these movements of charity reform and international mission were carried not so much by older dissenting groups such as the Quakers but by new charitable societies that formed in and on the margins of the Anglican Church. For the genealogy of these relationships, see Brunner, *Halle Pietists in England: Anthony William Boehm and the Society for Promoting Christian Knowledge*; Sames, *Anton Wilhelm Böhme, 1673–1722*; Wilson, "Continental Protestant Refugees and Their Protectors in Germany and London: Commercial and Charitable Networks"; and idem, "Halle Pietists in Georgia."

31. Ward, *Protestant Evangelical Awakening*; Schlenther, "To Convert the Poor People in America"; Wilson, "Public Works and Piety"; Van Horne, *Religious Philanthropy and Colonial Slavery: The American Correspondence of the Associates of Dr. Bray, 1717–1777*.

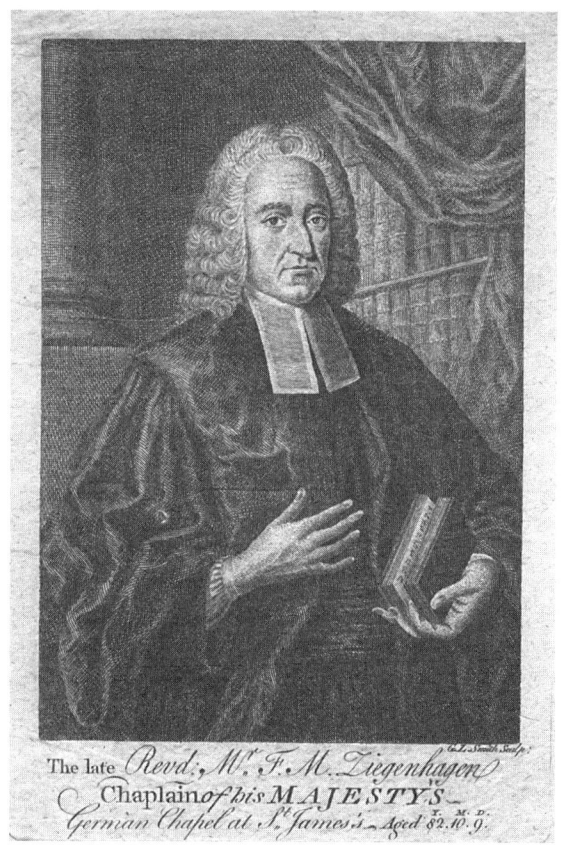

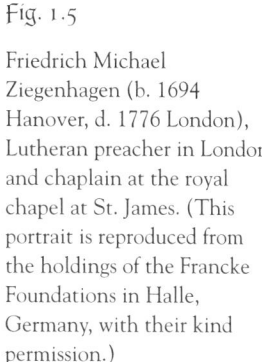

Fig. 1.5

Friedrich Michael Ziegenhagen (b. 1694 Hanover, d. 1776 London), Lutheran preacher in London and chaplain at the royal chapel at St. James. (This portrait is reproduced from the holdings of the Francke Foundations in Halle, Germany, with their kind permission.)

Part 3 of his program statement, *Der grosse Aufsatz,* "the true project, showing how those who have temporal property can lend a hand to the work of the Lord."

Yet another strand in the institutional history of the Halle enterprise, and one of particular importance in the context of this book, relates to the attempt to establish economic autarchy. In both social and economic respects, A. H. Francke and his followers exhibited a dynamic activism that was closer to the Dutch and English Calvinists than to the quietism often associated with German movements of evangelical conversion and repentance.[32] Although enjoying considerable protection by and privileges from the Prussian crown, the Halle Pietists

---

32. Ritschl, *Geschichte des Pietismus,* 2:2; Hinrichs, *Preussentum und Pietismus,* 77.

remained well aware of the sudden changes in patronage and similar dangers to institutional continuity that went with dependence on royal protection.[33]

Over the course of the three decades from 1698 to 1727, Francke and his supporters therefore developed an interlocking edifice of funding and labor, mainly by voluntary workers and students. A frugal and prudent household economy provided orphans, students, and instructors with nourishment supplied by the Orphanage's own agriculture and food-processing facilities such as bakeries and breweries. When ill, they were cared for in the Orphanage hospital. Francke's appeals for funding of both existing and contemplated institutions and objectives deviated specifically from traditional patterns of charitable giving. True, there were detailed suggestions for aggressively securing testamentary bequests, which aroused much objection on the part of the Lutheran orthodox clergy and at the court in Berlin. Some of the ensuing conflicts appear in the correspondence between Francke and one of his major associates and patrons among the Prussian service nobility, the Baron Carl Hildebrand von Canstein, who had to justify one large bequest to the King's ministers by presenting the funding efforts of the Foundations in contemporary mercantilist terms to distinguish them from traditional Catholic models.[34] There was a clear and open request to the Pietist public for financial investment, illustrating how the institutions in Halle could be promoted by the loan of secure capital for developing a large domestic and international commerce. This commerce was to include in particular medications and colonial goods. Potential investors were assured of careful and independent capital management and accounting to safeguard the stipulated use of funds, which were not to go for running expenses for the schools and Orphanage. Provisions for the recall of loans and interest at 5 to 6 percent per annum were stipulated.[35]

A variety of annuity schemes were offered, and there were continuous and open attempts to attract capital for commercial enterprises, ranging from cattle trading and mining in Hungary to the purchase of large agricultural properties

33. For these relationships, see, in particular, Schicketanz, *Canstein Korrespondenz* and *Carl Hildebrand von Cansteins Beziehungen zu Philipp Jakob Spener.*

34. "[D]en Stiftungen im pabstthum" (Schicketanz, *Canstein Korrespondenz,* 611, 320ff.). Canstein had been converted by Philipp Jakob Spener in Berlin and administered his estate. He also left much of his own estate to the Foundations.

35. The quotations are from Podczeck, ed., *Der Grosse Aufsatz* (*Handel ins gross,* 161): "Wie die Anstalten zu Halle durch Darleihung eines Capitals gefördert werden können, item II; Wie es mit den Capitalien soll gehalten werden, item IV." Wilson, "Development of Eighteenth-Century Voluntary Institutions."

in and around Halle.[36] The most successful of the schemes in Halle were the manufacture of *arcana* and other proprietary medications in the laboratory of the Orphanage pharmacy and their distribution through a wide network of agents, and the establishment of a large printing house and a Bible Institute named after the Baron Canstein (*Die Cansteinsche Bibelanstalt*) that mass-produced Bibles and religious literature in German as well as in a range of European vernacular languages. Until the middle of the century, the Foundations also published a local journal, the *Hallesche Nachrichten*, manufactured geographic globes, and above all acquired a large amount of local real estate and a number of mills and manufacturing units in the vicinity of Halle.[37]

Although not all the elder Francke's attempts at economic self-sufficiency and expansion were realized and only the trade in books and medications survived beyond mid-century, the universal appeal for charity reform and a shrewd use of local and regional patronage created considerable autarchy for a religious institution that practiced the new philanthropy of the eighteenth century—independent of the municipal poor laws and outside direct control by the state.

The Pietist Benefactresses—A Multitude of Women

This enterprise of social and religious reform held considerable attraction for women who had undergone and in turn had promoted evangelical conversion and revival. Since the Protestant Reformation and Catholic Counter-Reformation of the sixteenth century had developed their own and often overlapping agendas of social and religious reform, women throughout Europe and in all sectors of society had absorbed and acted on the call to practical and active piety. Although still circumscribed by the traditional constraints of the Christian role model of spousal subjection, motherhood, pious modesty, and passive acceptance of clerical guidance, increasing numbers of women were initiators and leaders in the central religious experience of the time: conversion and a new Christian life. In the case of German Pietism, and of its much contested successor, the

36. Some of them were reminiscent of the investment and reinvestment schemes described by Cavallo for Turin as part of the development of voluntary hospital financing. Cavallo, "Motivations of Benefactors," esp. 109ff.

37. Welsch, "Die Franckeschen Stiftungen als wirtschaftliches Grossunternehmen." Although the Baron Hildebrand von Canstein played a major role in funding and networking until his death in 1714 (Wilson, "Development of Eighteenth-Century Voluntary Institutions"), the Francke Foundations' finances appear to have remained firmly in the hands of the founding family until 1769.

Moravian or Herrnhuter movement founded by Nicholas Count Zinzendorf, the contribution of women was not only indispensable but determined the very fabric of the evangelical movements. Many of these women and their French, Dutch, and English sisters were famous throughout the seventeenth and eighteenth centuries. There were established scholars like Anna Maria van Schurmann in Holland and leaders of their own movements of Christian conversion, such as the Philadelphian Jane Leade in England and Eleanora von Merlau in Germany. The social leveling of the chiliasm and enthusiasm of the times found brief expression in a group of visionary maidservants and similar women of modest standing in Central Germany, who are known to history as "ecstatic females." And there were the much-maligned independent prophet-esses like Catharina Elisabeth Wetzel, Eva von Buttlar, and Eva Margareta von Frölich, who were blamed as much for their assumed or actual sexual proclivi-ties as for their Christian prophecy.[38]

However much these women differed from one another in background and in religious agenda, in social standing and in their persistence to remain outside the tenets of their social groups—to remain, as Witt calls them, "extraordinar-ies"—they shared their insistence on independent, direct, and intense religious experience and divine inspiration, as well as a sense of the end of time and the impending millennium. They also shared their reception. Both contemporary and later writers treated them with considerable gender and religious bias, if not contempt. Even in the movements of piety and reform that first embraced them, they were as often as not considered more of a liability than an asset because of their extreme, often chiliastic and separatist positions and associations. Philipp Jakob Spener insisted on female discretion and abstention from religious lead-ership both in the privacy of his original conventicles in the Frankfurt of the

38. For the so-called founding period (1692–1727), I rely on the new and critical study by Witt, *Bekehrung, Bildung, und Biographie*, which deals with the female teaching institutions of the Francke Foundations and contains a good survey of the still-sparse literature on the subject. But with few excep-tions, there continues to be a lack of fuller studies and of even the most basic biographical work. For recent individual treatments, see Andersson, "Die Autorität der Prophetin: Eva Margaretha Frölich und der prophetische Diskurs"; for Eleanora Merlau Petersen, see Ritschl, *Geschichte des Pietismus*, vol. 2, and Matthias, "Enthusiastische Hermeneutik des Pietismus, dargestellt an Johanna Eleonora Petersens Gespräche des Herzens mit Gott." For Anna Marie Schurmann, see Wallmann, *Philipp Jakob Spener*, chap. 4; and Becker-Cantarino, *Der lange Weg zur Mündigkeit: Frauen und Literatur in Deutschland von 1500 bis 1800*, 110–29, and the literature cited there. The German literature in this field is constantly expanding, however, and the seminal work by Wunder, *Er ist die Sonn, sie ist der Mond: Frauen in der Frühen Neuzeit*, is now available in English translation. See also Wunder and Vanja, *Wandel der Geschlechterbeziehungen*.

1670s and in the growing Pietist network in Berlin, where he had settled as senior preacher of Saint Nikolai in the 1690s.[39]

A. H. Francke seems to have been far more open to the enthusiasm and visions of many of his female parishioners and followers, even when they included his own wife.[40] In his institutional policies, however, he eventually accepted the social realities and constraints of female participation in the Foundations, both in terms of female education and of the place of women in the institutional hierarchy.[41] On the other hand, Francke well realized that his political network and his economic plans could not do without the financial and social support of well-connected women—the Pietist benefactress or *fundatrix*. Among these women, few were on the fringes of separatism, and many were empowered by their social standing and the financial and legal independence that often—although by no means generally—was conferred by noble birthright or widowhood.[42] They brought to the Pietism of August Hermann Francke the large regional networks that joined the nobility and the well-connected urban matrons of the period; in turn, Francke offered them opportunities to be influential beyond the traditional roles of face-to-face local charity and individual piety. At the same time, this network sheltered their reputations and, in anti-Pietist locations like the Electorate of Hanover, their political standing behind the wall of Pietist caution and eighteenth-century discretion. It is this smaller group of influential women that concerns us in the following.

Attempting to trace their specific role requires casting a wide if shallow net. That there have been few studies of the philanthropic role of women in this Pietist group, or for that matter of their untitled sisters in the bourgeoisie and the

---

39. For Spener, see, for instance, Wallmann, *Philip Jakob Spener*, and Witt, *Bekehrung, Bildung, und Biographie*, 23ff. and notes.

40. Francke's position was indeed far more ambiguous and not fully resolved. See de Boor, "Pietismus, Enthusiasmus, und Separatismus an der Wende des 17./18. Jahrhunderts," and Zäpernick, "Johann Georg Gichtels und seiner Nachfolger Briefwechsel mit den hallischen Pietisten, besonders mit A. M. Francke," on the relationship between Francke's wife and the radical Pietist Johann Georg Gichtel.

41. For the schools for girls and the ladies' chapter (*Damenstift*), see Witt, *Bekehrung, Bildung, und Biographie*. The lack of acknowledged—although not actual—female leadership in the Foundations is obvious from the official institutional histories.

42. That noble women often enjoyed independent use of their dowries and inheritances in the eighteenth century is evident in many sources. As noted by Becker Cantarino, *Der lange Weg zur Mündigkeit*, there is an almost complete lack of newer studies on the agency of women in the German nobility, although in their case the poverty of source material is at least partly relieved by the availability of archival material; see Becker Cantarino's Introduction, note 36. See also Paletschek, "Adelige und bürgerliche Frauen, 1770–1870."

working population,[43] is in good part due to the fact that the primary sources themselves reflect the patriarchal role distribution between men and women and the discipline and caution of the Pietist enterprise. Although there are a number of reasonably new studies of the *femmes savantes* to whom the Enlightenment paid selective attention,[44] our access to them and to the lesser noblewomen of the period is still often obscured by the condescending or indeed apologetic tone in which nineteenth-century historians transmitted their stories.[45] Although they count among the most important allies and supporters of the Francke enterprise, women like the Baroness Henriette Katharina and her daughter Charlotte Justine von Gersdorf lack their own biographies and are discussed mainly in the context of their famous relative, the Count Nicholas von Zinzendorf. The same goes for their numerous cousins and friends, whether reigning countesses like Henkel Donnersberg zu Pölzig and Stolberg-Wernigerode, or indispensable diplomatic intermediaries like Wilhelmine Sophie von Münchhausen in Göttingen.[46] But

43. As noted by Witt, none has received full treatment since German Pietism returned to the attention of historians after 1945. The central journal of Pietist studies, *Pietismus und Neuzeit*, in twenty-one volumes to 1997, contains a number of articles dedicated to religiously prominent women leaders (see in particular vol. 17), but despite a number of studies on the self-expression of Pietist women, there is no attempt at a larger view. On the American side, Roeber has covered in detail and for the lower social strata an entire German geographic territory that was one of the eighteenth-century Pietist population centers (Roeber, "In German Ways"; idem, *Palatines, Liberty, and Property*). For the far more overt role of women in the Moravian communities, see Fogleman, *Hopeful Journeys: German Immigration, Settlement, and Political Culture in Colonial America, 1717–1775*, and Smaby, *The Transformation of Moravian Bethlehem: From Communal Mission to Family Economy*.

44. Dismissively from Leipzig in 1736, Louise Adelgunde Victoria Gottsched, *Die Pietisterey im Fischbein-Rocke*; brief entries are in several eighteenth-century literary encyclopedias, for example, *Lobrede des Frauenzimmers in gebundener Rede* (Leipzig, 1716); Georg Christian Lehm, *Teutschlands galante Poetinnen . . .* (Leipzig, 1715); Amaranthes (G. S. Corvinus), *Nutzbares, galantes, und curiöses Frauenzimmerlexikon . . .* (Leipzig, 1715). (All quoted after Witt, *Bekehrung, Bildung, und Biographie*, Part I.) More recently, Woods and Fürstenwald, *Schriftstellerinnen, Künstlerinnen, und gelehrte Frauen des deutschen Barock: Ein Lexikon*.

45. A comparison of the biographic information in Zedler's *Universallexikon* and the *Allgemeine Deutsche Biographie* of 1879 is instructive. Zedler uses the term "femmes savantes" without hesitation; the ADB entry for the Gersdorf family, written by Gustav Kramer, one of the directors of the Francke Foundations and its major nineteenth-century biographer, describes the two learned baronesses Gersdorf—Henriette Katharina and Charlotte Justine—as "*nonetheless honestly pious, genuinely humble, and despite all not assertive about their knowledge*" (emphasis added). By contrast, August Hermann Francke's earlier treatment of female education in his 1698 introduction to Fenelon's *Tractätlein von der Erziehung der Töchter* is concerned only with a Christian education, and he fully included women in his ambitious plans, which included Greek, Hebrew, and the arts and sciences in addition to reading, writing, and arithmetic (Kramer, *August Herrmann Francke*, Anhang, 2:9–13).

46. Becker-Cantarino, *Der lange Weg zur Mündigkeit*, provides a fuller account than heretofore available of Erdmuthe von Zinzendorf. For the Baronesses Gersdorf in their relations to A. H. Francke

as elsewhere in our sources, the less accessible business correspondence of the Francke Foundations provides evidence that where commerce and philanthropy were involved, the bounds of discretion, caution, and anonymity could be transcended.

The Gersdorf women and their in-laws, most notably Erdmuthe von Zinzendorf, born a Countess Reuss, were in fact models of the evangelical reformer and benefactress. By the beginning of the eighteenth century, Henriette Catharina Gersdorf née Friesen (1648–1726) was a wealthy and well-connected widow whose voice was heard at the courts at Dresden and Berlin. She reformed the manners and morals of her tenants and improved the religious and secular instruction of the enserfed population on her Lusatian estates around Gross Hennersdorf to better their skills. She was a generous contributor to the Francke Foundations on behalf of several female students and of Silesian refugees from Catholic persecution. Her son-in-law reported that "she had constructed and supported a series of poor houses and orphanages, and as well extended her generosity to the Orphanage in Halle and contributed much to its foundation and development."[47] Although this comment barely suggests the conflict between several philanthropic obligations, her refusal to submit to Francke's urging for continuing financial support when her own obligations stood in the way eventually led to a cooling of relations with Halle.[48] She at last so overcommitted her resources that her unmarried second daughter, Henriette Sophie, was forced in the 1740s to sell a large part of the estate to a male cousin. This cousin, in turn, left a moderate legacy to the Salzburger settlement in Georgia, and at least one Baroness Gersdorf continued to figure prominently in the American contributions of the Foundations.

---

and Zinzendorf and the evangelical revival, see the summary references in Hinrichs, *Preussentum und Pietismus*, and Ward, *Protestant Evangelical Awakening*, 33ff. A fuller treatment of Henriette Katharina, based on primary sources in the Francke archives, is in Witt, *Bekehrung, Bildung, und Biographie*, in particular Parts III and IV, chap. 1. A doctoral dissertation on the Baroness Münchhausen by Elisabeth Quast is in progress, from which I have drawn information on her Göttingen circle. I thank the author for sharing this information with me.

47. Hinrichs, *Preussentum und Pietismus*, 196, quoting a letter from 30 October 1714, in Gneomar Ernst von Natzmer, *Lebensbilder aus dem Jahrhundert nach dem grossen deutschen Kriege*, 200. Gersdorf wrote 179 letters to G. A. Francke. According to Zäpernick, to whom I owe this information and the reference to the letters to the Baroness von Münchhausen cited below, most dealt with her ward, the Count Zinzendorf, and only a few with the financial transactions implicit in the references by her son-in-law. Only one explicitly mentions her financial difficulties and her loss of Rth 80,000, arising from mismanagement of her estate.

48. Witt, *Bekehrung, Bildung, und Biographie*, 131ff., 157ff.

This network of active and politically indispensable Pietist benefactresses paralleled and was connected to the men in the Pietist network by marriage and family connections. It ranged from intermediaries at the Russian court who had estates in the Baltic provinces to Göttingen and Hanover.[49] Women from this pious nobility participated in Halle domestic charity, education, and support of foreign missions. They selected and supported candidates for the mission clergy and their schoolmasters, chose and paid for the shipment of edification literature and educational material, sent clothing and medications to "their" American congregations and to the orphanage at Ebenezer in Georgia, and supported the building of its three churches and at least as many in the middle colonies. They set priorities and manipulated their own resources and their influence to secure the right of Pietist clergy to make collections on behalf of the colonies.[50] Their donations and bequests—many small but given on a regular basis—contributed to the export of German books and medications to Georgia and Pennsylvania. And they transcended the older role of local charity and shared vicariously in the attempt to establish God-fearing societies in the transoceanic colonies, whether by conversion among native populations as in India, or, as in North America, by settling European fringe groups and expecting them to replicate European models of social reform.[51]

One example of particular interest in our context is Wilhelmine Sophie von Münchhausen née Wangenheim (b. 1701), and her husband, both Pietist leaders in the Hanover Electorate. She sponsored Heinrich Melchior Mühlenberg after he left his vicarage at the estate of the younger Baroness Gersdorf, and her influence is reflected in the mandatory visits paid by Pietist pastors on their way to North America before her early death in 1750. She was married to Gerlach Adolph von Münchhausen, whom George II of England and Hanover had

49. For the Baltic nobility and their connections to the Russian court and to both Halle and Herrnhut, see Amburger, *Geschichte des Protestantismus in Russland*.

50. For instance, a letter of 24 March 1747 by G. A. Francke to H. M. Mühlenberg, in Korrespondenz Mühlenberg (KM) 1:275.

51. The most famous English example among eighteenth-century titled ladies with a foreign evangelical mission was Selina, Countess Huntingdon. Taking over from the evangelist George Whitefield in the latter half of the eighteenth century, she may well have been representative of a less well known cohort of women. Although probably more outspoken in her plans and extravagant in her losses and enjoying direct access to the North American colonies, she represents the assumption of leadership in the evangelical movements by women, in particular widows, of the requisite social and financial standing. See Schlenther, "To Convert the Poor People in America." For an earlier instance, see Kuppermann, *Providence Island, 1630–1641: The Other Puritan Colony*. For Halle's Indian mission in general, see Jeyaraj, *Inkulturation in Tranquebar*.

entrusted with the founding charter of the University of Göttingen in 1732, and was well connected to the Hanoverian court in London. Despite her social prominence and political connections, however, one must dig hard and deep to piece together even a sketchy outline of the Baroness's active involvement in the affairs of Halle.[52] She was apparently not a *femme savante* but came from an old noble family. She left a good-sized but by no means ample legacy for the Pietist foreign missions at the time of her death, which is recorded in the India archives of the Francke Foundations. She made a number of contributions to Ebenezer through her American protégé, the Baron von Reck. She sponsored catechists for "my schools" in Pennsylvania, and, as noted, her house was among the obligatory stopovers for missionaries on their way to North America.[53] And she seems to have stood as well in a female tradition of medical charity that involved active endorsement and dispensing of specific remedies.[54]

But in all this, there is little to prepare us for the extraordinary perception and acknowledgment of agency by Friedrich Michael Ziegenhagen, Lutheran chaplain at the Court of Saint James and the linchpin of the Halle missionary network in India and North America. In 1743, after thanking her for her letters about the young Heinrich Melchior Mühlenberg recently arrived in Pennsylvania, Ziegenhagen expressed his satisfaction with her approval of the pending church and school construction and her efforts on behalf of the North American mission. He continued:

> The death of the blessed Mrs. Francke surely has deprived the work of the Lord in the East and West Indies of a faithful and industrious mother and helpmate. But behold the ways of the Lord. He goes abroad and calleth

52. Ward was content with a parenthetical reference that "([she] had been converted under Francke's influence and . . . linked the Pietist networks of Schaumburg Lippe and Wernigerode)." Ward, *Protestant Evangelical Awakening*, 110, quoting Ruprecht, *Der Pietismus in den Hannoverschen Stammländern*.

53. See KM 1, for example, Letter 6. There are two letters to Mme. von Münchhausen by Mühlenberg, full of grateful drivel (Letters 60 and 70); another to Francke mentions a black powder against epilepsy she had sent (Letter 17); but there are few letters by or to the Baroness in the general correspondence section of the Francke archives at Halle. A fuller treatment of her letters in the Francke Nachlass in Berlin is forthcoming by Quast.

54. The traditional dissemination of medical knowledge by noblewomen as part of their charitable obligations persisted to the early modern period and only slowly receded in this class. Leibrock-Plehn, *Hexenkräuter oder Arznei: Die Abtreibungsmittel im 16. und 17. Jahrhundert*, 169ff., and the literature cited there. Also Getz, "Charity, Translation, and the Language of Medical Learning in Medieval England." For the lesser nobility in Germany, see Vanja, "Aufwärterinnen, Narrenmägde, und Siechenmütter-Frauen in der Krankenpflege der frühen Neuzeit."

other workers to the vineyard, and among them he calls His dear daughter in H[anover] and says to her: You shall be the nursing mother, be content, I shall be with you and bless your work. Many have worried, and not without cause, over the great loss of our dear Mrs. Francke, but be comforted, for the Lord lives, and He know how to make up for this loss and is indeed ready to make up for it. And what remains for me to say? Dear Lady, must I not congratulate you from the bottom of my heart and in the name of the Lord on your new position in the Kingdom of the Lord? And on the blessing that has flown from your work for the Philadelphia cause? For has not God through His rich blessing (*I refer to the 250 ducats from Legal Counselor Surland*) sealed your work and shown that it pleases Him well. . . .

And thus He intends that in the future I shall not only regard you, count on you, and honor you as an honest disciple and friend of Jesus Christ, but a co-worker, helpmate, and nursing mother in the Kingdom of the Lord.[55]

Even given Michael Ziegenhagen's single-minded dedication to the task of Pietist mission, this letter is surprising in its full acknowledgment of Sophie Münchhausen's importance. In its use of biblical metaphor, it provides a good example of how active female agency could be turned into a passive vessel of the Lord's will, so as to be acceptable to both writer and recipient within the bounds of a multilevel relationship. But we should note that men as well were part of this very Pietist discourse of humility, which has fooled many readers of eighteenth-century German documents in America. The addressee, a highborn woman of many connections, was not only expected to understand and accept her role as defined by early modern biblical metaphor. She would gladly shoulder the task previously carried by a commoner (Gotthilf August Francke's first wife, Johanna Henriette, who died in 1743, was the daughter of Henriette Rosine Goetze and came from an urban untitled family) in accordance with the conventions of social equality in the closed Pietist community at Halle.[56] She would be the "nursing mother" of the missions, harking back to the metaphorical usage of the English prophetesses of the mid-seventeenth century[57] and apparently reserved for those giving beyond the call of female duty and piety. In short, her status and

55. MAFSt I (India) E 7, 31, letter by Friedrich Michael Ziegenhagen to the Baroness Münchhausen, Kensington, 12 January 1743. My translation and emphasis. I thank Gertraud Zäpernick for this reference. Unfortunately, no picture of the first Baroness survives.

56. See in particular Hinrichs, *Preussentum und Pietismus*, 184ff.

57. Hobby, *Virtue of Necessity, English Women's Writing, 1649–88*.

connection, indispensable in obtaining legacies and sponsoring collections on behalf of the American and Indian missions, admitted her to the inner sanctum at Halle.

Her communications with G. A. Francke, although both a bit more down to earth and conventional in their form of address, reflect this position. In January 1744, she discussed the planning of "my schools in Pennsylvania," suggested a schoolmaster for Ebenezer in Georgia, and warned of a lack of planning regarding church construction.[58]

Care for the colonial missions, however, was not confined to the collecting and giving of money and the patronage of its ministers. Ebenezer in Georgia in particular and its refugee population both needed and received continual material support. The Ebenezer diaries twice annually, both in anticipation and retrospect, deal extensively with substantial gifts of clothing, medicines, linen, books, and sundries that were put together in Halle and Augsburg, crated, and dispatched through Hamburg and London to Savannah. The value of these shipments and the costs of transport ran to several hundred pounds sterling for each shipment, reflecting donations in cash and kind. They were largely marshaled under the guidance of the women in the Francke circle, both untitled and titled, although many remained cloaked in anonymity or proffered their regular donations through clerical or other intermediaries. This was true not only for noblewomen, but for the many contributors from the middle and even the serving classes whose donations appeared in the ledgers of the missions. A Mrs. Büsing, the widow of the Inspector of Churches in Oldenburg, was a faithful contributor and collector of donations to Ebenezer. In several instances, she assigned collections "on behalf of the institutions in Ebenezer and in particular the orphanage at that place" and forwarded her own gifts and those of her maid, giving careful instructions on how to split between the widow of Reverend Gronau and the wife of Reverend Boltzius. A female servant and convert from Catholicism, Katharina Hake, who worked as a caretaker for severely and dangerously ill charity patients in Halberstadt, made several substantial donations (ranging from 20 Reichthaler [Rth] to 25 Rth or the equivalent of £5 sterling each) on behalf of the Salzburgers. The minister transmitting her bequest apologized

58. The moneys that so impressed the Reverend Ziegenhagen had apparently gone directly to England: "I have already transmitted to England the considerable gift forwarded by Mr. [Syndicus] Surland as 150 [sic] ducats for the church." Letter from Frau von Münchhausen to Francke, under 4 January 1744, Hanover, MAFSt 4 G 1 (?), fols. 15–18. Despite the difference in the amount, the reference is probably to the same donation.

profusely for this "obstinacy," probably to explain these very substantial sums given beyond her station, but noted also that when barred from communion for ignoring church discipline, she would abstain from attending services altogether.[59]

Closer to home, the labor and shrewd sense of their women were indispensable to the commercial success of the Francke Foundations. According to an intimate if not unbiased observer, Inspector Georg Neubauer, much of the early success of the pharmaceutical business was due to the women in the Francke circle.[60] During the 1740s and beyond, these women often went against the preferences of Gotthilf August Francke and Michael Friedrich Ziegenhagen in their patronage of specific candidates and staff of the transatlantic missions and congregations. Some used their position to lend continuous support to Georg Ernst Thilo, the Georgia mission physician who fell out of favor almost immediately after his passage through London, where he had refused to bleed Court Chaplain Ziegenhagen according to the patient's instructions. An overly "enthusiastic" disciple of Johann Juncker, fired from his North American duties by G. A. Francke on several occasions and disdained by the senior pastor of the Salzburger settlement, he nonetheless for three decades received most of the medical supplies needed for his eventually successful practice in Georgia.[61] Many of his orders carry the intriguing notation, "Free of charge as a gift"; in fact they seem to have been paid for in large part by the daughter of the founder, the widow Freylinghausen, who like many of her family and of the immediate Francke circle worked in the management of the pharmaceutical business of the Foundations.[62]

But however closely involved, these women, both noble and untitled, continued to pursue their agenda from Europe, in contrast to many of the marginal prophetesses and inspired women among the separatist sects. In North America, the constraints of social status and political caution were less obvious. But although the eventual wives of the Pietist ministers in North America—both

59. For example, letter from Conrad Schmid in Halberstadt to G. A. Francke, 9 April 1744, MAFSt 5 E 2, Items 1–2r/v, fols. 16–18.

60. Most prominently, the mother-in-law of Gotthilf August Francke, Henriette Rosine Goetze, and although not well known but clearly a major contributor to the *Medikamentenexpedition*, a niece of the elder Francke, the "Jungfer Francke." Henriette Rosine Goetze, née Böse, was the widow of Christian Gottfried Goetze, judge and member of the faculty of law, Leipzig. She died in 1749, aged sixty-eight years and much honored at her death by poems and memorials.

61. Christian Ernst Thilo's professional practice is described in greater detail in Chapter 7 of this volume. His enthusiasm seems to have included, as was often the case, intimations of sexual contact during sessions of prayer and repentance; Wilson, "Hallesche Waisenhausmedikamente."

62. AFSt Wirtschafts und Verwaltungsarchiv, Repertorium ii, ix.

immigrant and American-born—were strong and active participants in the development of German Pietist settlements and congregations in North America,[63] the barriers against full reporting on the role of the distaff side have remained largely intact.

The Medical Institutions of the Orphanage

That August Hermann Francke's reforms also included changing the provision of medical care to the poor should not come as a surprise. Attempts to link the reform of charity and of health care pervade post-Reformation European history. In an almost unbroken chain of tradition, most medical charity—financial and in kind—had been received and administered through the established churches and through municipal governments that relied on Catholic orders of mercy or, in most Protestant jurisdictions, on appointed reputable citizens who coordinated the financing and administration of long-term shelter and care of the chronically ill and impaired and the acutely ill in the case of epidemics.[64]

By the end of the sixteenth century, the link between charity, medical care, and the housing of the poor and undomiciled in institutional settings was a recognized and large undertaking in most European towns of any size. But in the course of the seventeenth century, medical charity on a voluntary basis became a vehicle for religious reformers who remained outside or on the fringes of the churches. In England, this was in large part due to the exclusion of dissenting groups from clerical and judicial tenure after the Restoration.[65] In Central Europe, traditional mechanisms developed after the Middle Ages were no longer able to deal with the immense displacement of civilians and families of soldiers during the century of wars that ravaged Protestant and Catholic territories alike from 1620 onward. The new philanthropy of Pietism and similar movements tried to address these needs and to further its own agenda. These movements harnessed medicine to their schemes of reform to gain a foothold in settings formerly closed to them.

63. Roeber, "In German Ways"; Fogleman, *Hopeful Journeys.*
64. Imbert, *Le Droit hospitalier de l'Ancien Regime;* Jones, "The Constitution of the Modern Hospital Patient"; Jütte, "Die medizinische Versorgung einer Stadtbevölkerung im 16. und 17. Jahrhundert am Beispiel der Reichsstadt Köln"; Kinzelbach, *Gesundbleiben, Krankwerden, Armsein in der frühneuzeitlichen Gesellschaft: Gesunde und Kranke in den Reichsstädten Überlingen und Ulm, 1500–1700,* 241ff.
65. Shoemaker, "Reforming the City: The Reformation of Manners Campaign in London, 1690–1738"; Fissell, "Charity Universal? Institutions and Moral Reform in Eighteenth-Century Bristol"; Porter, "The Gift Relation"; Craig Rose, "Politics and the London Royal Hospitals, 1683–1692."

In urban areas, medical reforms were often furthered by the traditional links of charity practice to academic centers, as in Italy and France.[66] This link was particularly close and exceptionally fruitful in the case of the Halle Pietism and its institutional core. In addition to their schools, the Orphanage Foundations had planned and built a hospital by 1710 and, after 1715, a large associated dispensary. The growth of these medical facilities coincided with the swift rise of the medical faculty, which quickly assumed a prominent role among Central European medical schools.[67]

A voluntary hospital on the grounds of the Orphanage, including a dispensary serving the poor and the lower-middle-class population of the city of Halle and beyond, was intended to improve access to medical care, support the financing base and the reputation of the institutions, and last but not least, find a new and extensive outlet for the supplies from the Orphanage pharmacy and eventually the commercial drug business. The first hospital, built in 1708, was of moderate size, with no more than thirty beds designed to provide care for resident students and orphans, for a selected general public, and for religious expatriates.[68] This infirmary, and its slightly larger successor, saw a total of 10,973 patients from 1730 to 1798. More important, the ambulatory care dispensary established in 1718 treated and dispensed medications to roughly 12,000 patients a year, or about 30 patients a day, until the 1760s.[69]

Unlike most municipal hospitals, the Orphanage facilities were not confined to an urban catchment area but took in patients from rural areas; just as important, they attracted patients from all social strata. Both hospital and ambulatory

66. In particular France and Italy, which have been well studied. See Jones, *Charity and Bienfaisance: The Treatment of the Poor in the Montpellier Region, 1740–1815*; Cavallo, "Motivations of Benefactors"; Henderson, "The Hospitals of Late-Medieval and Renaissance Florence: A Preliminary Survey."

67. For the medical school, see above all the series by Kaiser and Krosch, "Zur Geschichte der medizinischen Fakultät der Universität Halle im 18. Jahrhundert." A recent overview in English is by Konert, "Academic and Practical Medicine in Halle During the Era of Stahl, Hoffmann, and Juncker."

68. Helm, "Der Umgang mit dem kranken Menschen im halleschen Pietismus des frühen 18. Jahrhunderts."

69. I here follow Piechocki, "Gesundheitsfürsorge und Krankenpflege in den Franckeschen Stiftungen in Halle/Saale," and Konert, "Academic and Practical Medicine." More recent work by Helm, "Kinder und Lehrkrankenhaus," takes a more critical look (see note 72 below) and confirms that the hospital in fact served only the sick in the Orphanage institutions by 1730. The bed size is normal for the period. Although Bonner, *Becoming a Physician: Medical Education in Britain, France, Germany, and the United States,* does not discuss the Halle institutions, he gives similar examples for the German territorial hospitals of the period.

facilities were run on a mixed charitable and fee basis,[70] and both drew on the medical faculty of the University and its students and teachers to treat patients. In turn, this arrangement offered students a setting for clinical instruction and experience. Students of theology who worked as instructors at the Orphanage in return for modest stipends provided supervision and care to both hospital patients and those confined at home, supervised the distribution of medications on behalf of the Orphanage pharmacy, and acquired some medical knowledge that was to serve them in their future posts as parsons in rural areas and missionaries abroad. Here, among other students of theology, Heinrich Melchior Mühlenberg acquired his understanding of medical practice.

The reputation of the Orphanage, the large number of patients, and the opportunities for close and closely supervised patient care it offered to selected medical students made it indeed attractive as a clinical teaching facility. As noted by its long-term director, Johann Juncker: "[U]nd die Studiosi haben den grossen Vortheil, dass sie in jungen Jahre alte Practici werden; denn da sie in einem Jahr bei 12,000 Patienten mit helfen expediren, ist solches eine Anzal, die gar mancher alter Practicus nicht ausweisen kann" (and the students have the considerable advantage of becoming seasoned practitioners while still young in years. For they help to manage over the course of one year as many as 12,000 patients, and that is surely a number that goes well beyond the patients seen by many experienced medical practitioners).[71]

In the far-reaching if not fully realized hospital plans developed by A. H. Francke in his *Project von der Verpflegung der Kranken* in 1709, Francke summarized many of the major strands in the physical, patient care, and hygienic aspects of hospital development at the cusp of the eighteenth century.[72] Many new hospitals of this time were dedicated to patient care of selected social groups defined by the need of the state—as in the large army hospitals in Vienna and Berlin—or by the patronage of subscribers, as in the hospitals of London, Birmingham, and eventually Edinburgh. Halle occupied an intermediate

70. Konert, "Academic and Practical Medicine," and idem, "Caritas est viva: Gedanken zu einem Forschungsprojekt über den Einfluss des Pietismus auf die Entwicklung von Medizin und Pharmazie"; Wilson, "Pietist Universal Reform."

71. Wirtschafts und Verwaltungsarchiv Franckesche Stiftungen ix/ii/1, 1718ff., fols. 78–83.

72. Porter, "Gift Relation"; Rose, "Politics and the London Royal Hospitals"; Risse, "Before the Clinic Was 'Born': Methodological Perspectives in Hospital History"; Fissell, *Patients, Power, and the Poor in Eighteenth-Century Bristol.* Helm assumes, probably correctly, that this statement was written largely by the Orphanage physicians of the period, most notably Christian Friedrich Richter ("Der Umgang mit dem kranken Menschen im halleschen Pietismus").

position. Although firmly in the voluntary and philanthropic sector, it did not rely on personal patronage in fact or in intention. More than others, it used unpaid voluntary labor, including student interns. But in most other respects— care for chronic versus acute patients, hygiene, nutrition, housekeeping, use of resources, and staff arrangements—it reflected mainstream trends.

The population to be served was defined to include both unspecified groups of the sick poor without domicile and those persecuted or ridiculed for their religious beliefs and abandoned in time of illness.[73] Contagious cases were not to be excluded, although admitting patients with chronic conditions was not considered prudent or advisable. Financial prudence was reflected in the insistence that services correspond to patient need: Students, itinerant artisans, and similar patients might require only lodging, nursing care, and medications; poor local day workers or married women might prefer to be house patients staying at home but receiving free medications and some modest financial support. The preference for dispensary care for the sick who were not inmates of the Orphanage and its schools reflected the preference for outside relief, generally considered a cost-saving alternative in charitable settings.[74] Making optimum use of the manpower constellation at the Francke Foundations, the home visitors for these housebound patients were to be students of theology, who would be able to observe the poor in their homes and to learn charity and humility while exercising sufficient authority and a measure of judgment. Students were to secure receipts for material assistance rendered and to provide careful accounting to the administrator. As in other charitable settings, the abuse of charity care by patients and families able but unwilling to provide for their own support was a perennial theme and turned out to be manifold, particularly in the dispensary.[75]

As befitted a progressive eighteenth-century institution, hygiene received considerable emphasis.[76] The infirmary was to be distant from the Orphanage

73. The Pietist sense of persecution and isolation had apparently remained strong despite a decade of acceptance and protection by the Prussian monarchy. Rose discusses a similar pattern for England in "Politics and the London Royal Hospitals."

74. See also Lindemann, *Patriots and Paupers: Hamburg, 1712–1830*; for the nineteenth century, Lettsom, "Hints Designed to Promote the Establishment of a Dispensary, for Extending Medical Relief to the Poor at Their Own Habitations."

75. Cavallo, "Conceptions of Poverty and Poor Relief in Turin in the Second Half of the Eighteenth Century"; for the nineteenth century in North America, see Hatfield and Roswell, "Report of the Special Committee of the Medical Association of the District of Columbia, on the 'Hospital and Dispensary Abuse in the City of Washington.'"

76. For cross-national exchanges in environmental medicine leading to hospital improvements, see Riley, *The Eighteenth-Century Campaign to Avoid Disease*.

accommodations proper, outside the walls of the city, exposed to crosswinds, and with spacious grounds for both patient exercise and a graveyard. The original plans foresaw two wards of six to eight beds each for men and women, as well as a number of separate smaller rooms for contagious or mentally disturbed patients; isolated quarters were suggested for those with skin and venereal diseases. Ventilation of the wards was a major consideration, with stoves and strategically placed chimneys in each room; ceilings were to be sufficiently high. Housekeeping and personal cleaning services were to be provided on a daily basis. Patients who arrived without clean linen were to be provided with shirts and sheets, and their own clothing was to be cleaned and kept until discharge. The bedding of discharged patients was to be thoroughly cleaned and changed.

Diet was to be healthy, nourishing but frugal. Most provisions were to be bought at wholesale prices from the Orphanage's own supplies, including beer and baked goods, thus introducing economies of scale. The medical director from 1718 to his death in 1755, Johann Juncker, took special charge of this task and thirty years later proudly reported his accomplishments in reining in the brewmaster, securing the purchase of quality hops and malt, and providing brewing instructions yielding a considerable increase of beer from the same raw materials.

Patient care was to be provided at three levels, using as little paid labor as possible. Students of medicine from the University worked under the supervision of a salaried physician. In the infirmary, the physician was to make daily visits of all wards and to prescribe treatment. The Orphanage pharmacy provided large volumes of free medications to both the infirmary and the dispensary.[77]

Caregiver and administrative staff were the major exceptions to the reliance on voluntary and unpaid labor. A salaried administrator, the housefather, kept both financial and medical records, hired and discharged caregivers, and supervised the administration of medications. Female caregivers under a matron were occasionally supplemented by men hired for the seriously ill in isolation or for controlling people with seizures. But extraordinary care was exercised to retain paid staff only for periods of actual need. In contrast to Catholic societies, the Protestant philanthropy of the eighteenth century, with its emphasis on charity infirmaries and dispensaries, could attract voluntary labor only for tasks that carried less onerous duties than care of the sick in hospitals[78] and was forced to

77. This contribution remained substantial beyond 1740, when the pharmacy became a separate commercial unit (see Chapter 3). See also Welsch, "Die Franckeschen Stiftungen."

78. Risse, *Hospital Life in Enlightenment Scotland: Care and Teaching at the Royal Infirmary of Edinburgh*.

rely on paid caretakers from the very bottom of the social heap. The poor reputation of these paid caretakers is evident from many contemporary documents and reform proposals. Low wages and the refusal to engage all but the matron on a continuous basis contributed to shortages, complaints, and high turnover. In one of many administrative memorandums, the hospital administrator pointed out that some women thought they could make better wages by taking in laundry. Even at a medically progressive institution like the Halle Orphanage, therefore, nursing arrangements remained mired in early modern tradition, using a housefather and housemother, usually a married couple who were prone to leave the hospital without leadership when one or the other was fired.[79]

Capital and major running costs were to be obtained through the system of charitable donations and bequests that also financed the Orphanage institutions proper. However, the patient's ability to pay was not ignored. The *Project von der Verpflegung der Kranken* required that patients be distinguished both according to their specific needs—shelter, care, food, and medications—and by ability to pay; those requiring only lodging and personal care might contribute from their own means. In the case of itinerant artisans, for example, some reimbursement might be obtained from their fraternal brotherhoods or mutual sick funds.[80]

Patients dying penniless were to be granted a burial site, a free coffin, and a shroud; for all others, burial costs were to be taken from the sale of their remaining possessions, with the balance going into the Orphanage funds. However, where possible, the next of kin was to be notified both of the course of the disease and the burial. In this Christian and voluntary setting, autopsies were frowned on, although they did occur, and the hospital regulations at mid-century in fact provided for the attendance of the hired women caregivers to prepare and clean the dissection room.[81]

---

79. The apparent inability to develop a corps of trained and motivated caregivers for the infirmary and the associated dispensary is surprising, as the Halle Orphanage was at the center of the very Pietist tradition of reform that eventually created the Lutheran deaconess movement and reintroduced secular nursing orders. See Vanja, "Aufwärterinnen, Narrenmägde, und Siechenmütter"; Fritschi, *Schwesterntum*.

80. *Grosse Aufsatz*, item XIII. The full text is in Wilson, "Pietist Universal Reform." The existence of artisan mutual funds funded by participants and even employers as an alternative to coercive charity care is well recognized in European accounts of the early modern period. See, for example, Riley, *Disease Without Death*. There is little information on attempts to transfer this type of mutual or fraternal insurance to North America before the nineteenth century. In Central Europe, such organizations were the indispensable forerunners of more general insurance mechanisms imposed from above. See Labisch, *Homo Hygienicus;* Schoultz, *Stadt und Gesundheit im Ruhrgebiet.*

81. Piechocki, "Gesundheitsfürsorge und Krankenpflege," 39. Piechocki has detailed the debate over the availability of corpses for dissection in "Die hallesche Anatomie im 18.–19. Jahrhundert," 67–105.

In summary, until mid-century, the Francke Foundations could claim that they had breached the traditional municipal monopoly of charity care. A complex and interlinked set of voluntary institutions independent of the traditional Lutheran establishment and local charity had been set up and supported through a variety of funding mechanisms, from testamentary bequests to capital invested against interest. Acutely aware of the limits of their institutional resources, the Foundations and their medical administrators had promoted the more cost-effective alternative of home or domiciliary and of dispensary care over the inpatient hospital model and had carefully singled out their preferred needy populations, leaving the less rewarding oversight of the idle poor, beggars, and malefactors incumbent on the secular magistrate. Also, and in contrast to at least the English model, the dispensary served not only the poor but also a middle-class clientele. Eventually, the reputation of the dispensary and its pharmaceutical regimens grew so much as to attract paying patients. This permitted the institution to provide a growing volume of free care to the poor and yet to realize a profit:

So lange die Apothecke wenig unter die Armen ausstreute, hatte sie jährlich einen grossen Verlust, und man hätte sie beynahe gäntzlich lassen eingehen, je mehr sie aber hernach gegeben, desto mehr hat sie eingenommen, und kann nun nicht allein seit vielen Jahre die Waysen und Armen frey halten, sonder auch jährlich einen guten Überschuss haben. Denn die Reichen kommen häufig neben ein, und die Apothecke behält doch das allgemeine Zeugniss, dass die Medicamenta wohlfeiler, als anderswo gegeben werden. (As long as the pharmacy gave little to the poor, it ran a large deficit every year, and it was close to being shut down. But later, the more was given of charity, the greater the sales for profit, and we have now for many years not only been able to distribute medications freely to the orphans and the poor, but the pharmacy has shown a good annual profit. For the rich now stop in freely, and the pharmacy is still known for its low prices, which are less than elsewhere.)[82]

But the lack of municipal support and interference achieved in Halle eventually posed a delicate dilemma. Although the Orphanage pharmacy was subject to visitation from University physicians, first under municipal rule and after

---

82. Juncker, "Instructions," App. B 5, in Piechocki, "Gesundheitsfürsorge und Krankenpflege."

1725 under the tightening net of Prussian health legislation, both the infirmary and the dispensary remained self-contained until the 1760s. This independence was gained at a price: There would be no municipal subsidy when costs escalated, as they invariably did in the hospital infirmary, and prolonged independence shut the facility off from the University's need for beds. The hospital early on restricted its intake to the large student and teacher population of the Orphanage Foundations, and by the 1750s, like the educational institutions, continued as an in-house facility, eventually coming under state regulation.[83]

83. As such, they existed until 1945, when the Foundations were deprivatized. They are now returned to voluntary status but no longer run as medical facilities.

A Radical 2

Heritage

Tempered

The seventeenth century and its movements of religious dissent were a fertile breeding ground for both a new medicine and the structure of medical care. It is a matter of historical perspective whether one assumes that these reforms carried over to the medical Enlightenment of the eighteenth century or were discontinuous and looked backward to the calls for more general reforms of society during the early modern period. English medical historiography speaks of a medical revolution for the seventeenth rather than the eighteenth century. This claim derives not only from the concomitant changes in scientific and medical thought but from the call for a change in the corporate monopolies of the medical professions, the rejection of traditional academic learning and medical hierarchies, and a reform of the materia medica.

These calls for a reform of medicine and medical practice were part and parcel of the reform of religious belief and lifestyles. They did not originate in one country or society. Rather, they were inspired by a community of reformers of many religious persuasions, professional backgrounds, and cultural origins, who traveled throughout continental Europe to escape war and religious persecution. By the middle of the seventeenth century, their places of refuge were centered in the Protestant Netherlands and England, where the Puritan interregnum in particular encouraged a wide spectrum of reforming proposals.[1] Many of these proposals linked their antiestablishmentarian and antimonopolistic tendencies to the practice and philosophy of medicine. They were carried over into the period after the Restoration of the Stuart monarchy by pragmatic and utilitarian reformers like Samuel Hartlib, and we find their echo in the medical plans of Pietist reformers.

In England as on the continent, the antecedents of these movements and the tenor of the times made it inevitable that much of this discourse of medical reform and of medicine continued to be in religious terms, whether carried on by the proponents of a new experimental science, by religious radicals and separatists, or by their opponents in the established professional bodies and churches.[2] The whole reservoir of religious emblematics, with choices determined by the writer's medical and political predilections, was used to invoke agendas and arguments. The virtues of the new Christian medicine of the Swiss physician Paracelsus (Theophrastus von Hohenheim, 1493–1541) and the Dutch Jean-Baptiste van Helmont and their followers were invoked by more radically inclined physicians. These were often proponents of a heavily chemiatric materia medica embedded in a tradition of alchemy, hermetics, and spagyrical medicine; their opponents tended to consider them both medical and religious heretics, which may say more about the place of alternative medical systems and beliefs in political polemics than about the intrinsic value of their therapeutic approach. The chemiatrists in

1. Among the numerous works on radical Protestant medical thought and practice and its manifold relations to the natural history of the seventeenth century, Webster, *The Great Instauration: Science, Medicine and Reform, 1626–1660*, remains the most important and comprehensive. For a recent discussion of the medical relevance of seventeenth-century utopias by natural philosophers and religious reformers alike, from Francis Bacon to Johann Andreae and Johann Comenius, see Berns, "Utopie und Medizin: Der Staat der Gesunden und der gesunde Staat: Utopische Entwürfe des 16. und 17. Jahrhunderts."

2. Webster, *Great Instauration*. For England, see Cook, *The Decline of the Old Medical Regime in Stuart London*; the essays collected in Roger, French, and Wear, eds., *The Medical Revolution of the Seventeenth Century*, in particular, Elmer, "Medicine, Religion, and the Puritan Revolution"; Wear, "Religious Beliefs in Early Modern England," and in his own collection (Wear, ed., *Health and Healing in Early Modern England: Studies in Social and Intellectual History*). The difference between the more pluralist Netherlands and Restoration England has recently been emphasized by Cook, "Natural History and Seventeenth Century English and Dutch Medicine," although Cook carefully skirts a full discussion of the link between the new sciences and physico-theology (255). See also Grell, "Plague in Elizabethan and Stuart London." Dutch studies on this topic remain fragmented; see van Lieburg, "Religion and Medical Practice in the Netherlands in the Seventeenth Century," which concentrates on early seventeenth-century Reformed Pietism and the vibrant and mutual reception of Pietist and revival medical-religious literature to 1700. The reception of this revival literature in Germany is well described by Sträter (*Sonthom, Bayly, Dike, und Hall*), but much work remains to be done on its medical components.

turn argued that their medical philosophy—and by inference, practice—would and should replace that of the Roman heathen Galen and his classical mentors, whose school continued to be the bedrock of scholastic and university medicine, derived from classical and medieval transmission of a largely but by no means exclusively botanical reservoir of simples and *composita*.[3] Battle was joined not only on therapy but on issues like hierarchical access to medical care and medical knowledge and the use of the vernacular in new medical texts accessible to a larger population, with the Paracelsians usually on the side of a more popularly accessible medical literature.[4]

Over time, the new piety of German Pietism that arose in the 1670s embraced a slightly different type of medical reform. By the beginning of the eighteenth century, the link between chemiatric and Paracelsian medicine and medical reform was no longer the unique hallmark of—although it often remained a stigma attached to—the medical reformer. But some of the links to this earlier tradition remained. Although Pietist academic physicians at Halle were as concerned as their peers with experience, experiment, new knowledge, and careful reasoning in medicine, Pietism like its seventeenth-century English predecessors continued to reject the vain display of book or worldly learning.[5]

---

3. For a magisterial overview of the interaction of European traditions from Greek medicine to our period, see Nutton, *The Western Medical Tradition*. The daunting literature on Paracelsus, one of the catalysts of the debate between Galenists and chemiatrists, generally reflects the trends of this debate in overwhelming detail, but is much obscured by ideology even when it addresses questions of politics and social conflict. Debus (*The English Paracelsians*, and idem, *The French Paracelsians: The Chemical Challenge to Medical and Scientific Tradition in Early Modern France*) and Pagel ("Helmont-Leibniz-Stahl," and idem, *Paracelsus: An Introduction to Philosophical Medicine in the Era of the Renaissance*) focus on the implications of chemiatric and alchemical medicine for the history of chemistry and philosophy of medicine and are the most dispassionate contributors to this discourse.

4. Whether these writers were in fact accessible to their contemporaries is not at all obvious. In medicine as elsewhere, sects calling for an opening of barriers to knowledge tend also to be protective of their own hierarchies. See, for example, Nicholas Culpepper, Gent. Student in Physick and Astrology, *The English Physician enlarged, with 369 medicines made of English herbs, that were not in any impression until this, being an astrolog-physical discourse of the vulgar herbs of this nation*; and the much later and controversial approach to open knowledge by Samuel Hahnemann (most recently, Dinges, *History of Homeopathy*). For the disdain of academic tradition and the use of the vernacular, see Elmer, "Medicine, Religion, and the Puritan Revolution," and Webster, *Great Instauration*. Much of this debate in fact can be traced back much farther than the seventeenth century; the assumption that the battle of the vernacular versus Latin (Webster, *Great Instauration*, 265–73) was joined only in the seventeenth century is contradicted by the work of Getz, "Charity, Translation, and the Language of Medical Learning in Medieval England," and other medievalists.

5. See Elmer, "Medicine, Religion, and the Puritan Revolution," 25, for England. For the mental framework of the German Pietist physician, see above all the work of Habrich, "Therapeutische Grundsätze pietistischer Ärzte des 18. Jahrhunderts," and "Characteristic Features of Eighteenth-

This central behavioral tenet of Pietism and many other radical sects under-
lies the traditional but erroneous assumption that Pietism was hostile to science and that its medicine was oriented to a religiously motivated passivism.[6]
On the contrary, Pietist medical tradition was firmly rooted in a biblical and
Christian doctrine of health and of the means of curing disease as divine gifts.
God had entrusted the physician with the power to heal,[7] and only the practice
of medicine, not academic dispute, was the proper way to discharge this oblig-
ation. As in seventeenth-century England, many German Pietist physicians dis-
trusted apothecaries as venal and insisted on their own chemical learning and
on a form of practice that would permit them to prepare their own medications.[8]

The Pietist Physician

But even the Pietist emphasis on abolishing social hierarchies, at least in the
framework of Christian discourse, did not relieve all its physicians—or at least
the less radical among them—of the need to make a living, and the more comfortable and prestigious livings remained uncomfortably dependent on a university reputation or noble patronage. Most German universities, Halle being
the singular exception, did not welcome radical reformers on their faculty, and
noble patronage remained indispensable. This patronage was most generous in
the tolerant small territories of Southwest Germany, such as Sayn-Wittgenstein

Century Therapeutics in Germany." For the evolution of medical thought in the Pietist setting, see
Geyer-Kordesch, "Passions and the Ghost in the Machine," although her argument still remains
uncomfortably close to the dichotomy between reason and reasoned experiment on the one hand and
mystical enthusiasm and holistic insight on the other hand. A more recent and more searching chain
of argument is presented in a series of essays in *Reading the Book of Nature: The Other Side of the Scientific
Revolution* (Debus and Walton, eds.), in particular, Newman, "Alchemical and Baconian Views on the
Art-Nature Division," 81–90, which takes this debate back well before the 1660s and the Restoration
in England. The rhetorical linkage of either medical and religious orthodoxy or enthusiasm tends to
obscure the implicit realities of the constraints of knowledge, however obtained, on the medical practice of the seventeenth and eighteenth centuries. For an elegant argument on this long-standing debate,
see Wear, "Medical Practice in Late 17th and Early 18th Century England: Continuity and Union."
    6. These older views are represented by Szindely, *Krankheit und Heilung im älteren Pietismus*; see
also Lindberg, "The Lutheran Tradition."
    7. Fritz Krafft summarizes this injunction for the early modern period in his introduction to
Dehmel, *Arzneimittel in der Physikotheologie*.
    8. Legal reformer John Cook for example had proposed that physicians make their own med-
ications and disclose their use and their contents in the vernacular. Webster, *Great Instauration*, 262.
Medicinae pauperum were proposed throughout to reduce the materia medica to a few carefully chosen
substances to ensure that the poor had access to appropriate medicinals. For the persistence of this
debate in England, see also Cook, *Trials of an Ordinary Doctor*.

and Ysenburg, and the court towns of Berleburg and Büdingen. Here and in the strongly Lutheran and much less tolerant duchy of Württemberg, whole networks of well-trained and often outstanding medical men—we know of no women—clustered around independent and radical scholars. There was Johann Conrad Dippel, chemist, physician, and author of numerous religious and medical polemics under the pseudonym Christianus Democritus. Johann Samuel Carl, whose influence we encounter later in this book, was an early student of Friedrich Hoffmann and an adherent of Georg Ernst Stahl's medical philosophy. And there were many competent but uncomfortably sectarian physicians like Johann Philipp Kämpf.[9] The reigning counts often ended their patronage abruptly, letting go even of well-regarded physicians in the interest of maintaining religious peace in their territories. The newly displaced formed yet another medical-religious diaspora, living and practicing precariously in the Netherlands, Denmark, and Sweden, and some emigrating with radical groups into the North American colonies.[10] Johann Samuel Carl's position in Berleburg and Ysenburg-Büdingen and at the court of Sayn-Wittgenstein was vastly improved by the patronage of the reigning counts, although his marriage to a noblewoman was not well regarded.[11] In 1736, he was called to Denmark to become physician to the Pietist King Christian VI and to modernize the Danish

9. With the exception of Johann Samuel Carl, there is not much literature on most of these physicians other than in regional studies, many of which date back to the 1890s. Some of this material is summarized in *Geschichte des Pietismus*, 2: Sections I–IV.

10. According to unpublished work by Habrich, Dippel was a competent chemist who first expressed the structure of a famous chemical dye, Prussian blue. He took a medical doctorate at Leiden in 1711. Kaempf was well regarded as a medical practitioner and appears to have been one of the teachers of George de Benneville, a French Huguenot who emigrated to Pennsylvania in 1740. See Chapter 7.

11. Intermarriage between noblewomen and Pietist scholars was not uncommon, although rarely accepted by the families of the bride. The physician Johann Juncker married a Countess Waldeck and had to leave the territory, surfacing in Halle several years later. In describing Carl's medical career and thought, I rely above all on Christa Habrich's work, most importantly her still-unpublished monograph "Untersuchungen zur pietistischen Medizin und ihrer Ausprägung bei Johann Samuel Carl und seinem Kreis," which offers a wealth of contextual detail and medical and pharmaceutical insight. I am much indebted to Dr. Habrich for sharing her work with me. Carl's appointment in Büdingen was in 1708, and he went to the court of Sayn-Wittgenstein in 1728. His career and medical thought, as well as his Pietist and medical network, offer a full case history of a prominent Pietist physician and parallels and overlaps the Halle developments in many ways, not least in the manner in which their lives and teachings touched that of many American practitioners of medicine. Carl played a major role in Inspirationalist circles, from which several men and women emigrated who were to become of crucial importance to the development of a German-language print culture around Christopher Sauer. See Schrader, *Literaturproduktion und Büchermarkt des radikalen Pietismus: Johann Heinrich Reitz: "Historie der Wiedergebohrnen" und ihr geschichtlicher Kontext.*

system of health care. He resigned, again for political reasons, and returned in 1740 to Halle, where he spent the rest of his life and died in 1757.

Even in the more staid environment of Prussia, patronage was a tender issue for the reforming Pietist physicians in their relationships with aristocratic and influential patients. Stahl wrote a critical little tract on the physician's duty to make house calls, and the dictates of medical fashion among the Pietist aristocracy at the court of Berlin are mirrored in correspondence between the brothers Richter and the Baron Hildebrand von Canstein. Canstein had little if any hesitation to second- or even first-guess his medical correspondents on a variety of diagnoses and treatments.[12]

In Pietist and bourgeois Halle, the opportunities offered by access to a new and progressive university also called for prudent accommodation rather than confrontation with medical monopolies. Although Pietist views on the proper role of the Pietist physician continued to draw on the spiritual precedents of seventeenth-century medical reform, as did their approach to the linkage of charity care and poor reform, medical issues and medical practice had to transcend this precedent. Relationships between the Orphanage Foundations and the University medical faculty were thus based on mutual self-interest, which subsumed radical tendencies. But the conflicts or differences in medical philosophy that distinguished avowedly Pietist physicians at Halle do not support the traditional assumptions about Enlightenment rationalism versus religious enthusiasm. Local sensitivities concerning the patient's right to his or her own body and the persistent revulsion against dissection of deceased members of the community were at least overtly honored by the Foundations, despite the wish for a more lenient or medically enlightened policy on the part of the medical director of the Orphanage hospital and dispensary, Johann Juncker, himself a devout Pietist. Thus, despite collaboration between the medical school and the dispensary of the Orphanage, there is only ambiguous evidence for the medicalization of charity care that has been proposed as a major reason for the growth of clinical facilities during the eighteenth century.[13]

---

12. A striking example in our context is the correspondence between the brothers Richter and the Baron Canstein during 1699–1708 (Hauptarchiv Franckesche Stiftungen [HAFSt] C 285). See, for the English setting, the arguments proposed by Jewson, "Medical Knowledge and the Patronage System in Eighteenth-Century England."

13. In her attempt to place this medicalization debate into a comparative framework, Loetz, "Medikalisierung in Frankreich, Grossbritannien, und Deutschland, 1750–1850: Ansätze, Ergebnisse, und Perspektiven der Forschung," observes the low priority placed on this phenomenon by researchers

Academic Medicine and Medical Education at Halle

By 1720, the department of medicine at the Friedrich University, under its founders Friedrich Hoffmann and Georg Ernst Stahl, had grown from small beginnings to a medical magnet rivaling Leiden in terms of both faculty and number of students. Both Stahl and Hoffmann were reformers of medical education as well as proponents of two of the great explanatory schemes of early eighteenth-century medicine: Stahl's vitalism and iatrochemical concepts of illness and healing—the marshaling of the body's defenses under the guidance of the soul—and Friedrich Hoffmann's iatromechanics within a Cartesian framework.[14]

Hoffmann and Stahl were close contemporaries, and their lives and work bridged two centuries. Hoffmann lived from 1660 to 1742, Stahl from 1659 to 1735. Although Stahl left Halle in 1717 to practice as physician at the Hohenzollern court in Berlin, Hoffmann returned from that court after a brief period (1709–12) to head the medical faculty until his death. Georg Ernst Stahl developed his philosophy of medicine, the *theoria medica vera*, while in Halle and had many followers among the Pietist medical community and the students, in particular with regard to the restoration of Hippocratic medicine and his insistence on the healing forces of nature. But Hoffmann was not rejected among Pietist students because of his more rationalist approach. On the contrary, he was a highly popular teacher and practicing physician who early in his career had published a major elementary text of largely Cartesian orientation, which explained the main functions of the human body in mechanical terms in the context of the new mathematics and physics.[15] But he too required a *primum movens*, and

---

like Roy Porter and his associates. For a full study of an eighteenth-century German setting, see Lindemann, *Health and Healing in Eighteenth-Century Germany*. For France, most recently Brockliss and Jones, *The Medical World of Early Modern France*.

14. There is a very large body of work on the University in Halle, its medical faculty and students, and the orientation of its medical minds, most of it in German. Much of this work is based on primary sources mined and published by Wolfram Kaiser and his associates, in particular Arina Völker (a selection of titles is in the composite bibliography at the end of this volume).

15. *Fundamenta Medicinae ex principiis naturae mechaniciis ad usum Philiatrorum succincte proposita* (1695). The major English-language work on Hoffmann's theories remains Lester King's studies; King places him in the accepted European medical context. See King, "Stahl and Hoffman: A Study in Eighteenth-Century Animism," and idem, *The Road to Medical Enlightenment: 1650–1695*. See also French, "Sickness and the Soul: Stahl, Hoffmann, and Sauvages on Medical Pathology." A recent summary of the respective contributions of Hoffmann and Stahl in terms of conflicting ideas but parallel practice is by Konert, "Academic and Practical Medicine in Halle During the Era of Stahl, Hoffmann, and Juncker."

he postulated an "aether" as the driving but entirely material force of all physiological processes, centered in the brain and distributing itself over the entire body through the nerves, through which it regulated the tone of the fibers.[16]

As for many of the medical theorists of the period, Hoffmann's success as a physician and teacher was due to the fact that in the therapeutic setting, he preferred experience and reason over theory and disposed of a wide and highly popular therapeutic armamentarium ranging from diet and the use of mineral waters to a large reservoir of materia medica.[17] Stahl opposed Hoffmann's iatromechanical concepts with a more holistic approach, in which the ancient concepts of body and soul were more intricately linked by mechanisms of reciprocal affect, which he described in considerable detail.[18] But although he considered the soul as the first cause of all movement, he did not regard the body simply as God's machine, and his own and his students' insights into the chemical determinants of physiology and pathology remain part and parcel of the history of chemistry independent of their philosophical underpinnings. At the level of therapy, Stahl, like Hoffmann, was an eclectic or synchretist, sharing with iatrophysicists fairly traditional ideas from humoral pathology and using a materia medica similar to Hoffmann, the exclusion of cinchona bark and opium being notable exceptions. Physician reliance on traditional and known remedies, which was the prudent course of the conservative practitioner then as now, was linked to a proper concern for reliable income. Like their European medical peers, Stahl and Hoffmann, Johann Samuel Carl, and Johann Juncker developed their own medications, and Hoffmann derived a lifelong substantial income from them. At least in the early stages, alchemical and chemiatric traditions were still part and parcel of this development.[19]

But at the same time, at the University and elsewhere among medical innovators and teachers, the change to a more discriminating pharmacological therapy was advocated. Again, regardless of medical philosophy, Stahl and Hoffmann, and

16. King, "Stahl and Hoffmann"; Lanz, *Arzneimittel in der Therapie Friedrich Hoffmanns (1660–1742): Unter besonderer Berücksichtigung der Medicina consultatoria (1721–1723)*, chap. 4.

17. Lanz, *Arzneimittel in der Therapie Friedrich Hoffmanns*, chap. 5.

18. The works of Johanna Geyer-Kordesch on Stahl and of Christa Habrich on Johann Samuel Carl and his circle ("Untersuchungen zur pietistischen Medizin") have provided a larger philosophical, anthropological, and medical context for Stahl's medicine and the Pietist patient and physician. See Geyer-Kordesch, "Georg Ernst Stahl's Radical Pietist Medicine and Its Influence on the German Enlightenment," and idem, "Die Medizin im Spannungsfeld zwischen Aufklärung und Pietismus: Das unbequeme Werk Georg Ernst Stahls und dessen kulturelle Bedeutung."

19. Lanz, *Arzneimittel in der Therapie Friedrich Hoffmanns*, refers to a number of chemiatric arcana manufactured by both Hoffmann and Stahl. For a fuller discussion, see Chapter 3.

later Juncker, Carl, and Christian Friedrich Richter, another Stahl pupil, inveighed against polypharmacy and indiscriminate prescribing. The chemiatric enthusiasm of the seventeenth century had yielded to a more sober view that recognized the dangers inherent in heroic chemiatric or, for that matter, botanical treatments.

If eighteenth-century medicine, Enlightened or otherwise, remained in a state of speculation and transition, its major innovations were in new approaches to both patient and physician education, often for purposes beyond traditional medical practice. Medicine as taught at Halle University was progressive and not only productive of several iatrogenic schemes, but for several decades may be said to have been at the forefront of medical education in Central Europe. Both during and after Stahl's and Hoffmann's tenures, the medical faculty performed many educational and clinical functions for the Orphanage, whose medical institutions in turn were a place for men promoting the reform of hierarchies, medical education, and a new approach to medical ethics and to access to care. This was true in particular of Johann Juncker, who was a late student of Stahl, and of the forensic physician Michael Alberti (1682–1757), a student of Hoffmann. Among the second generation of Halle medical talent, Johann Juncker was an eminent practical physician before joining the faculty in 1727. He led the Orphanage medical institutions from 1718 to 1753.

Until mid-century, for reasons related to both denominational politics and the breadth of its faculty, Halle's medical school attracted a wide range of students. They came from Sweden, Denmark, the Baltic regions returned to Russian sovereignty in 1709, and Moscow and Saint Petersburg, where Peter I had fostered an international medical team with strong German and Scottish influences.[20] Students from the Protestant territories of the empire, which included the Reformed communities in Hungary, provided a reservoir of practitioners accustomed to negotiating the shoals of teaching and working in multicultural and multidenominational settings. Overall, until the 1740s, the medical school educated more students than the other German medical schools combined.[21] By 1750, the army medical and surgical college in Berlin drew an increasing number of students but lacked the academic standing to dispense a full medical degree, for which many of its students subsequently went to Halle.[22] The only other medical school of com-

20. Kaiser and Völker, "Repräsentanten der Ars medica halensis in der russischen Medizingeschichte des 18. Jahrhunderts."

21. Konert, "Academic and Practical Medicine," table 1, citing Oehme but excepting Vienna; for Vienna, see Lesky, *Österreichisches Gesundheitswesen im Zeitalter des aufgeklärten Absolutismus*.

22. This school was a practical army training college later attached to the Charité at Berlin.

parable size in the German-language areas was Strasbourg, which had remained a Protestant institution after the seizure of the Alsace by Louis XIV in 1681 but by mid-century was slowly being incorporated into the French system. Both in terms of teaching and student potential, therefore, the academic medical environment at Halle offered a rich mine of talent waiting to be tapped by a philanthropic institution that had put the reform of charity and charity care on its banner.

Care of the poor, and the clinical teaching opportunities they offered, was one result of this interaction. In return for free care, charity patients (*die Armen*) had to agree to be examined and treated in the presence of students. This proved a successful teaching strategy over several decades, despite original objections, particularly among women.[23]

In a retrospective of his work, which was embedded in instructions to his successors, Juncker did not deal expressly with the relations between the Francke Foundations and the Friedrich University, which after Christian Wolff's return in 1740 had ceased to be the undisputed preserve of the Pietist professors of theology.[24] But Juncker had made full and innovative use of the opportunity for intensive and interactive medical education that the linkage of Orphanage clinic and medical school offered.[25] From 1717, even before Juncker had joined the medical faculty, the "Collegium Clinicum Halense" offered an outstanding training opportunity. Clinical facilities for inpatient care were an early feature of the Halle Orphanage, where the brothers Richter repeatedly permitted medical students to accompany them on their rounds, resembling the instructional patterns at Leiden. By 1718, the dispensary for the poor where patients were treated free of charge and provided with medications and other necessities grew rapidly in popularity (see Chapter 1). Juncker as the head of service soon drew in the so-called *provectiores*, students working with physicians of university standing, who thus obtained the knowledge and experience that, in other places, were available only to practicing physicians. In turn, Juncker's eventual standing among the medical faculty[26] confirmed the rise in status of the ordinary or salaried

23. Piechocki, "Gesundheitsfürsorge und Krankenpflege in den Franckeschen Stiftungen in Halle/Saale," 45.

24. Hinrichs, *Preussentum und Pietismus*, chap. 5.

25. Kaiser, ed., *Johann Juncker und seine Zeit*; Konert, "Academic and Practical Medicine."

26. The holdings of the National Library of Medicine in Washington, D.C., include 125 doctoral dissertations under Juncker's guidance, including the famous case of a woman physician, Dorothea Erxleben, who graduated in 1754. See Kaiser and Krosch, "Zur Geschichte der medizinischen Fakultät der Universität Halle im 18. Jahrhundert (VIII): Zum 250. Geburtstag von Christiane Dorothea Erxleben."

physician, which, as elsewhere in Europe, prefigured the change from the restrictive physician of the poor to the eventual gatekeeper of the teaching hospital.

Juncker pointed with pride to his abandonment of private practice and insisted on the autonomy of the clinical physician in relation to both patients and students. As the head of a teaching infirmary and dispensary, he provided to the heads of the Foundations assurance of effective and profitable patient care and enhanced the reputation of the institution in the outside world. He assured the medical faculty that its students would receive appropriate clinical teaching opportunities and the theological faculty that work in the dispensary was appropriate Christian preparation for the ministry. He advised brevity and control of discussions in student conferences without interfering with proper teaching ("by friendly insistence, the medicus must limit the students' tendency to stray from the subject, without, however, neglecting to explain in an appropriate fashion, the true fundamenta sanitatis conservandae").[27] He instructed his successor (who in the event was his son) that even where the patients on the wards did not require constant medical attention, daily attendance was necessary to control the administrator and nursing staff and to prevent medical students from adopting their preferred treatment plans or even carrying out surgical interventions. But he claimed as a distinguishing feature of Pietist medical education the close bond between teacher and student that is apparent also in the writings of other Pietist physicians: "I often think with great delight of this hidden blessing. For in the last 37 years many a student has left here who are now united with me in a bond of love and praise the Lord for the gift that they received during their time in being permitted to assist in providing medical service."[28] The conjunction of religious philanthropy and a progressive medical school led by distinguished medical faculty yielded many well-prepared medical practitioners of a Pietist bent, both in the German territories and abroad. But this conjunction ended in the late 1750s and never fully revived. The cohort of great Pietist physicians had been exhausted by attrition; Stahl and Hoffmann died in the 1730s, and Juncker and Carl died in the 1750s. The Friedrich University saw a severe decline in resources during the Seven Years' War (1756–63), and when it recovered in the 1770s, the Halle Orphanage Foundations were well beyond their prime as an

27. This and the following quotations are in Wirtschafts und Verwaltungsarchiv Franckesche Stiftungen, ix/ii/1, 1718ff., fols. 78–83. See also Piechocki, "Gesundheitsfürsorge und Krankenpflege."

28. "Mit Erquickung dencke ich öfters an diesen heimlichen Segen; Denn es sind in verwichenen 37 Jahren gar manche studiosi ausgegangen, welche nun im Bande der Liebe mit mir stehen, und Gott für die ehemalige allhier genossene Medicinische Handreichung bey aller Gelegenheit preisen."

institution of reform. The new greats of the Halle medical school, among them Wilhelm Hufenagel and Christian Reil, although former Halle students, had not gone through the Orphanage facilities for their clinical training, and care for the poor returned to the control of the municipalities and the Prussian state.[29]

Lay Medical Education and the Printed Word

Patient education as well found a fruitful environment at Halle. Juncker and his colleague Carl were prolific publishers of textbooks, in both Latin and the vernacular, which specifically addressed lay needs and imposed, on both patient and practitioner, explicit requirements that went beyond traditional dietetics.[30] This trend, which was part of the genre of *Populärmedizin*, came over the course of the eighteenth century to differ substantially from the self-help medicine treatises of earlier periods, whether in the Italian tradition of *secreta* or the English precedent of the seventeenth century, from Baxter to Culpeper.[31] In the Central European setting, popular medical instruction and assignment of personal responsibility for health became in many ways medicine from above and were favored by enlightened absolutists from the Hohenzollerns and the late Hapsburgs to the Romanovs. Much of the historical emphasis has been on cameralist administrative initiatives and has been described in terms of medical policing of health.[32] But here as elsewhere, the dichotomy between secular and religious spheres is misleading. Even the most enlightened absolutist counted on the

29. Seils, *Friedrich Albrecht Carl Gren in seiner Zeit, 1760–1798*; Bonner, *Becoming a Physician: Medical Education in Britain, France, Germany, and the United States*, 36, for the Halle medical curriculum and its brief monopoly in the natural sciences.

30. Presentation of practical issues rather than medical philosophy made Juncker's works popular as textbooks, which were published in numerous editions. The German version of a *Conspectus chirurgicae* had been published in 1722 and offered instruction to the surgeon not well versed in Latin. The second and third editions of the *Conspectus Medicinae Theoretico-practicae*, devoted to the theory and practice of medicine, were published in 1724 and 1732. A *Conspectus Formularum* was published in expanded form in 1730. Here as elsewhere, pharmacotherapy was discussed repeatedly in relation to expectant treatment and nonpharmacological stimulation of the "motus naturae." J. S. Carl published extensively in the journals of natural history and observation and contributed to the Nuremberg *Commercium litterarium*. According to the bibliography compiled by Christa Habrich, almost 50 percent of his twenty-eight monographs were in German.

31. Eamon, *Science and the Secrets of Nature: Books of Secrets in Medieval and Early Modern Culture*; Webster, *Great Instauration*; Smith, "Prescribing the Rules of Health: Self-Help and Advice in the Late 18th Century."

32. Rosen, "Cameralism and Medical Police"; Lesky, ed., *A System of Complete Medical Police: Selections from Johann Peter Frank*; Lindemann, *Health and Healing in Eighteenth-Century Germany*, chaps. 2 and 3.

clergy to promote reform—whether of agriculture or public health, including variolization. Even in conditions of secular administrative dominance, pastors could hardly have been expected to promote such measures bereft of biblical reference or injunction.[33]

Again, conditions in Halle were fortuitous and quickly exploited by the astute Pietist leadership. Prussian administrative reforms had begun under Frederick III (I) Hohenzollern, and public health reforms were initiated in 1725 under his son, Frederick William I, a relentless promoter of domestic reform. But the Orphanage Foundations had already gone into the business of popular medical instruction by the first decade of the century, when they started promoting their new medications with the help of numerous publications, in particular several self-help texts that provided lay instruction in illness and health, followed by another set of instructions on how to use which Halle medicines for what ills. The titles of these manuals (*The Highly Necessary Understanding of the Body; A Brief and Explicit Account of the Body*) clearly suggested an educational message, and the link to the Pietist framework was established in the prefaces to Christian readers in these and other printed materials. The title page of the longest and most frequently republished text, *Die Höchstnöthige Erkenntnis* or *The Highly Necessary Understanding of the Body,* by Christian Friedrich Richter, pointed to the importance of understanding man and woman (*des Menschen*) in regard to both to the body and the natural, that is, nonspiritual, life, promised a clear instruction concerning health and how to preserve and maintain it, and provided "the causes, signs, and names of diseases so as to ensure that everyone, even the unlearned, might even in the absence of a physician use this treatise to cure most, even serious disease"[34] (see Figure 2.1). Despite the invocation of the "unlearned" reader, the intended audience was clearly both literate and educated. It encompassed students and teachers of medicine and, expressly, the middle and upper classes

33. Lindemann, *Health and Healing in Eighteenth-Century Germany,* chap. 2; Dehmel, *Arzneimittel in der Physikotheologie,* illustrates this in the work of Johann Jacob Schmidt's *Biblicus medicus,* part of a multivolume work published in 1743 and written during Schmidt's tenure of an isolated rural parish in Pomerania. Schmidt, formerly a student at Halle, forced Old Testament references into an early modern medical and natural history framework, ranging from a categorization of the healing professions to a description of pharmaceuticals and therapeutic interventions. His work even found an audience in North America. See Chapter 7.

34. *Seeligen Hn. D. Christian Friedrich Richters Höchst-nöthige Erkenntnis des Menschen, sonderlich nach dem Leibe und natürlichen Leben, oder ein deutlicher Unterricht, von der Gesundheit und deren Erhaltung* (1708, 1712, and subsequent reprints).

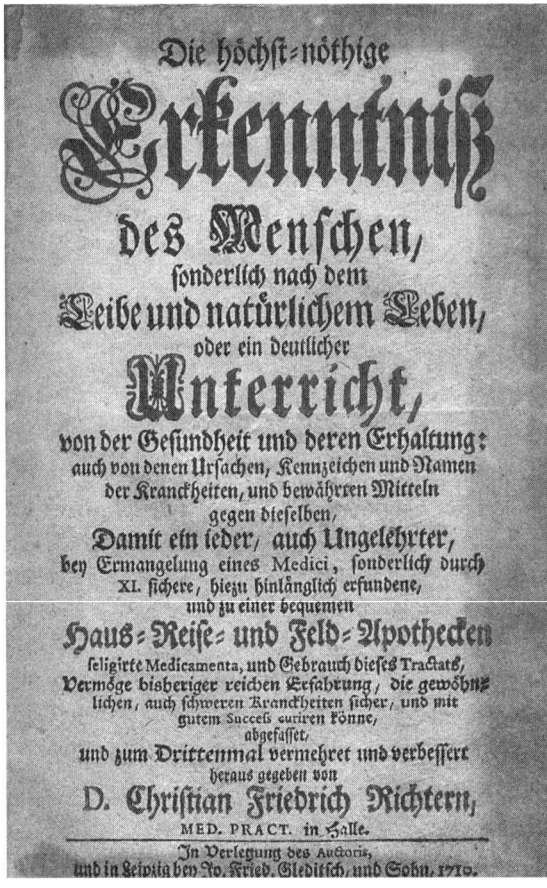

Fig. 2.1

Title page of *Die Höchst-nöthige Erkenntnis* by Christian Friedrich Richter (1710 ed.), a 1,200-page self-help manual on the causes of health and illness and on the uses of the Halle Orphanage medications. (Courtesy, Francke Foundations in Halle, Germany.)

among the lay public. In structure, the *Höchst-nöthige Erkenntnis* remained in the heterogeneous but still recognizable tradition of the Institutes of Medicine.[35] Part I laid out in detail anatomy, nonmorbid physiology and its interface with disease, pathology, followed by instructions on lifestyle and dietetics. Part II was dedicated to diseases, their causes, therapies, and outcomes, and to an appendix on prenatal, maternal, and infant care.

35. For the slow but pervasive changes in these texts in the teaching institutions of Italy and then Central Europe during the early modern period, see in particular Bylebyl, "Teaching Methodus Medendi in the Renaissance," and King, *The Road to Medical Enlightenment*, on Hoffmann and Boerhave.

In terms of medical philosophy, Part I reflects much of the transitional and syncretic thinking of the period and was heavily influenced by the author's mentors, Stahl and Hoffmann. Stahlian principles of the animus or soul as the sole and direct mover and controller of bodily and mental functions were joined to Friedrich Hoffmann's anatomy of the nervous system, although the Stahlian system was emphasized over Hoffmann's Cartesian paradigm, and the centrality of the soul as the final *movens* was emphasized. Overall, however, the medical framework remained embedded in classical and early modern concepts and terminology. In particular, the continually resurrected Hippocratic principle of the body's ability to heal itself was stressed as the first requirement for care and cure.[36]

This combination of an introduction to medicine and health, coupled with a practical nosography in Latin and German and a long list of practical therapeutic suggestions—although concentrated on the Halle Orphanage medications—made this text a vehicle for self-instruction that incorporated mainstream medical teaching. It found a market not only among its original target audience in the Pietist community but also in the Southeast European and Russian areas with large German components. It established the reputation of a large set of medications prepared at and sold through the Orphanage. Its origin and stated purpose—to promote a Christian medicine and to fund the charitable goals of this famous philanthropic enterprise—seem to have added rather than detracted from its appeal. Despite its clear roots in the seventeenth-century tradition, the Richter manual was no longer freighted by hermetic or Paracelsian baggage, but tied explicitly to current therapeutic and academic practice.

Also, although not central to the therapeutic section, the Pietist message was reasserted. The introductory sections to Parts I and II provided a decidedly Christian reference framework. God reigned over health and illness, but as announced in the title, imposed on patients and physicians the duty to preserve, maintain, and reestablish health: "[A]nd such are the body and its members, being equipped with such form and structure as enable the soul to fulfill [His] final purpose. . . . But what shall I tell you, oh Reader, of your own body and of how it and your material nature is abused. . . . For it is abundantly clear that *reason* is much used against the spirit of the Lord, and while your

36. For a recent discussion of the implications of this principle for therapy and assumptions of therapeutic efficacy of the materia medica, see Estes, "Changing Fashions in Therapeutics."

reason is designed to understand His Being from His works, you perversely deny Him."

Another avenue of lay instruction was the *Wöchentliche Hallische Anzeigen*, a weekly published by the Francke Foundations. The journal carried articles by many of the Halle faculty on matters of lay concern, including advice on nursing and infant care.[37]

The Outcomes of Reform

The outcomes of this favorable conjunction deserve more than a passing glance, both in terms of the content of medical care and the modes of practice. As observed in many other settings, we have almost too much material documenting physician education, program statements illustrating the meshing of academic and government objectives, and the philosophies of the small number of physicians who had the inclination, the opportunity, and the time to see their work into print. In Halle, as amply described by Wolfram Kaiser and his associates, there are lists of students both enrolled and graduating, a vast corpus of doctoral dissertations, publications of the professors, and some studies of individual practitioners.[38]

But how do we know whether what students learned and eventually practiced was in fact a new medicine embodying Pietist reform? Halle physicians, like most others, left few casebooks and similar documents, although the evidence preserved in the institutional setting of the Orphanage is richer than customary in general ambulatory practice and permits some glimpses into whether and how medical reform occurred and whether it should be ascribed to Pietist incentives. Fortunately, this evidence includes diagnostic and therapeutic counsel sent across the Atlantic during the first half of the century, and it affords, if not a full body of material on medical practice and the content of care, then the

37. Konert, "Practical and Academic Medicine." These developments occurred well before mid-century and prefigure the summary of German developments in Bonner, *Becoming a Physician*, chaps. 1 and 2.

38. For instances in another German territory, see Lindemann, *Health and Healing in Eighteenth-Century Germany*, note 8, chap. 2. For Halle, see the work of Kaiser, "Der Lehrkörper der Medizinischen Fakultät in der hallschen Amtszeit von Georg Ernst Stahl"; Kaiser and Krosch, "Zur Geschichte der medizinischen Fakultät der Universität Halle"; and Kaiser and Völker, "Repräsentanten der ars medica halensis." The lack of more recent work on the primary sources is noted by Helm, "Der Umgang mit dem kranken Menschen im hallschen Pietismus des frühen 18. Jahrhunderts," note 12. But see Konert, "Academic and Practical Medicine."

opportunity to look at widely different locales of practice by Pietist physicians and other medical providers. We turn to these in Part 2.

In terms of guild monopolies, the Orphanage Foundations were most successful in breaching that of the apothecaries and used the proceeds of their manufactures to finance seventy years of missionary activity and charity care. But they relied for the continuation of royal privileges on visitations of its production facilities by University committees and on the academic standing of the heads of its pharmaceutical enterprise, first the brothers Richter and after 1740, David Samuel von Madai. There was less success in terms of surgical reform, that is, the inclusion of surgical in medical training, which had been promoted by Laurenz Heister and others and was part of Juncker's and Carl's agenda as well. In the Halle setting, the guilds won out until mid-century.

From 1720 to 1750, the Halle link between charity practice and clinical education was at the forefront of European reforms. Selected medical students did ward duty and practiced medicine under the supervision of the medical director of the Orphanage hospital and outpatient clinic, with a large body of charity patients providing opportunity for demonstration in return for free care. The therapeutic practice in Halle differed from the more selective use of the *medicina pauperum* practiced elsewhere—and even by Johann Samuel Carl on the urging of this noble but frugal patron—by using the whole range of Orphanage medications rather than a reduced version consisting of simple and inexpensive preparations.

Although here as well Halle medicine was not unique, both medical ethics and the trend to the reform of pharmaceutical practice led to a turn to expectant medicine, which in the event conflicted with the more aggressive use of pharmaceuticals advocated in the Richter manual; in North America, one Halle transplant, the *medicus* Ernst Thilo, rejected English and French surgical practices urged on him during his stay in London. He was a very sparing practitioner of venesection once in Georgia and abstained from amputations and similar procedures.[39] The conscientious among Halle practitioners followed Stahl's early injunctions against the use of opium and cinchona, not so much for the religious reasons later attributed to this practice but for reasons in line with their own medical and physiological precepts.[40] Similarly, they rejected variolization for the attendant dangers from adverse effects and infection from carriers of

39. Wilson, "Hallesche Waisenhausmedikamente."
40. The best and most inclusive work on this subject remains the still-unpublished work of Christa Habrich, "Untersuchungen zur pietistischen Medizin."

variolated bacteria.[41] More important, they increasingly rejected heroic courses of therapy. Several of the Orphanage medications were slowly reformulated over time, replacing older chemiatric substances such as mercury sulfide and crude antimony in their violent and cathartic forms. Nonetheless, even Pietist practitioners were unable or unwilling to cease administering excretionary and depleting medications, whether of botanical or mineral origin. Carl in particular favored bitter substances for regulating the mixture of the humors, and in general Pietist therapy remained within the moderately inclined mainstream of eighteenth-century European medicine.

With the slow excision of older chemiatric preparations from the materia medica came the increasingly obvious rejection of hermetic traditions in medicine, despite the roots of Pietist medical reform in Paracelsian circles. Whether radical Pietists or the increasingly staid Halle physicians, they advocated the eradication of superstitious and magic practices among the lay public as part of modern and Christian patient education. On the other hand, Carl in particular, in his *Armenapotheke* of 1713, conceded the possible value of a number of so-called folk or herbal medicines. Medicine under Pietist auspices, therefore, was neither monolithic nor an entirely distinct body of medical practice. Its practitioners had their own medical disagreements although they were united in the need to reform patient and physician behavior within the framework of the new evangelical piety. As noted, many Halle medical students went on to practice in the countries of Eastern and Southeastern Europe; a few went to North America, where they found a good number of radical Pietists already practicing in German communities. But all were well aware of the reputation of Halle as a medical magnet, and the Pietist clergy who came to these shores after 1740 had little doubt that their medical sophistication was at least equal to that of their English colleagues.

---

41. For similar American objections, see Duffy, *Epidemics in Colonial America*, chap. 1.

3

A most useful way to relieve the costs of running the
pharmacy and, in particular, [its] laboratories, would be
to establish a wholesale trade in the necessary materials
and obtain these from Amsterdam without having to rely
on middlemen. This would have the advantage that
materials which we must now purchase dearly here, particularly in Leipzig, could be obtained directly and without
spoilage and tampering or adulteration after having passed
through many hands. And it cannot be denied that such
a wholesale trade, once it is well established, could yield
significant profits for the support of our institutions.

—*Wirtschafts- und Verwaltungsarchiv Franckesche
Stiftungen, ix/ii/1ff, presumably a 1702 note by
August Hermann Francke*

The Halle Orphanage Foundations began their
pharmaceutical manufacture in the early 1700s,
after receiving a special exemption to establish a
pharmacy as part of their larger charter of privileges
from the Elector, Frederick III Hohenzollern. That
exemption from guild and corporate regulations was
granted in the context of a larger set of exemptions
for the operation of a charitable enterprise, such as
release from taxes and fees.[1] The stated reason for

1. *Churfürstlich Brandenburgisches Privilegium Über das
Waysenhaus zu Glaucha an Halle, Anno 1698* (reprint, Halle, 1998),
item 10.

the pharmacy privilege was to enable the Orphanage to obtain medicines without having to rely on the town pharmacies "at night and during the winter," because the Glaucha district did not have its own apothecary shop. However, the government in Berlin prudently insisted on the customary fees and taxes for any sales transacted. As for his other enterprises, Francke's goals were far larger than the creation of a simple local pharmacy for the sick of the Orphanage and the resident population. After several pious benefactors had bequeathed a number of secret recipes to August Hermann Francke in the furtherance of his goals, he spent considerable sums on securing skilled laboratory workers and equipment to develop these recipes and made extensive plans for securing raw materials and opening up sales networks.[2]

Both manufacture and trade took off in earnest with the development in 1702 of *essentia dulcis* or "sweet essence," a potable tincture of gold marketed as a general fortifier and tonic; by the 1720s, the pharmaceutical component of the Halle enterprise had become highly profitable, supporting as much as one-third to one-half of the Foundations' total expenditures over time. It remained profitable until the latter third of the eighteenth century.[3] Although a good number of unsung laboratory workers participated in the development of the Orphanage medications,[4] major credit is usually given to the brothers Richter, a family of medically trained brothers (who had come to Halle in the 1690s) from Sorau in Lusatia, a border province of Silesia. They were, in order of birth, Christian Sigismund (1672–1739), Christian Albrecht (1674–99), Christian Friedrich (1676–1711), and Christian Erdmann (1680–1710). Among the brothers, the best known is Christian Friedrich Richter, a student of Georg Ernst Stahl and a writer of considerable gifts, who is remembered both for his hymns and as the author of the manuals accompanying the Halle medications.[5] After C. F.

2. Poeckern, *Die Halleschen Waisenhausartzeneyen;* one of the testators was Superintendent Fischer, a major Lutheran figure in the Baltic areas whose family had close Pietist connections since the 1680s; see Wallmann, "Beziehungen des frühen Pietismus zum Baltikum und zu Finnland." The report on Fischer's communication of recipes is in the Wirtschafts-und Verwaltungsarchiv der Franckeschen Stiftungen, Halle (VAFSt) ix/Repertorium ii/16, fols. 185–94, and letter by David Samuel von Madai of 28 May 1742, ibid.

3. Sales at home and abroad in fact continued throughout the nineteenth and until well into the twentieth century.

4. The most careful study of the personalities involved and their relative pharmaceutical and chemiatric contributions remains Poeckern, *Die Halleschen Waisenhausartzeneyen,* whose findings I follow in this account.

5. The title of his twentieth-century biography refers to Richter as the physician, apothecary, and hymn writer of Halle Pietism. See Altmann, *Christian Friedrich Richter (1676–1711): Arzt, Apotheker, und Liederdichter der Halleschen Pietisten.*

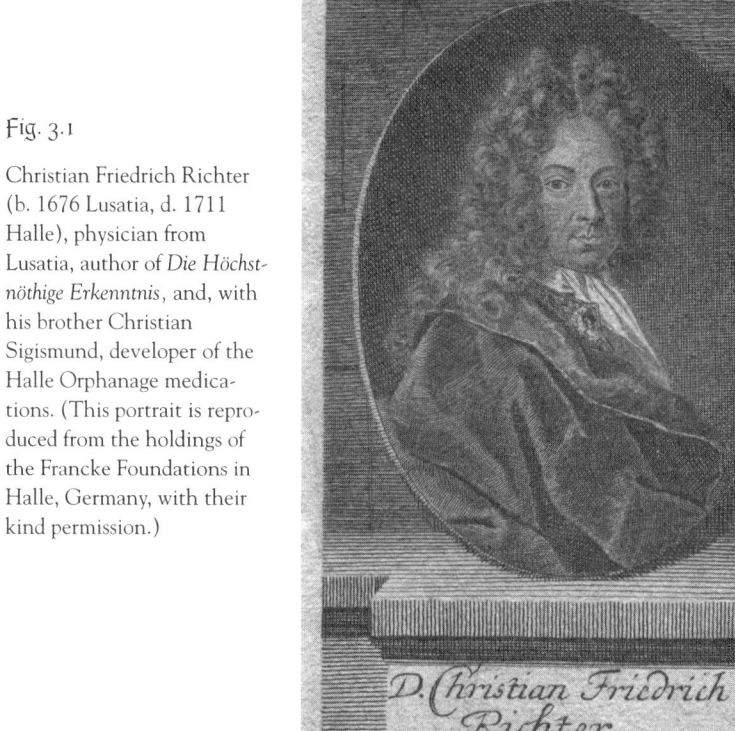

Fig. 3.1

Christian Friedrich Richter
(b. 1676 Lusatia, d. 1711
Halle), physician from
Lusatia, author of *Die Höchst-
nöthige Erkenntnis*, and, with
his brother Christian
Sigismund, developer of the
Halle Orphanage medica-
tions. (This portrait is reproduced from the holdings of
the Francke Foundations in
Halle, Germany, with their
kind permission.)

Richter's death in 1711, the pharmaceutical business was continued by his
brother Christian Sigismund and, after the latter's death in 1739, by his son-in-
law, David Samuel von Madai, a Hungarian physician trained in Vienna and a
respected author on fevers.[6]

After a period of experimentation and laboratory development from 1699
to 1703, a selection of eleven medications combined in various quantities in
physic chests and an additional selection of roughly a dozen individual items
had become a standard Halle commercial offering by 1708 (see Tables 3.1 and

6. Kaiser, "Der Lehrkörper der Medizinischen Fakultät in der halleschen Amtszeit von Georg
Ernst Stahl."

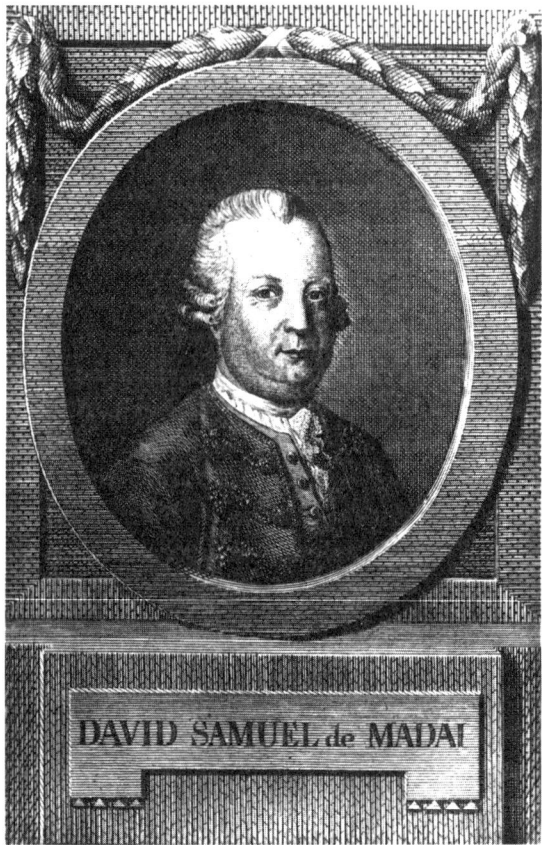

Fig. 3.2

David Samuel von Madai (b. 1709 Pressburg, d. 1780 Halle), Hungarian physician and son-in-law of Johann Sigismund Richter. He was head of the *Hallesche Medikamenten Expedition* during its most profitable period, from 1740 to 1770. (From a private German archive.)

DAVID SAMUEL de MADAI

3.2). These offerings remained fairly stable in price during the entire eighteenth century (see Tables 3.3 and 3.4), although the composition of some of the chemiatric medications continued to change over time.[7] Exceptions to price stability were several of the chemiatric preparations, most notably the *essentia dulcis*, a potable tincture of gold recommended as a general tonic and strengthener for a wide range of conditions in men and women, children and adults. That tincture, by its very claim to contain gold in solution, was linked by many

7. For physic chest prices, see Wilson, "Die Halleschen Waisenhausmedikamente und die 'Höchst-nöthige Erkenntnis' im Kolonialstaat Georgien, 1733–1765," table 2, adapted in this study as Table 3.3; see also Table 3.4. For the composition of the medications and changes over time, see Poeckern, *Die Halleschen Waisenhausartzeneyen*, "Kommentar," and personal communication. The

critics of the Halle medications to an alchemical tradition that was slowly losing its academic respectability, although by no means its appeal to the public. And the public ensured that it would remain a prominent remedy throughout, from early shipments to Russia in the first two decades of the century to North American orders at the end of the century. Its price was halved in the 1720s to counteract accusations of undue profit, although most chemiatric preparations remained high-priced items.[8]

Many of the Halle products, particularly if sold singly through outside commercial agents, were accompanied by single product sheets. However, Pietist emphasis on a framework that would integrate Christian reform through faith and the proper use of the natural and spiritual gifts of God demanded a more thorough approach to lay medical instruction than single-product advertising. The whole set of Orphanage medications was promoted, with their uses explained in considerable detail, in several popular medicine texts addressed to the public and interested medical practitioners. These texts, in particular the 1,200-page *Höchst-nöthige Erkenntnis vom Leibe und natürlichen Leben* (see also Chapter 2), continued to be published throughout the century in multiple editions and translations. The texts were sold separately and as components of a range of multiproduct physic chests developed as a major vehicle of the Halle trade. The Richters' successor, Samuel von Madai, took over the pharmaceutical trade fully in 1740 and published a condensed and largely commercial text, which was translated into many languages (including Latin, French, Dutch, and modern Greek) and was sold throughout Europe and the North American territories until the end of the eighteenth century and beyond.[9]

Both domestic and foreign trade operated through associated apothecaries and commercial houses as well as private agents, university professors, Pietist clergy, and Lutheran missionaries in the Baltic territories, Russia, and India. Early successes abroad were obtained through Pietist partners in the Russian

---

medications on the B list (Tables 3.2 and 3.4) appear as additional medications throughout the century, both in the *Höchst-nöthige Erkenntnis* and in the 1784 *Brief Account*. See Chapters 6 and 7 for orders from North America. This large assortment contradicts the assumption by Beisswanger, *Arzneimittelversorgung*, 156, based on Kaiser and Piechocki ("Die pharmazeutische Industrie von Halle in der zweiten Hälfte des 18.Jahrhunderts," *Münchener Medizinische Wochenschrift* 110 [1968]: 120–30).

8. Poeckern, *Die Halleschen Waisenhausarzeneyen*.

9. David Samuel von Madai, *Kurze Nachricht von dem Nutzen und Gebrauch einiger bewährten Medicamenten, welche zu Halle im Magdeburgischen in dem Waisenhaus dispensiert werden* (Halle, 1746). A Greek version bearing the autograph of Redman Coxe is at the College of Physicians, Philadelphia. A late version in German was published in Halle in 1808 by C. F. Düffer.

Table 3.1 The Halle Orphanage medications, as provided in standard medicine chests, composition, and indications for clinical use (A list)

Medication[a]	Composition[b]	Clinical Uses
Essentia dulcis, or sweet essence (4 oz)	Tincture of gold (*aurum potabile*). Arcanum. Effective ingredient is a subtly purple-hued gold dissolved in *spiritu vini*. Further distilled and concentrated to reduce *sp. vini* content to obtain *ess. dulcis concentrata* (1 lot of *ess. d. ord.* reduced to 1 drachm). Less concentrated preparations available for use as ointment (*e. d. extenuata* and *e. d. ad oculos*).	Panacea. Tonic, especially for the nerves. Fortifier and strengthener, beneficial to nervous system, increased vital spirits. Anodyne (*sine* opium), antispasmodic, induced sleep. Wound balsam, useful in women's illnesses, epilepsy, other seizures, labor, palsies (strokes, where external application was suggested), arthritis, gout. Reduced premature fetal activity in last 6 weeks of gestation and useful for problems arising during and after delivery.
Essentia amara, or bitter essence (6 oz)	Extract (infusion or tincture) of bitter herbs. Exact composition unknown.	Antiscorbutic and blood purifier. Used alone or in combination with polychrest pills (see below) once or twice weekly, for running sores and ulcers, French pox, gonorrhea, apoplexy, upset stomach, fevers, rheum, and cough.
Essentia antihypochondriaca (Milz-öffnende Essenz) or spleen-opening essence (4 oz)	Resin of jalap, extract of black hellebore and aloe, dissolved in rectified *spiritus frumenti* and in *spiritus vitrioli*.	For agues, quartan fevers, plague, burning or malignant fevers. Anthelmintic. Chief use in hypochondriac diseases (sickness of the spleen) in either sex, melancholy, fury of the womb, hysteric passions, palpitations, madness.
Pilulae polychrestae, or pills of many virtues (3 oz)	Scurvy grass, lesser centauri, fumitory, black hellebore, gentian, aloes, myrrh, ground ivy, resin of juniper, and terebinth. Also pistacia and Scotch pine.	Cathartic and emmenagogue. Mainly for female use to purify the blood, head, and stomach and to open the spleen, to evacuate noxious matter via the stool or urine. May be given with *ess. amara* or *pulv. antispasmodicus* (see below) for anxiety, vomiting, looseness of the belly, bloody flux, edema, jaundice, reduced or

Medication	Composition	Uses
(continued)		excessive menstruation, against miscarriage, and during labor. Counterindications: Painful hemorrhoids or blood in phlegm or urine and in patients with chronic menstrual problems.
Pilulae contra obstructiones, or antiobstructive pills (1 oz)	Panchimagogum extract, containing colocinth, agaric, scammony, black hellebore, and soccotrine aloe.	Cathartic for excessive costiveness, when obstructions cause headaches, giddiness, tinnitus, flatulence, vomiting, shortness of breath, etc. More effective than purges and sometimes used with glysters (enemas). Exercise and plenty of liquids recommended.
Pilulae purgantes, or cathartic pills (1 oz)	Panchimagogum extract, containing ingredients similar to the *pilulae contra obstructiones*, with jalap added for stronger effect.	Cathartic dissolving gastric mucus. Less aggressive than and replaced *pulvis laxans* (see Table 3.2).
Pulvis contra acredinem, or powder against acrimony (5 oz)	Powdered oyster shells with red currant juice.	Absorbed and neutralized acrimony. Gentle diaphoretic and diuretic. Used for many febrile diseases, stomach complaints, diarrhea, urinary difficulty, and skin eruptions, including measles, smallpox, and purple fevers (*purpura*).
Pulvis antispasmodicus, or antispasmodic powder (5 oz)	Arcanum similar to *pulvis bezoardicus*, although without *antimonium diaphoreticum*. Later mixtures substitute *cinnabaris nativa* for c. *praeparata* and add Glauber's salt.	Anodyne, cathartic, and diuretic. Strengthened stomach, corrected abnormal bile, relaxed spasmodic contractions, dissolved viscous humors and coagulated blood. Used for diarrhea, vomiting, blood spitting, stone problems, excessive menses, diarrhea and vomiting, hemorrhage, chest pains, shortness of breath, palpitations, and gout.
Pulvis bezoardicus, or bezoar powder (6 oz)	Mineral bezoar made of varying compositions of potassium sulfate, potassium nitrate, and *cinnabaris praeparata*. Previously contained *antimonium diaphoreticum* and *cinnabaris nativa*.	Antidote against poisons; promoted sweating without perturbing the blood. Used in arthritic inflammations, for evacuating abnormal bile, and in upper respiratory illness.

Table 3.1 (continued)

Medication[a]	Composition[b]	Clinical Uses[c]
Pulvis vitalis, or life-giving powder (96 doses)	Admixture of powdered oyster shells and four chemiatric recipes of varying composition over time, including *magisterium diaphoreticum*, *sulphur veneris et martis*, and *materia grisea*. Camphor was a constant ingredient.	Gentle sudorific, tonic, and antiscorbutic. Used in fevers, diarrhea, dysentery (red and white fluxes) to quiet cramps and promote excretion. Also in venereal diseases, putrid sores and boils, and fistulae. Claimed to be a very different tonic from other medications. Patients should remain quiet and warm. Safe and reliable also in case of upper respiratory diseases and prevented return of skin diseases in children.
Balsamus cephalicus, or balsamic nerve strengthener (6 drachms)	Balsam of Peru, camphor, beef suet, and *spiritus vino* with distilled oils.	Applied to head, stomach, and limbs to strengthen nerves and other parts and to dissolve obstructing humors. For diseases of head, toothache, apoplexy, palsy, swellings, and wounds. Occasionally taken internally.

SOURCES: Adapted from Wilson, "Traffic in Medicines and Medical Ideas." The listing and the information on clinical use are based on Richter, *Höchstnöthige Erkemtnis* (1715 and subsequent eds.) and Madai, *Brief Account* (1784, English ed.). Information on composition is from Poeckern, *Halleschen Waisenhausarzeneyen* (1984), who transcribed the secret formulary of David Samuel von Madai and successors compiled in 1740–1840.

[a] Latin names according to Richter 1715 and Madai; *Brief Account*, 1784, with English equivalents from Madai 1784. Weights adjusted to oz troy; quantities as sold in a large physic chest for Rth 30 or £ sterling 6/-.

[b] Changes in composition over time are only partly captured, for reasons of space.

Table 3.2   Additional Halle Orphanage medications, by composition and indications for clinical use (B list)

Medication[a]	Composition[b]	Clinical Uses
Pulvis solaris, or golden powder	Like pulvis vitalis, but without materia grisea (i.e., camphor) (see Table 3.1).	Like pulvis vitalis.
Pulvis laxans, or softening powder	Calomel (mercurous chloride), scammony, and powdered oyster shells.	Cathartic and anthelmintic. Dissolved mucus and purifies blood. Used for diseases of the skin and venereal disease. Not to be used more than twice in any given illness.
Pulvis niger, or black powder	Chemiatric byproduct of making essentia dulcis.	Tonic. Used first in cases of pediatric consumption and dysentery (bloody fluxes). To be used in very small doses, in patients who do not respond to other medications, or in case of very sudden and dangerous symptoms. Can improve effect of other medications.
Pulvis polychrestus	Chemiatric medication made of ens veneris, sulphur auratum antimonii, copper sulfate, and powdered oyster shells. Replaced in physic chest by essentia antihypochondriaca.	Strong laxative. Used in all fevers (except those beginning with diarrhea, cough, or congestion of the chest, smallpox, or measles). Given with forced liquids and discontinued when stools appear.
Pulvis stomachicus (Resolvierendes Magenpulver), or stomach powder	Cinnabar and potassium sulfate.	For gastric complaints and fevers.
Pulvis uterinus griseus or nigricans, gray or black uterine powder	The gray powder was composed of niter and materia grisea (fired or carbonized camphor) and powdered oyster shells. In the black powder, the camphor was carbonized by sulfuric acid.	Not specified but generally used as a refrigerant, diuretic, antiseptic, diaphoretic, and mild cathartic, often for female fevers.
Elixir polychreston	Panchimagogum extract, containing colocynth pulp, agaric, scammony, black hellebore, juice of aloe, and a mixtura simplex.	Strong laxative, with indications similar to pilulae polychrestae on Table 3.1. Given with forced liquids and discontinued once stools appeared.

Table 3.2 (continued)

Medication[a]	Composition[b]	Clinical Uses
Magisterium diaphoreticum, or sweat-inducing powder	Early chemiatric medication (a bezoardicum lunare), containing metallic antimony and silver. Later versions used iron and ferrous sulfate instead of antimony.	Mildly diaphoretic without causing weakness. Used in skin diseases including excema and syphilis, where it should be used together with ess. amara and dulcis. Also for diarrhea, ear- and toothaches, and fevers with chills. Patient should drink warm tea and coffee until sweat appeared, keep quiet and out of drafts.
Balsamus mineralis, or mineral balm	Byproduct of essentia dulcis, dissolved in spiritus vino rectifissimus.	Mild diaphoretic anodyne. Used for fevers, consumption, wounds, and other external applications.
Electuarium antiphtisicum, or lozenge for phtisis	Powdered herbs and flowers of liverwort, sage, rue, common nettle, garden hyssop, mint, and clarified honey.	Strengthened and healed lungs by promoting expectoration. Used for hoarseness and dry cough, probably in cases of consumption.
Tinctura salina, or saline mixture	Potash, root of gentian, and unripened oranges.	Not specified, but generally used as a cooling diaphoretic and gastric sedative.
Tinctura corallina, or coral tincture	Juice of lemons mixed with ammonium carbonate to produce ammonium citrate. Spiritus frumenti added.	Not specified, but probably used as an absorbent for gastric complaints and as an astringent.

SOURCE: Adapted from Wilson, "Traffic in Medicines and Medical Ideas." The listing and the information on clinical use are based on Richter, Höchstnöthige Erkemtnis (1715 and subsequent eds.) and Madai, Brief Account (1784, English ed.). Information on composition is from Poeckern, Halleschen Waisenhausarzeneyen (1984), who transcribed the secret formulary of David Samuel von Madai and successors compiled in 1740–1840.

[a] For unit sizes, doses, and prices, see Table 3.4. Latin names according to Richter 1715 and Madai, Brief Account, 1784, with English equivalents from Madai 1784.

[b] Changes in composition over time are only partly captured, for reasons of space.

Table 3.3 Prices of Halle Orphanage medications, 1712–1784, as advertised in various Halle texts and brochures (A list)

| | Price per Lot, Richter, Höchst-nöthige Erkenntnis, 1712–37 eds. | | Price per Lot,[a] Madai, Brief Account, 1764 ed. | | Price per Ounce, Madai, Brief Account, 1784 ed.[b] | | | | |
| | | | | | German | | Dutch | | English |
Medications	Reichsthaler	Groschen	Reichsthaler	Groschen	Reichsthaler	Groschen	Florins	Stüber	Shillings/Pence
Essentia dulcis[c]	2		1		2		4		7/4
Essentia amara		4		4		8		14	1/3
Essentia antihypochondriaca		4		4		8		14	1/3
Pilulae polychrestae		16		16	1	8	2	16	5/-
Pilulae contra obstructiones		8		8		16	1	8	2/6
Pilulae purgantes		12		12	1		2		3/8
Pulvis bezoardicus		4		4		8		14	1/3
Pulvis contra acredinem		3		3		6		10	-/11
Pulvis antispasmodicus		4		4		8		14	1/3
Pulvis vitalis (Dosis)		2		1		12[d]	1		1/10
Balsamus cephalicus		6		6	2		4		7/4

SOURCES: Based on Wilson, "Hallesche Waisenhausmedikamente," table 2. Prices are from Richter, *Höchst-nöthige Erkenntnis* (1712–37), and Madai, *Brief Account* (1764 and 1784). The rates of exchange are as stated in Madai, *Brief Account* (1784). Reichsthaler at 24 groschen throughout. See Table 3.1 for English names.

a 1 Lot = 4 drachms or 0.5 oz.

b Rates of exchange are stated in Madai (1784) and also in the Halle ledgers, as Rth current 5/£ sterling. Price differences over the course of the century are small except for the *essentia dulcis* and the *pulvis vitalis*, which decreased by 50 percent between 1729 and 1737. (See John McCusker, *Money and Exchange in Europe and America, 1600–1775* [Chapel Hill: University of North Carolina Press, 1978], 61–80, tables 2.11 and 2.12, for moneys of account and the agio on Hamburg bank money. In view of the variability of Pennsylvania currency rates over the period under study, no attempt has been made to calculate equivalent values based on commerical rates for the colonies.)

c The *essentia dulcis* is the *ess. d. ordinaria* throughout. According to the 1784 *Brief Account*, the *ess. d. concentrata* sold for Rth 8/oz. Other preparations were the *ess. d. externa*, an ointment, at 16 gr/oz, and the *ess. d. ad oculos*, an eye medication, at 16 gr.

d In 1784, advertised in unit sizes of 1 packet containing 12 doses.

Table 3.4   Additional Halle Orphanage medications (B list) and selected prices

Medication	Unit Price, Reichsthaler/groschen, 1784 (1705)
Pulvis solaris (12 doses at 4 grains)	/12
Pulvis niger (12 doses at 1 grain)	4/
Pulvis laxans (lot)	/5
Pulvis stomachicus, or stomach (fever) powder (12 doses at 0.5 drachm each)	/6
Pulvis polychrestus (12 doses at 1/4 grain each)	/12
Pulvis uterinus griseus or *nigricans* (1705 dose at 8 grains), 12 doses	/12
Balsamus mineralis (oz)	2/
Balsamus apoplecticus (lot)	(/12)
Magisterium diaphoreticum (8 doses at 1 groschen each)	(/8)
Elixir polychreston (half lot)	(/6)
Electuarium antiphtisicum (16 oz)	1/-
Tinctura salina (lot)	/4
Tinctura corallina (lot)	/4

SOURCES: For dose sizes and 1705 prices, *Madai Formulary*, as transcribed by Poeckern, *Hallesche Waisenhausarzeneyen*; Richter, *Kurzer und deutlicher Unterricht*; 1784 prices and unit sizes, Madai, *Brief Account*. The Reichsthaler is equal to 24 groschen in all prices.

trade to Riga, Moscow, Saint Petersburg, Tobolsk, and Archangelsk, which peaked between 1709 and 1715.[10] Beginning in the 1720s, the trade extended throughout continental Europe and England. Through agents in Amsterdam and Rotterdam, it went as far as the East and West Indies, and at least after 1730, to the Lutheran missions in North America.[11]

Clerical and commercial agents were usually protected by local privileges and patents. These included an imperial privilege in Catholic areas under Austrian rule where like-minded Pietists had established a market in the Hungarian provinces, the duchy of Siebenbürgen, and the Banat. Strict quality control ensured that the pharmaceutical privilege of the Francke institutions and the reputation of their products remained intact in the face of falsifications and of continual opposition by guild apothecaries and outside agents. In many

10. Winter, *Halle als Ausgangspunkt der deutschen Russlandkunde im 18. Jahrhundert*.
11. Wilson, "The Traffic in Halle Orphanage Medications: Medicinals, Philanthropy, and Colonial Mission." Also Lehmann, *Hallesche Mediziner und Medizinen am Anfang deutsch-indischer Beziehungen*.

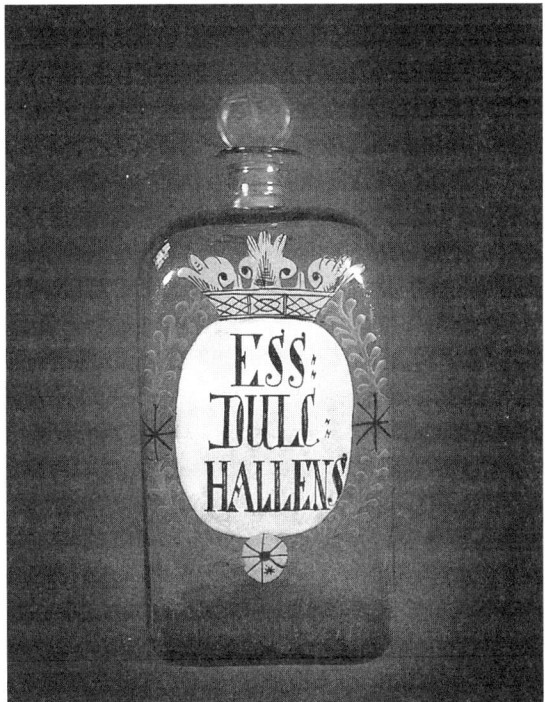

Fig. 3.3

An 18th-century imitation of the container of the *essentia dulcis*, the famous tincture of gold and the star of the Halle Orphanage medications, probably from a glassworks in Thuringia. (Photograph from a private collection and Museum für Thüringer Volkskunde, Erfurt.)

areas of Germany, the Halle medications were an accepted part of pharmaceutical offerings by pharmacies, dry goods merchants, and itinerant salesmen.[12]

The Product and the Discourse of Pharmaceutical Reform

What then were these medications? What made them famous, how were they similar or different from other pharmaceuticals of the period, and how and for

12. Beisswanger, *Arzneimittelversorgung im 18. Jahrhundert: Die Stadt Braunschweig und die ländlichen Distrikte im Herzogthum Braunschweig Wolfenbüttel,* 152ff., 198ff., describes this trade in a neighboring territory, the duchy of Braunschweig-Wolfenbüttel. The territory was highly regulated in terms of its pharmaceutical trade throughout the century, but the patterns of distribution and demand described by her are probably quite typical of a medically well-provided small territory with many pharmacies and itinerant but licensed salesmen. Older studies, like that of Peickert, *Geheimmittel im deutschen Arzneiverkehr: Ein Beitrag zur Wirtschaftsgeschichte der Pharmazie und zur Arzneispezialitätenfrage,* still classify the Halle products as *arcana* in the traditional sense. For an authoritative pharmaceutical classification, see the work by Schneider, *Lexikon zur Arzneimittelgeschichte,* "Geheimmittel und Spezialitäten," C 73, vol. 4.

what diseases did they work? With one obvious exception, we can answer these questions at least in part on the basis of archival and empirical work and by historical comparison.[13] The exception is the central question for what therapeutic purpose these medicines were prescribed and used, but it is one that cannot be validly addressed, let alone answered, from our very different medical knowledge base. It is generally accepted that the materia medica of the late seventeenth and early eighteenth centuries drew from both the chemiatric school, loosely attributed to Paracelsus and his followers, who since the sixteenth century had increasingly relied on chemical procedures to produce distilled or otherwise refined pharmaceuticals from metals and minerals, and from an even more loosely defined Galenic tradition, which used a vast store of botanical, mineral, and animal substances that had been part of the medicine of Christian Europe since the early Middle Ages. This central pharmaceutical tradition is apparent also in the Orphanage medications, despite the claims for medical and therapeutic reform made by the Richter brothers as authors of the popular medicine texts discussed in the context of lay medical education in Chapter 2.

Richter's treatises have been noted by a number of medical historians, but comment is usually restricted to Part I, which is used to demonstrate the pervasiveness of Stahlian and Christian thought in Pietist medicine.[14] The second part has received less attention, although it is of considerable interest for an understanding of the pharmaceutical and therapeutic thinking of the period. Part II not only departed from the standard academic format for the exposition of therapy, but in several respects broke new ground in pharmacotherapy—despite or because of the fact that its author implicitly linked the rationale of reform to the commercial objectives of a philanthropic enterprise.[15] This framework was entirely tied to the therapeutic and academic practice of the period,

13. I refer in particular to the work done under the supervision of Rudolf Schmitz in Marburg and Erika Hickel in Braunschweig, although this work has been suspended after the death of Professor Schmitz and the retirement of Professor Hickel. The contributions of their students have been essential to my own understanding of German patient and provider preferences in North America. See in particular the work of Leibrock-Plehn, *Hexenkräuter oder Arznei: Die Abtreibungsmittel im 16. und 17. Jahrhundert*, and Lanz, *Arzneimittel in der Therapie Friedrich Hoffmanns (1660–1742): Unter besonderer Berücksichtigung der Medicina consultatoria (1721–1723)*, on the materia medica of Friedrich Hoffmann.

14. Geyer-Kordesch, "Georg Ernst Stahl's Radical Pietist Medicine and Its Influence on the German Enlightenment," and idem, "Die Medizin im Spannungsfeld zwischen Aufklärung und Pietismus"; Helm, "Der Umgang mit dem kranken Menschen im halleschen Pietismus des frühen 18. Jahrhunderts."

15. This study uses the more extensive and definitive of the Richter texts, the *Höchst-nöthige Erkenntnis*, mostly in the 1715 edition. I also proceed on the assumption, which has not been fully

however, and bears little if any resemblance to the truly popular texts of the period, including John Wesley's *Primitive Physic*, which embraced a very different and antiacademic perspective more in the tradition of the antiestablishment tracts of the seventeenth century.[16]

Much of the introduction addressing lay readers of Part II is dedicated to a closely reasoned discourse on the current state of the materia medica, suggesting the influence of Georg Wedel and his students, Georg Ernst Stahl and Friedrich Hoffmann, in their attempt to reduce polypharmacy, set reasonable standards of product safety, and reduce the use of complex *composita*.[17] A recent and detailed study of the pharmaceutical preferences of Hoffmann, derived in particular from his *Medicina Consultatoria* (1721–23), affords a modern benchmark and an opportunity to assess Richter's premises in an empirical perspective. That study also provides insight into the overlap of several arcana developed and sold through the Orphanage pharmacy by the Halle medical establishment, including Hoffmann, Stahl, and Johann Juncker. Hoffmann's practice in particular, as was customary in the period, included local practice and consultations with distant patients and their physicians.[18]

In his treatise, Richter pilloried the redundancy of most traditional *composita* from the so-called Galenic materia medica and the resultant inability to nail down the efficacious component; he deplored the general lack of reliability and effectiveness, and the frequent adverse effects, of most pharmaceuticals, whether simples or *composita*. Although the major thrust was directed against this vast Galenic armamentarium and its multiple accretions during various retransmissions into the European materia medica, the text fell short of full support for the chemiatric tradition. This tradition had inspired the early stages of pharmaceutical development at Halle, but it is clear from the medications in Table 3.1 in particular that traditional botanical mixtures of herbs and antacids like powdered oyster shells still held their place and in some cases even replaced earlier chemiatric preparations with similar names. But overall, traditional

---

examined, that Christian Friedrich Richter was indeed the sole or main author of this work. This generally held assumption is supported by the fact that subsequent editions are simple reprints typical of the period, up to and including page numbers.

16. John Wesley, *Primitive Physick: or An Easy and Natural Method of Curing Most Diseases*, various eds. A recent study of Wesley's medical views is in Abelove, *The Evangelist of Desire: John Wesley and the Methodists*.

17. Konert, "Academic and Practical Medicine in Halle During the Era of Stahl, Hoffmann, and Juncker."

18. Lanz, *Arzneimittel in der Therapie Friedrich Hoffmanns*, "Arzneimittelliste," 187ff.

materia medica from both the Galenic and chemical armamentarium—for example, the *alexipharmacae* or precious stones used as antidotes for poisoning—was relegated to one brief and late chapter. The so-called *Dreckapotheke* of the period was entirely disregarded.[19] Traditional domestic remedies were likewise given limited space. Item 67, for instance, provided recipes "which in common diseases can also be used with good effect. They too are formulated in such a manner that the body will not thereby become unduly agitated, as is the case with many so-called domestic remedies."[20]

Instead, Richter dedicated most of the text to an extensive discussion of the development, clinical indications, and therapeutic use of the Halle Orphanage medications. Their benefits were extolled in particular for their safety as tested in the clinical settings of the Orphanage, and for their purity and lack of adulteration because of close quality control during manufacture. Those advantages, he argued, justified their treatment as arcana or trade secrets, the traditional and persistent venue for protecting the profit of trading on one's academic or clinical reputation by selling a proprietary medication.[21] Underlying the pervasiveness of this practice, of course, was not only immediate profit but the equally persistent and ancient debate about whether the physician himself should closely supervise, if not manufacture himself, the production of pharmaceuticals or divide his labor and his profit with the apothecary.[22]

But by 1700, and in an academic setting, carrying the argument of efficacy absent full disclosure of ingredients demanded a deft sense of balance. Richter maintained that balance by linking the social usefulness, the charitable purpose, and the recognized rectitude of the Foundations to his own medical expertise and academic credentials. The conscious marshaling of current medical issues in the development of the final set of medications chosen for the physic chest was evident throughout. Each remedy was discussed in considerable detail as to

19. For a recent treatment of this body of remedies, which included dung and other excreta, see Cowen and Wilson, "The Traffic in Medical Ideas: Popular Medical Texts as German Imports and American Imprints."

20. Richter, *Höchst-nöthige Erkenntnis*, 565–66.

21. For Hoffmann's and some Stahlian arcana, see Lanz, *Arzneimittel in der Therapie Friedrich Hoffmanns*, 158, 170; for the persistence of the *secreta* tradition, see Eamon, *Science and the Secrets of Nature: Books of Secrets in Medieval and Early Modern Culture*.

22. Again, it is interesting to look at the generic similarities of these arguments in other medical settings. For our period, see the work of Cook, *Trials of an Ordinary Doctor: Joannes Groenevelt in Seventeenth Century London*, and idem, *The Decline of the Old Medical Regime in Stuart London*. For a larger overview, see Wolf, *Über die Anfänge der Pharmaziegeschichtschreibung: Von Johannes Ruellius (1529) bis David Peter Hermann Schmidt (1835)*.

intended effects for specific morbid conditions, providing a coherent account of therapeutic intentions.

All other considerations aside, the primary therapeutic objective motivating the Halle physicians was the lack of effective medicines, particularly during epidemics. (The German term used throughout by Richter was *kräftig*, which is rendered in the following as *potent* or *effective*, although the latter term in particular is devoid of the physiological and methodological implications of modern usage.) As noted, the Richter brothers practiced at the hospital of the Halle Orphanage Foundations, which in its early years admitted some of the city's poor as well as the orphans and students residing at the Foundations. In a large and fairly constant clinical setting, they had examined all classes of simples and *composita* in the attempt to obtain a small and safe armamentarium with predictable and reasonably specific effects. Despite Richter's awareness of nature's self-healing processes and a nod to Hippocratic principles, however, he rarely questioned the traditional linkage of specific symptom relief and cure, obtained largely through the well-tried mechanisms of purging, excreting, and otherwise eliminating noxious substances and cleansing the blood while fortifying the body with additional medications.

In Tables 3.1 and 3.2, Richter's clinical indications are matched by a modern transcription of the Halle formulas to illustrate the results of product administration, patient observation, and subsequent elimination and substitution of remedies in an eighteenth-century large pharmaceutical manufacture. For the purposes of developing the Halle medicine chest, Richter and his associates had accumulated an armamentarium of thirty items that combined the necessary attributes in the right strength. Eleven items were eventually selected for the chest. The advantages of the new assortment were said to be particularly noticeable for fevers and gonorrhea, white flux, *lues venerae*, consumption, and old running sores. Contents were graded in type and quantity, and the amounts in each chest, regardless of price, were proportionate to the expected frequency of use. Medications not included in the physic chests were sold separately on request.

Notable are continuous recommendations of dosage and specific dosage instructions by patient age. Although tied in part to the patient population of the Orphanage Foundations, which provided the clinical subjects for medication development, these dosages must have been considered sufficiently relevant to general therapeutic needs for the larger user population of the medicines in the physic chests. Not only effectiveness but also safety of administration in the absence of a physician were important considerations. For instance, the *essentia antihypochondriaca* was found to contain all properties adhering to the older *elixir polychrestum* but to be safer in use, less obnoxious in taste, and requiring less care in administration and dosage. An early antifebrile essence required judicious application in cases where the fever did not tolerate hot remedies, and it was considered unsafe for a physic chest. Another exchange was made in the case of the *pulvis laxans*, which had encountered problems of compliance in the case of distant patients or isolated providers, and was replaced by *pilulae purgantes*, which acted as both a purge and a sudorific. There was in fact considerable evolution in several of the remedies over the course of the century. Because these changes were not reflected in corresponding changes in product names and the composition of the medications remained a trade secret, it is unclear whether changes were driven by safety reasons, price of raw materials, or manufacturing considerations. A major thrust was in the replacement of native or crude antimony by a number of processed cinnabar preparations by 1740; for example, *antimonium diaphoreticum* and *cinnabaris nativa* were replaced by *cinnabaris praeparata* in the *pulvis bezoardoicus*. Botanical mixtures also underwent changes in composition.[23]

But the star of the set remained the so-called *essentia dulcis*. Its description in the *Höchst-nöthige Erkenntnis* ran nearly fifteen pages, and it was the biggest potential moneymaker. At the stage of product development, and despite its initial success, however, the effects proved difficult to reproduce reliably, apparently because frequent administration was needed, which in turn required substantial amounts of gold for large-scale preparation. *Essentia dulcis* was used continually in the early charity practice, however, and seems to have drawn in enough support to permit the manufacture of larger amounts and distribution among most patients in need.[24]

The development of the *essentia dulcis* led to several side or byproducts. By 1703, when a strengthening tonic was needed for three children devastated by consumption, the Orphanage physicians produced a mineral balsam and a *pulvis*

23. Poeckern, personal communication.

24. According to Item 19: "Though we now had this remedy [the *ess. dulcis*], it would have been of little benefit if we had not quickly observed this one advantage that in many cases the strength of this medication lay in its repeated application, which could be as often as every half hour" (Richter, *Höchst-nöthige Erkenntnis*, 531). What the author and his successors failed to mention was the extraordinary financial support required for *essentia dulcis* and the bitter fight over rights of production, sales, and profits that ensued between them and August Hermann Francke and his successors over the course of the entire century; see Poeckern, *Die Halleschen Waisenhausartzeneyen*, "Kommentar," and Wilson, "Die Halleschen Waisenhausmedikamente."

nigrus or "black powder," which was administered to one of the children in a dose of as little as one grain. The medicine was claimed not only to have restored the child's strength but to have improved the effect of other medications. A final addition to the Halle armamentarium was the *pulvis vitalis*, found to be far superior to other medications in *affectionibus lymphae* and in most fevers. *Pulvis vitalis*, however, one of the more expensive items in the physic chest, was difficult to manufacture and counseled to be used only as a last resort. It nonetheless proved to be one of the mainstays of both Russian orders at the beginning of the century and North American orders until 1795; it and a sister substance, the *pulvis solaris*, were apparently recommended and used in small doses for lying-in women.[25]

The need for potent medicines for female problems—fortifiers, blood purifiers, and medicines to restore the menses—is reflected in a number of indications given for several of the medications, both those containing traditional botanicals and chemiatric preparations. The attractiveness in particular of the *pilulae polychrestae* was evident throughout our period, in orders from Russia in the first two decades of the century and from North America beginning in 1750.

Opposition to the whole range of the Halle medicines, in particular the *essentia dulcis* with its alchemical genealogy, came from the Lutheran establishment. Both medical and religious orthodoxy raised objections to the linkage between alchemy and Paracelsian mysticism, a charge routinely levied against the medical reform proposals of dissenting elements in the seventeenth century.[26] Technical objections centered on a number of issues, competition for the pharmaceutical market being an underlying and occasionally overt motive. Although the *Höchst-nöthige Erkenntnis* refrained entirely from astral or sidereal medicine, its signatures, or any of the other early modern paraphernalia of Paracelsian or hermetic texts, its authors did attribute the first breakthrough to the bequest of several chemiatric manuscripts to the Foundations. The *essentia dulcis*, in particular, was attacked by chemical distillers on the grounds that gold could not provide a distillate.[27]

25. For example, by Anna Maria, née Weiser, wife of Heinrich Melchior Mühlenberg. Several of her orders are in the Mission Archives of the Francke Foundations (MAFSt 4 [Pennsylvania]; see Chapter 6).

26. See in particular Shackelford, "Rosicrucianism, Lutheran Orthodoxy, and the Rejection of Paracelsianism in Early Seventeenth-Century Denmark"; Gunnoe, "Erastus and Paracelsianism"; and the collection of essays in Grell and Cunningham, eds., *Religio Medici: Medicine and Religion in Seventeenth-Century England*.

27. Stahl also parted company with his student Richter on the question of suspending gold in a tincture; see Stahl, *Wider die Goldmacherei*, 1706, and unpublished correspondence between Christian

The Richter brothers cited numerous testimonials by physicians and clients in support of the safety and usefulness of their medications. Above all, with the possible exception of the claims for the *essentia dulcis*, Richter was careful to maintain a medically conservative attitude that would not run counter to the criteria of medical and pharmaceutical reform. He claimed never to have extolled the superiority of the Orphanage products to the exclusion of all others and above all rejected the charge of a miraculous cure. Instead, he argued, his own clinical observations indicated cures and relief in serious as well as non-responding diseases. Conversely, where he and others lacked success, there was no evidence that other remedies in fact worked. Nor had it been possible to show that the Orphanage medications caused harm, whereas it was all too well known that ordinary medications—and often the physicians themselves—harmed the health of many. Ill effects were ascribed to excessive doses and patient error in cases of self-medication.[28] Likewise—although that argument was rather spurious in view of the ongoing trade in German territories—the Richters claimed that there was no intent to compete with local practice; it had been a condition of the pharmaceutical privilege granted to the Foundations that sales outside licensed pharmacies be restricted to locations where no physicians and pharmacists were available.

The traditional issues of secrecy and the refusal to publish the formularies were argued from well-known premises established in the debate for pharmaceutical reform.[29] Refusal to reveal the recipes was intended to protect patients from having to rely on pharmacists or others for preparation, which could give rise to dangers of adulteration and abuse. For the honest physician who wished to use the medications because of their superior strength and potency, lack of knowledge of the composition and modus operandi was no obstacle because

---

Sigismund and Christian Friedrich Richter and Hildebrand von Canstein, Hauptarchiv Franckesche Stiftungen (HAFSt), C 285. The chemical process is fully described in the manufacturer's formulary in Poeckern, *Halleschen Waisenhausartzeneyen*. It is worth noting that in rejecting the claims for this medication, the issue was not one of alchemy (the production of nobler metal from a more common metal), but a serious question of technical feasibility apart from medical efficacy. Nonetheless, the Richters felt the need to publish a series of testimonials, which appeared in a series of treatises (see, for instance, *Ausführlicher Bericht von der essentia dulcis. . . .* Im Verlag des Waisenhauses, Halle, 1708).

28. Richter, *Höchst-nöthige Erkenntnis*, 541. For the growing concern with precise dosage instructions enabling patient compliance, see, most recently, Crellin, "How Shall I Take My Medicine?"

29. For *arcana* and *secreta*, see Eamon, *Science and the Secrets of Nature*; Müller-Jahncke, "Astrologisch-magische Theorie und Praxis in der Heilkunde der frühen Neuzeit"; Beyerlein, *Die Entwicklung der Pharmazie zur Hochschuldisziplin (1750–1875): Ein Beitrag zur Universitäts- und Sozialgeschichte*, chaps. 1 and 2; Cook, "Henry Stubbe and the Virtuosi-Physicians."

physicians rarely prepared their own medications and instead relied on apothecaries. Likewise, although physicians might insist on knowledge of ingredients for reasons of safety, the known usefulness of the Halle medications over the course of several years was sufficient reassurance.

With the rhetorical skill that at the beginning of the eighteenth century was still a virtue rather than a vice in academic discourse, Richter claimed that yielding the monopoly of preparation and packaging would contravene the very purpose of the original bequests and the investment of time and financial resources. If well-off people were given access to having the medications prepared for themselves, there would be no margin of profit to be diverted to charity. And charity had to become more firmly grounded and self-sufficient in an age where people quickly tired of appeals to their purse.[30]

The Market: Privileged Trade and Trading Privileges

The trade in Orphanage medications was intended for both local or domestic and larger international markets. We know something about some of these markets and very little about others, aside from hints in the archives and in archive correspondence about their existence.[31] But there is no question that the trade was extraordinary both in terms of profit and of geographic scope.

By 1720, the Foundations had developed a domestic and Central European network linking licensed commercial and diverse private buyers and distributors. Individual orders went directly to clients in Germany, the Protestant areas of Eastern and Southeastern Europe, and the Protestant cadres at the Russian court. Trade during the reign of Peter I (the Great) of Russia relied heavily on previously established medical and diplomatic connections. The medical connections involved German physicians who had come to Russia under Peter's father. The diplomatic connections were established through Heinrich Wilhelm Ludolf, a far-ranging diplomatic agent in the service of George of Denmark, who went on a Russian mission in the early 1690s and in turn relied on Pietist associates in the formerly Swedish Baltic regions for some of his contacts in Moscow.[32]

---

30. For the difficulties of appeals to charity, see Owen, *English Philanthropy, 1660–1960*.

31. Archival sources used are "Externa des Medikamentenhandels von 1725–1799," VAFSt ix/ii/22, 28, 30, 32, 33, and 37. For some of the literature on licensed German sales, see Beisswanger, *Arzneimittelversorgung im 18. Jahrhundert*.

32. Wilson, "Heinrich Wilhelm Ludolf, August Hermann Francke, und der Eingang nach Russland."

Commercial attempts to trade into Southeast Russia and the Levant were made by early emissaries of the Foundations under Dutch and English trading and missionary auspices, but these early attempts apparently did not lead to a continuing trade.

What we know of the northern Russian commerce, however, shows that it was surprising in scope;[33] existing records for the years 1708 to 1717 contain substantial orders reflecting a relative preference for chemiatric medications. Orders for fortifiers or tonics, such as the *essentia dulcis* and *pulvis vitalis*, head the list, but there are large orders for the *pulvis contra acredinem*, diaphoretics like the *pulvis bezoardicus*, and cathartics containing substances often found in female emmenagogues, such as the *elixir polychrestum*. The trade appears to have been in full fling by 1709, and quantities were in fact substantial, running to as much as several thousand drachms at the equivalent of gold Roubles 6,481 or Reichthaler (Rth) 11,084 per year for the period 1709–19. One summary of pharmaceutical orders for 1712, for instance, is headed by purchases by a merchant in Archangelsk and by a pharmaceutical storage house and distributor (*Magazin der Medikamente*) in the same town, running to a total of Rth 5,342 (roughly one thousand pounds sterling), or one-third of total long-distance sales from Halle for the year.

We do not know the characteristics of the user population, but they included both Russians and foreigners. We have some names indicating the persons involved in the trade, much of which went through a few trusted associates in Moscow and the network of Pietist clergy and tutors at the estates of the Baltic nobility and in Moscow, and through the newly opened Baltic port at Saint Petersburg. Several merchant families trading between Amsterdam and Archangelsk acted as intermediaries, as did the body physicians of Peter the Great, among them the famous Blumentrost sons, heirs to an old German physician tradition in Moscow.[34] Much of the trade to Moscow apparently escaped the strictures of Russian customs and other pharmaceutical controls.[35] However,

33. The first large and still valid description of this trade in its historical context is by Winter, *Halle als Ausgangspunkt der deutschen Russlandkunde*. The orders cited in the following are from VAFSt, Rechnungen der Medikamentenexpedition, 1712–15, VII, Repertorium ii, *Fach 296*.

34. Dumschat, "Deutsche Ärzte im Moskauer Russland"; Trokhatchev and Wilson, "Laurentius Blumentrost, Scion of a Russian-German Medical Family."

35. Foust, *Rhubarb: The Wondrous Drug*; Pele and Pickhan, *Zwischen Lübeck und Novgorod: Wirtschaft, Politik, und Kultur im Ostseeraum vom frühen Mittelalter bis ins 20. Jahrhundert*. Foust in his book on the rhubarb trade from China through Russia has described a sophisticated regulatory and customs environment. The *Aptekarskij Prikaz*, which served as a central import and distribution point

this may well have been due to political reasons: Part of the trade from 1709 to 1719 benefited the Swedish officers confined in Tobolsk, Siberia, after the Battle of Poltava in 1708.

Early on, therefore, we encounter two significant factors that facilitated this cross-national trade by a philanthropic institution and explain the relative ease with which Halle was later able to transfer goods and moneys to North America during the colonial and the early republican periods. One was the use of a political network to gain access to areas without having to submit to burdensome customs and other regulations; the other was the use of merchandise as a means of transferring moneys in areas lacking a financial infrastructure and banking system. As noted, the Francke Foundations channeled considerable help to the Swedish officers in Siberia between 1709 and 1719, much of which came from Swedish sources.[36] It appears from some of the Halle business records that this money was channeled into Russia in the form of medications sent on credit. These were then sold by a variety of Halle agents and the proceeds returned to Halle through drafts and similar transfers, making Halle a political and financial intermediary.

That this was not an isolated instance of how medicines—and the parallel Halle book trade—formed an indispensable transfer mechanism for handling philanthropic finances can be illustrated over the course of the eighteenth century. Before 1720, for instance, we have correspondence with an aide to Field Marshal and Count F. W. von Seckendorff, a General Barner, who was apparently a member of the large expatriate officer corps of the period. From camp in Belgrade, he placed several orders for physic chests, in particular for *essentia dulcis* and *amara, pulvis antispasmodicus*, and *pulvis vitalis*, for friends in the Protestant nobility in Vienna, for himself, and for other army officers in the 1717 campaign against the Porte. These orders came to Halle with some rather acerbic comments on dried-up bottles and unopenable chests and the sharpness of the *essentia dulcis*, but these defects did not deter Barner from

---

for domestic and imported materia medica and medicinals, goes back to the seventeenth century. Although its service area probably did not extend much beyond the urban centers and its staff was largely foreign, this very Russian institution was the forerunner of a large system of military and private pharmacies instituted by Peter I and Tsarina Anna Ivanovna between 1700 and 1740.

36. Hermann Golz, "Repertorium Epistolarum Sibiriacum, aus Curt Friedrich von Wreechs 'Wahrhafter und umständlicher Historie von denen Schwedischen Gefangenen in Russland und Siberien . . .' (Sorau 1725) zusammengestellt"; Curt Friedrich von Wreech, *Wahrhafte und umständliche Historie von denen schwedischen Gefangenen.*

placing further orders on his return to Germany. At that time, he apparently placed a capital loan with the Foundations, the interest of which he received in an annual supply of medications.[37]

I emphasize here not a singular instance of commercial involvement but the fit of the pharmaceutical trade by a voluntary institution into existing patterns of international trade. Much of eighteenth-century large-scale commerce, in pharmaceuticals, dry goods, and other merchandise, included financial services—bills of exchange honored, discounted, and placed.[38] This function seems to have been assumed in Halle from the outset. It continued over the course of the century, in very different trading and national environments, and we discuss the evidence for North America in Chapter 5.

When August Hermann Francke died in 1727, there was a period of relative instability in the pharmaceutical enterprise as the surviving Richter brother and his and his brother's heirs fought with Gotthilf August Francke and among themselves for control.[39] With Samuel David von Madai's final assumption of that control in 1740, which included the transfer of net profits to the Foundations, a long period of extraordinary and sustained growth occurred that terminated only with Madai's death in the 1770s.[40] Figure 3.4 shows in aggregate form the rise and eventual fall of annual net profits from the pharmaceutical trade from 1728 to 1798. The total volume of this trade must surely have placed it in the top league of most European and English commerce in pharmaceuticals during mid-century.

But success came at a price. From the outset, local, regional, and national tariff and other trading restrictions had to be overcome again and again by petitions and the use of the network of former Halle pupils and associates in the nobility and the administration. In Prussia, there was the continuing if largely unsuccessful attempt by the Prussian medical and hygiene establishments to gain

37. HAFSt, F, letters by Major General Barner, for the years 1713–18.
38. As noted by Porter and Porter, "The Rise of the English Drugs Industry: The Role of Thomas Corbyn" (284ff. for capital investments and profits, 289ff. for the colonial trade).
39. The battles over the right to manufacture and sell all or some of the medications had started even in the 1710s, but had been settled by a series of compromises under the elder Francke. They resumed in the 1730s, and for a while both Madai and the son of Christian Sigismund Richter acted as company distributors, for instance in Braunschweig-Wolfenbüttel. See Beisswanger, *Arzneimittelversorgung im 18. Jahrhundert,* 157. For a chronological account based on Francke archive sources, see Poeckern, *Halleschen Waisenhausartzeneyen.*
40. Our knowledge of this growth in quantitative terms is in part due to this ongoing legal battle, because it split off the pharmaceutical trade from the Foundations proper and only the net profits went into Foundation accounts.

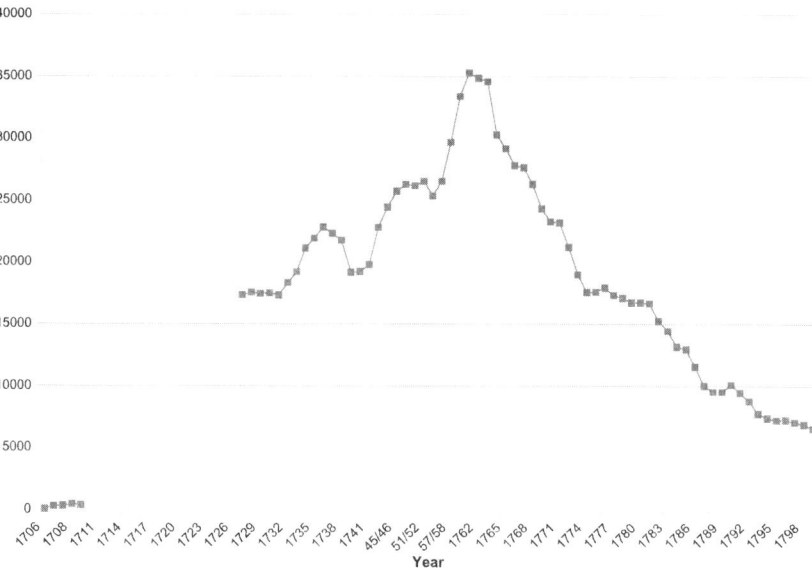

 g. 3.4

et profits from the Orphanage pharmaceutical business, 1728–1798, five-year moving
erage. No data available for 1710–26, 1732, 1784. (Source: Administrative Archives,
anckesche Stiftungen, Repertorium vii/ii.)

ntrol over pharmaceutical manufacture through restriction and visitations,
ginning in 1725.[41] Confessional and dynastic barriers continued to be of
portance in the German territories until the Napoleonic period. In Catholic
xony and the Austrian territories, where the Protestant areas around Pressburg
d in Siebenbürgen were major markets and army physic chests in some of the
lian campaigns were stocked with Halle medications,[42] trade continued to be
lnerable to dynastic religious preferences but also was favored by special
emptions.[43] The imperial cities plowed their own furrow of market and trading

41. For the Prussian ordinances of 1725, see most recently Beyerlein, *Die Entwicklung der
armazie zur Hochschuldisziplin*, chaps. 1 and 2.
42. VAFSt ix/ii/30, Draft of a letter to "Imperatricem et reginam Hungariae," 1750.
43. VAFSt ix/ii/33, "Acta den Medicamenten debit im chursächsischen betrf.," letter to Baron
n Ende, with response by the King of Saxony exempting the Orphanage pharmaceuticals from cur-
t regulations, 17 July 1769.

rules, and there as well as in Holland, the colonial trading interest seemed to have won out despite increasing political obstacles.[44]

The most important commercial threats were falsification, local quackery (*Pfuscherei*), and unauthorized sale. The popularity of the medications and a loyal public made them an easy target for imitations both in Europe and abroad. This may have been one of the reasons that there was continued insistence in Halle on its own distributors among clergy, friends, and trusted traders. Apothecaries were suspected of imitation and charged with substitution of their own substances and inferior products that threatened the reputation of the Halle medications. Although ever present, these dangers seem to have been counteracted by the public's brand-name loyalty, here, insistence on the genuine article, in particular firmly sealed bottles with the Orphanage seal clearly displayed (see Fig. 3.3 for an eighteenth-century imitation of an *essentia dulcis* bottle). Even officially sanctioned imitations using approximate generic recipes did not sell well, as noted by the state laboratory in Braunschweig.[45]

In the West Indies, apparently a market hotly contested by English traders, Halle products had to be sold through Dutch trading connections. As early as 1705, as reported in an exhaustive study of the pharmaceutical trade to Curaçao by the West India Company, a German *medicus* called Horst ordered a quantity of gold foil, apparently because he intended to imitate the *essentia dulcis*.[46] Among numerous instances of the substitution of seals and goods (including the imposition en route of faked seals), a major case in the 1760s throws further light on this West Indies trade. In a complex scheme of falsification and downright piracy, a Dutch trader named Dreissiger, in collusion with a merchant from Halle, reprinted the Dutch version of the *Short Account* (commissioned in Amsterdam in 1760) and sent the pirated edition from Holland to the West Indies together with a large shipment of imitations of the

44. For Frankfurt on Main, see VAFSt ix/ii/32, "Acta des von dem Sanitäts Collegio der kayserlichen freyen Reichsstadt Frankfurt am Mayn gesuchte Verbot der hiesigen medicam. betr. 1761." WAFSt ix/ii/22, "Copeyen der in anno 1764 von hofr Madai an das collegium medicum zu Berlin eingesandten memoralien," for example, 14 August 1764.

45. Beisswanger, *Arzneimittelversorgung im 18. Jahrhundert*, 155. Discriminating brand-name loyalty was not restricted to the Halle medications but according to Beisswanger extended as well to the Augsburg Schauer balm, a famous universal produced and exported to the Salzburger colony by the manufacturer, one of the colony's benefactors. (See, for example, Jones and Wilson, *Detailed Reports*, vol. 6).

46. Imitation and substitution by medications resembling the Halle set have been suggested by Alfons Rutten for Curaçao in the first decade of the seventeenth century. See Rutten, "Drinkbaar goud voor zwarte slaven; de geneesmiddel farbriktie op Curaçao in 1707 en de Hallese piëtisten."

Halle medications.[47] Dreissiger had provided the reprint to hide the name of the Halle agent in Amsterdam, which was prominently displayed in the original Dutch text. Madai discovered the swindle when the house of Petri in Amsterdam complained, forwarding copies of invoices and bills of lading returned by customers in the tropics who had noticed the swindle and returned the merchandise unpaid. Petri demanded reimbursement, for the equivalent of £ sterling 600, which may well have been made, because Tuphorn and Petri remained trading partners until the 1790s.

In Europe, the threats arose from medical and institutional developments, in particular the growth of medical regulation under enlightened absolutism. Prussia and other territorial states increasingly offered to apothecaries protection against irregular competition and to the bureaucracy a tool of regulation, although Halle was able to fend off these threats until the end of the eighteenth century. In the early part of that century, the Francke Foundations had been a special favorite of Frederick William I, who placed a large order for physic chests for his army in 1734. We should note that the then medical head of the Foundations, Johann Juncker, cautiously argued against accepting this tempting offer, on the grounds that it was impossible to predict the specific needs for an army of 10,000 men, as well as the specific therapeutic preferences of the army surgical and medical staff.[48] It is unlikely that Madai would have made the same argument ten years later.

Although not sharing his father's unquestioning admiration of the Halle institutions, Frederick II of Prussia continued protection of Halle trade, which reflected his understanding that tariffs and postal revenues were accruing to the Prussian coffers and that the local economy of Halle benefited from the Foundations as a major employer.[49] We do not know whether Frederick's aversion to religion affected his own purchases, but sales and net profits from the *Medimentenexpedition* peaked during the two decades of wars over Silesia between Prussia and Austria, in which the *Medikamentenexpedition* sold to all sides. With the end of the wars, pharmaceutical profits fell from 34,000 Rth in 1765 to roughly 7,000 Rth in 1799.

The pharmaceutical trade itself was changed by the reforms of the entire medical system that, although they had begun well before the French Revolution, were continued into law under the French Republic and then carried into the territories under French control in the Napoleonic era. From the

47. VAFSt ix/ii/22, fols. 5ff.
48. VAFt ix/ii/17, 1733, relating to the order of physic chests for an army of 10,000 men.
49. Correspondence in "Copeyen der in anno 1764. . . ."

potent medicine developed at the brink of the seventeenth century under the banner of Christian and medical reform, the Halle products had become part of the commercial market in proprietary medicines. The erosion of their position but their eventual survival in this market niche is evident from correspondence with Holland. In 1790, the new *Ministre de la santé publique et de l' éducation nationale* was barred by statute from continuing the Halle trading privilege. Instead, a secret license was extended to the Foundations' commissary, Welling, based on personal intercession by the King of Prussia and, no doubt, the transatlantic trading community.[50]

In Napoleonic Denmark, sales networks fell victim to pharmaceutical regulation in 1807, when "sale of the so-called Halle Medications, previously permitted to all, is now restricted to apothecaries and chemists." In a final act of regulation in 1812, a letter over the signature of Frederick William IV of Prussia revoked the Halle trade from continued exemption from pharmaceutical regulation and withdrew permission to maintain agents in Brandenburg and Prussia, on the grounds that these privileges were contrary to statute and unwarranted in view of the large number of local pharmacies capable of undertaking continuing sales.[51]

In summary, the medical standing of the Halle pharmaceuticals had been eroded by a century of regulatory reforms. Public-health regulations relegated *arcana* and nonreproducible substances to the field of patent or proprietary medicines and restricted their sale even when recipes came from respected physicians. In an undated and unsigned memorandum reflecting conditions at the beginning of the British continental blockade against Napoleonic Europe, the then head of the *Medikamentenexpedition*, Carl August von Madai, summarized the drastic decrease in profits and thus in moneys accruing to the Francke Foundations as follows:

> 1. In some jurisdictions, our medications have been entirely forbidden, for instance in the Austrian territories, where the few articles permitted had to be renamed.

50. VAFSt ix/ii/37, letter from Frederick William III, 10 July 1799, supporting the Halle request for exemption. A letter from Jan Lodewig Gregory in The Hague argued that the medications were a special class of *allgemeine Genesmittel oder arcana*. This argument was repeated by Welling, who had been the Halle agent since 1793 ("these internal medicines from Halle do not fall under the new regulations . . . since the benefit and potency of the Halle Orphanage medications are well known both to members of the Commission and to the public in general, so that even men of known medical repute and experience do not hesitate to recommend them").

51. Ibid., ix/ii/28, 12 July.

2. Elsewhere, our medications have been placed under extremely high tariffs which would eat up all our profit if we were to assume this cost. If not, we would have to increase prices, and this would make them so expensive as to frighten off all buyers. This was the case in Russia, Sweden, and England, where formerly we had strong sales.

3. The French wars have caused much damage, for wherever the French have assumed control, all sales have ceased. In particular, this has been the case in Holland since the French occupation, where all our sales have ceased *and we have incurred considerable losses because we maintained a large storehouse in Amsterdam from where we shipped to the East and West Indies.* (The italicized portion was deleted in the manuscript.)

4. The wars have almost entirely interrupted our trade with Königsberg in Prussia and Danzig and into Poland, as we have been told by many of our friends in these places.

5. The Missionaries in East India [Tranquebar, Madras, and other stations] had been in the habit of buying considerable amounts from us, but this trade has decreased substantially.

6. There is much imitation of our medications, which destroys inventories and markets.

7. Prices [of raw materials] have risen and there is a dearth of cash.

8. The preferences of the public have changed both with regard to our Orphanage and our medications.[52]

In a related letter of 1804, these changes in preference were linked to new therapies (*neue Cur-Methoden*) to account for the joint influence of public demand and medical attitudes.

In wider terms, at the beginning of the eighteenth century, freedom of action and freedom of the pharmaceutical market were available to those with the requisite products and market networks, including well-placed philanthropic institutions. By the end of the century, medical and pharmaceutical reform had joined hands with state control, at least in the continental European market.

Although the first signs of this decline of Halle and its trade had set in at the end of the 1760s and had accelerated in the transition from the eighteenth to the nineteenth century, a continuous if limited trade to the new American republic saw a resurgence during the 1790s and remained constant until beyond

52. See VAFSt ix/ii (1), unpaginated. Material in brackets added by me.

the turn of the century. Here, pharmaceutical reform and regulation were distant phenomena in a flourishing market in self-help and eclectic medicines.[53] North America became one of the redoubts of the proprietary medicine trade and its imitations. American choices were made in a culturally competitive environment and were as much determined by and reflected cultural and language traditions as theoretical differences in therapy. In this market, we revisit some of the earlier characteristics of the trade in Halle medications, including a network of favored providers and the use of the pharmaceuticals as instruments of financial exchange in underdeveloped capital markets.

53. Young, "Patent Medicines: Early Example of Competitive Marketing." Young notes that English patent medicines popular before the Revolution did not return to favor, but were imitated, people even asking for labels in England.

PART two

German Medicine in

North America,

1730-1810

4

In most Protestant German territories of the eighteenth century, people were accustomed to modest
but pervasive levels of structured medical care. As
elsewhere in Europe, bedside medicine was largely
reserved to the moneyed classes in their homes and
to the charity population in poorhouses and municipal and religious hospitals. But the majority of
people had access to a wide range of formal and
informal ambulatory services, from the town *physici*
to barber surgeons and apothecaries to the whole
range of early modern providers. People of all walks
of life used these medical resources frequently,
selectively, and often judiciously, given the persistence throughout eighteenth-century Europe of
traditional classifications of symptoms and diseases
and treatment options. They turned to—or used
simultaneously—self-medication, physician care,
and the prescriptions of the so-called empirics—
untrained but often experienced men and women—
depending on severity of illness or urgency, failure
of previous treatments, predilection, and financial
resources.[1]

1. The most recent and comprehensive English-language
account of medical care in Germany is by Lindemann, *Health and
Healing in 18th Century Germany,* which centers on the duchy of
Braunschweig-Wolfenbüttel. Although the area she chose for her
comprehensive multilevel study may not have been representative

This wide range of available services and medical products gave rise to a fairly open medical market despite the ongoing public health and medical reforms in most German territories that attempted to extend traditional municipal health regulations to rural areas.[2] Patients could and did make choices, and there was competition for paying patients among the providers of care and the manufacturers and sellers of pharmaceuticals, despite the continued existence— and support by the territorial states—of traditional medical hierarchies.[3]

Once ashore in North America, often beset by the morbid sequelae of naval passage and soon attacked by a variety of local diseases, German immigrants found themselves in strange territory in more ways than one—climate, geography, languages, and medical flora. Exclusive reliance on familial self-help practices including the use of traditional remedies or the adaptation of Indian materia medica is easy to postulate in theory and has indeed often been postulated, but it is difficult to envision as a reality except in a few instances.[4] Apart from some treasured medical stores and recipe collections brought along as part of their baggage, and from the presence of women able or at least willing to assist in birthing or other female complaints, there was in most early settlements little in the way of trained medical and surgical help or knowledge, regardless of language or national background. Usually, this type of help did turn up within the first five or ten years of community growth and of a patient population that could support one or two practitioners. In German areas of settlement from New York

of the medical policies of all German territories, the practice of general medicine was not vastly different from other semirural and rural areas in terms of health and illness, of patterns of mortality, and of the struggle between the various layers of providers and bureaucracies. For a comparative perspective, see, for example, Porter, *The Popularization of Medicine*; Grell and Cunningham, *Health Care and Poor Relief in Protestant Europe*; Fissell, *Patients, Power, and the Poor*.

2. For the early seventeenth century, see, for example, Kinzelbach, *Gesundbleiben und Krankwerden*, and Grell and Cunningham, *Health Care Provision and Poor Relief*. For administrative reforms from Prussia and the free city of Hamburg in the north to Austria in the south, see Rosen, "Cameralism and the Concept of Medical Police"; Lindemann, *Patriots and Paupers*; and Lesky, *Österreichisches Gesundheitswesen*.

3. The model of an evolving medical market rather than of pervasive physician dominance has recently gained much attention. See in particular the work of Cook, *Decline of the Old Medical Regime in Stuart London*; Brockliss and Jones, *Medical World of Early Modern France*; and Porter, *The Popularization of Medicine*. For the pharmaceutical market, which is relatively rarely studied for this period, the detailed empirical work by Beisswanger, *Arzneimittelversorgung im 18. Jahrhundert*, shows the pervasiveness of proprietary medicines in the inventories of many German pharmacies despite a close system of regulation and visitation.

4. Cowen, "Impact of Materia Medica of the North American Indians"; Duffy, *The Healers*; Gevitz and Sullivan-Fowler, "Making Sense of Therapeutics."

to Georgia, trained medical providers were often former French, Swiss, or German military personnel such as field apothecaries or barbers left adrift after the European campaigns of the early part of the eighteenth century, who would stay on if there was a large and sufficiently prosperous catchment area to generate income.[5]

But as in New England, the most linguistically and socially cohesive of the English colonies in North America, there was one major source of medical care in the community possessed of both learning and local ties: the clergy. The specifically Pietist practice of medicine, and with it access to the medications from the Halle Orphanage, was brought across the Atlantic and into German and Swiss Lutheran and Reformed congregations by several generations of Pietist ministers beginning in the 1730s. These ministers practiced side by side with other German medical men and women of very different levels of training along the East Coast and in the back counties of Pennsylvania, Maryland, and Virginia.

In joining medical and clerical functions, these ministers resembled their Congregationalist colleagues in New England, the Presbyterians in the middle colonies, and their Anglican brethren, who had all practiced medicine since the seventeenth century.[6] Clergy had the classical training that gave them access to the outlines of traditional medical theory and therapeutics. Although not necessarily possessed of university training, many even among itinerant ministers had a fairly good understanding of Latin and some aspects of medical therapy, including access to medical texts, herbals, and other traditional literature.[7] They were willing to join medical and clerical practice for reasons of community cohesion and the need to augment their incomes, and they enjoyed some measure of respect and the confidence of their congregations.

In the eyes of the colonial authorities from New York to South Carolina and eventually Georgia, there can have been little doubt that clerical medical practice would ensure social cohesion and medical services and help to block

5. A French surgeon practiced in Purysburg, South Carolina, for instance, and an army apothecary from Hungary, Andreas Zwifler, served in Ebenezer. See Wilson, "Die Halleschen Waisenhausmedikamente." Bodo Otto (Gibson, *Bodo Otto and the Medical Background of the American Revolution*) also seems to have been an army surgeon first. These people normally were not part of religious immigrant groups, who usually opposed military service.

6. For New England, see in particular Watson, *Angelical Conjunction*; Cotton Mather, *Angel of Bethesda*; Gevitz and Sullivan-Fowler, "Making Sense of Therapeutics."

7. See Chapter 2 for the persistence of humoral pathology despite numerous new explanatory schemes of the seventeenth century. As noted by Watson, *Angelical Conjunction*, the New England ministers seem to have been drawn in particular to chemiatric materia medica.

itinerants of doubtful religious persuasions from peddling their messages. And given the general religious tolerance prevailing in the middle colonies, practitioners of more radical religious beliefs rarely posed a civil danger other than competition for the congregations of the more conservative denominations. The medical communities of colonial eastern Pennsylvania are a good example of the range of religious dissenters in this area and of the ascendance of quite sophisticated medical practitioners from Silesia, Huguenot France, the Palatinate, and Protestant Hungary.[8] Many came from private colleges—the medical dissenting academies that stood in opposition to the academic monopoly.[9] Some could not have practiced either their religion or their profession in Europe. In America, they provided a level of rural medical practice and pharmaceutic dispensing that, except for the academic trappings they rejected for religious reasons, was probably little different from European models.[10]

Medical Needs and Medical Markets

Medical markets developed in response to the need for services by a growing colonial population. Pharmaceuticals were prescribed and usually compounded and sold by local physicians and surgeons. The public bought proprietary compounds directly from dry goods stores and sought the attention of barber surgeons and midwives. Attempts to stratify and control medical practice in individual colonies go back to early years of settlement,[11] but most of these attempts failed, and open medical markets existed on a regional basis, served by multiple types of unregulated practitioners, including the untrained and inexperienced. Although the failed attempts at regulation are generally attributed to the lack of hierarchical structures and academic centers on American soil, this view ignores eighteenth-century colonial demography, in other words, the demand side of the medical equation. Quite apart from questions of religious and language

8. Berky, *Practitioner in Physick*; Meier, *Early Pennsylvania Medicine*; Savacool, "Illness and Therapy."

9. Habrich, "Untersuchungen zur pietistischen Medizin."

10. The Moravian communities clearly had their own medical networks. There is no systematic and reliable work on these, which may well have been modeled on the Halle precedent. The physick garden of Brother Ettwein in South Carolina (Bethabara) was established in 1757, and there was a pharmacy in Salem. A Sachse-Gotha physician owned and used Richter's 1740 edition of the *Höchstnöthige Erkenntnis*. See Cowen and Wilson, "Traffic in Medical Ideas."

11. Warden, "The Medical Profession in Colonial Boston," in *Medicine in Colonial Massachusetts*, 145–57; Cowen, *Medicine and Health in New Jersey*; Bell, "A Portrait of the Colonial Physician"; Duffy, *The Healers*, chap. 5.

differences,[12] the uneven influx of new and geographically mobile populations, mainly but not exclusively into the middle colonies, created a much larger need for services than could have been met even if European structures had indeed been replicated.

Altogether, the North American population more than tripled over the first half of the eighteenth century and then tripled again by the end of the century.[13] Few immigrant groups brought their own professional medical providers, although as in the seventeenth century, religious groups on the margins of their European societies were often an exception. The Mennonites and the Herrn-huters or Moravians and the small Salzburger settlement in Georgia are examples of this practice,[14] as was, if for different reasons, the concentrated provision of medical care to plantation slaves by utilitarian owners.[15]

But large masses of urban and rural Scots, Protestant Irish, and German-language arrivals were unprovided in medical terms; the growth, often imper-manent, in the number of dispensing pharmacies opening shop and advertising their stocks to medical providers and lay folk alike, and the relative popularity of printed or laboriously copied self-help manuals in the vernacular indicate that there was an unserved market waiting to be tapped. Who would tap it, and how those offering medical goods and services of whatever provenance gained access to this *mixed multitude*, the felicitous term used by Sally Schwartz for the middle colonies,[16] becomes an important skein in the story of the North American medical market.

What we know about attitudes to medical care among the German-speaking colonial population, which changed considerably in geographical and cultural origins and social and economic makeup over the course of immigration in the eighteenth century, is largely based on inference from scattered second-hand reports. Relatively well-trained or aspiring American physicians found a common professional voice only in the 1760s, with the founding of medical

12. See Roeber, "In German Ways"; Wokeck, "Harnessing the Lure"; Schwartz, *Mixed Multitude*, for the German populations in particular.

13. Bureau of the Census, *Historical Statistics of the United States: Colonial Times to 1970, Series Z: Prefederal Statistics*.

14. Meier, *Early Pennsylvania Medicine*; Berky, *Practitioner in Physick*; Wilson, "Die Halleschen Waisenhausmedikamente."

15. This practice was found mainly in areas with large slaveholdings and was not restricted to the North American continent. See Duffy, *History of Medicine in Louisiana*, vol. 1, pp. 126–38; Savitt and Young, *Disease and Distinctiveness in the American South*, esp. chap. 6; Rutten, "Slavenhandel, ziekten en mortaliteit."

16. Schwartz, *A Mixed Multitude*.

societies,[17] and their voices were biased in many ways. For ambulatory care, the almost exclusive form of care for the American population from all social strata until the end of the nineteenth century, physician journals and similar materials that could document actual use linked to age and diagnostic information are few and far between before the 1750s and usually contained only charges and payments next to patient names or the medication prescribed.[18] Published formularies or dispensatories that would indicate adaptation to American conditions in terms of climate and morbidity are relatively rare before the mid-century, because the colonies were amply served with European works.[19] Indirect evidence of patient willingness to consult medical providers, which at the time was equivalent to the request for medicinals of all kinds, comes from the newspapers and broadsheets of the period, in which all kinds of people offered medical services, some even making a good living.[20]

17. Using the founding years of American medical societies is not intended to locate the medical professionalization debate in this decade. For a recent and incisive overview for German physicians from 1750 onward, see Bromann, *The Transformation of German Medicine*. For the nineteenth-century United States, the classic work remains Warner, *Therapeutic Perspective*. For a survey of colonial American practitioners that is still valid in both questions asked and emphasis, see Bell, "A Portrait of the Colonial Physician," Garrison lecture, in particular 6ff., for the retrospective views of the medical care scene before the foundation of medical societies. See also his "Medicine in Boston and Philadelphia"; Estes, "Therapeutic Practice in Colonial New England"; and Cowen, *Medicine in New Jersey*.

18. See Estes, "Patterns of Drug Use in Colonial America," and, as an example from the middle colonies, two physician ledgers in the Rutgers Archives set up to document the financial aspects of the partnership between John Griffith and Moses Scott, 1774–76, continued by Scott only after 1776. Information in the entries and treatment notes becomes far more voluminous in the 1780s. The need for this type of information was acutely felt by Europeans and colonial officials alike, however. See Cassedy, "Church Record Keeping and Public Health in New England." This information was urgently demanded, but rarely obtained, by the Halle authorities from their only direct medical emissary, Ernst Georg Thilo in Georgia.

19. Among the exceptions are Benjamin Franklin's publication of John Tennent's *EveryMan His Own Doctor,* and an herbal published by Christopher Sauer. See Cowen and Wilson, "Traffic in Medical Ideas." The first North American pharmacopoeia was written during the Revolutionary War by William Brown, the army surgeon general. See Cowen, "The Edinburgh Pharmacopoeia," and Edward Kremers, *Badger Pharmacist* (1940), 27–30. For German texts, excluding almanacs and collections of family recipes copied, there are the Richter manuals (see Chapters 2 and 3), the German versions of Samuel Tissot's *Advice to the People,* and unpublished formularies like the *Medicina Pennsylvania* of George de Benneville and the formulary by Abraham Wagner (see Chapter 7). For unpublished English formularies, see Watson, *Angelical Conjunction;* Estes, "Therapeutic Practice in Colonial New England."

20. The role of eighteenth-century journals and gazettes of all types in spreading medical knowledge has been most cogently argued by Jones, "Great Chain of Buying." In North America, they constitute a rich if daunting source, and their German component, although accessible through the work of Arndt and Olson, has not been well exploited in the field of medical advertising. I have found rich material for Georgia while compiling a bibliographical note on James Ewell (*American Dictionary of Bibliography,* 1999), and some examples are included in this study.

In terms of numbers over time, potential patients and pharmaceutical customers in the German immigrant population started coming to North America at the end of the seventeenth century. Different authors have made different estimates of the flow of German immigrants to 1775, but a range of between 85,000 to 110,000 or just under 30 percent of total European immigration to 1780 is generally accepted.[21] Despite a largely mid-century burst, which reached its peak by 1760, the German element stood at just 9 percent of the total American population at the time of the first national census in 1790, making for a far less impressive share in the new republic.[22] A rough demographic profile of this potential patient population is likewise available for the middle and southern colonies.[23] This makes it possible to define the areas in which medical providers in general, German providers in particular, and the Pietist medical missionaries who are at the core of this study could and did offer their services to the German public.

More difficult to obtain—but obviously no less important for a medical history—is a reliable age and sex distribution for immigrant groups and for established settlers. These types of data, which would indicate different levels of risk and type of illness and of using care in the population, are only occasionally available until the first census of 1790.[24] In general, German immigrant patterns resembled those of other national and ethnic groups of European origin, although peaks and valleys of emigration differed, and groups who had arrived in large numbers during the seventeenth century, like the English, had more time to reach stable rates of marriage and reproduction and thus population growth.[25]

21. The most recent estimates come from Fertig, "German Migration"; Fogleman, *Hopeful Journeys*; and Wokeck, *Trade in Strangers*. Wokeck's is the most detailed count, and her work has yielded the high end of the estimate. For the period after the Revolutionary War, see Grabbe, "Besonderheiten der europäischen Einwanderung in die USA."

22. The census total is of course the baseline to which all estimates of population rather than immigrants must conform. See the estimates by Fogleman, "Migration to the Thirteen British North American Colonies," 701, and idem, *Hopeful Journeys*, appendix, 160, and by Fertig, "German Migration," 202. See the estimates by Cappon, *Atlas of Early American History*, 98, of a 1775 German population in excess of 200,000.

23. See in particular the work of Wokeck, "The Flow and Composition of German Immigration"; Fogleman, *Hopeful Journeys*; and the collection of essays in Canny, *Europeans on the Move*.

24. Bureau of the Census, *Historical Statistics of the United States: Colonial Times to 1970*, Table 1, Series Z.

25. These very general statements are based on the recent summary by Canny, *Europeans on the Move*, for different emigrant groups in Europe and their migration patterns. Fertig, "German Migration," provides some information over time (215). Although the planned settlements are some exception to this lack of data, particularly in the case of the Moravians (Smaby, *Transformation of Moravian Bethlehem*), they are too small and exceptional to permit generalization. In my own study of

Based on most available estimates, and except for the small radical religious groups, German immigrants in the eighteenth century were relatively young, but the fact that many arrived in family groups probably raised their median age and the proportion of females.[26] Overall child mortality and adult disease mortality, once immigrants were offboard ship and had survived the sequelae of shipboard disease, were probably slightly below European rates,[27] except in areas of endemic malaria and during epidemics such as smallpox, throat distemper/scarlatina, and yellow fever.[28] Widows and widowers did not long remain unmarried because of the need, respectively, for a female head of the household economy and the relatively high mortality of women of child-bearing age. Birth rates were high, and child survival improved as settlers integrated into their areas of residence and acquired stable income or at least sustenance.

Both for the end of the century and before, we must look as well at the geographic distribution of this population over the thirteen colonies. It is well known that German speakers (and for that matter the Scots),[29] even when not arriving in settlement parties, tended to locate in proximity to related communities in terms of language and confession and of landholding and familiar agricultural patterns if at all possible. This led to a very uneven distribution,[30] which did not include much in the way of German settlements in New England and on the Atlantic coast but resulted in heavy concentrations to the west of the Hudson River in New York, in New Jersey, Pennsylvania, and the backcountry

a Georgia settlement, the original immigrant populations of 400 people who came by 1745 and another 400 people who arrived between 1749 and 1750 had grown to 1,065 by 1762, despite the relatively high age of the first cohort of adults, heavy initial mortality from malaria and dysentery, and a relatively low birth and child survival rate from 1733 to 1741 (Wilson, "Land, Population, and Labor").

26. Wokeck, *Trade in Strangers*, 47–50.

27. German infant mortality was still between 40 and 60 percent at the end of the early modern period (Imhof, *Lebenserwartungen in Deutschland*).

28. Duffy, *Epidemics in Colonial America*; Cassedy, "Church Record Keeping and Public Health in Early New England." For early descriptions of throat distemper in North America, see Beck, *Historical Sketch*.

29. Wokeck, "Trade in Strangers"; idem, "Charting Courses."

30. Cappon, *Atlas of Early American History*, 98ff., 117ff. According to Cappon's work, which incorporates that of an earlier demographer, Paullin, for the religious groupings, the German-speaking share of the 1775 population was 30–50 percent in areas of high German population density. In regional terms, therefore, Germans were never a majority. I have included the Dutch population in Fig. 4.1 only as a point of reference. It is impossible to draw clean lines between the population speaking Dutch and that speaking Low German. As noted below, the split between High and Low German speakers was a European regional one.

of Maryland, and in defined regions of Virginia and North and South Carolina (see Fig. 4.1). Thus, from almost the beginning of German settlement, there were areas of considerable German population density; for their health care, this population tended to look to German providers regardless of levels of training, to German self-help texts, and, where available, pharmaceuticals—in short, a nascent regional and language-based medical market.

Market Determinants: Language and Religious Affiliation

This preference was due not to any inherent difference or specific medical features distinguishing German medical providers or products over those from England.[31] Rather, it was due to language-related and similar cultural characteristics such as familiarity with medical nomenclature, medicinal substances, and almanacs and medical self-help texts.[32] And this familiarity seems to have been crucial despite the fact that over the course of the century, the German immigrants came from very different regional backgrounds.[33] By the end of the seventeenth century, High German had finally and definitively won out over most regional German dialects as the language of literacy and printing. Remaining exceptions were the Alemanic of Southwest Germany and Switzerland and the "Low German" of the provinces bordering on the North Sea and the Baltic.[34] The persistence of the latter in the New Jersey Raritan congregations and in rural and urban New York was a major linguistic and class barrier encountered by many of the Lutheran clergy. New York and New Jersey parish records reflect

31. This is an important difference from the transmission of legal systems. Roeber, in *Palatines, Liberty, and Property*, and "In German Ways," described the persistence and reception of German legal traditions, which were radically different from English traditions.

32. George de Benneville, a Huguenot physician with a German medical education who practiced in Pennsylvania from 1741 to 1790, triangulated his large medical compendium by providing German, English, and Latin nomenclature (Savacool, "Illness and Therapy"). As late as the last decade of the nineteenth century, Friedrich Hoffmann, the noted German-American pharmacologist and editor of *Die Pharmazeutische Rundschau*, published a list of German botanical and other medications for recent settlers in Wisconsin and other heavily German areas to assist pharmacists in providing service (*Popular German Names of Drugs and Medicines*).

33. The literature on the regional background of German immigrants is extensive. For recent summaries, see Roeber, *Palatines, Liberty, and Property*, Wokeck, *Trade in Strangers*, and Häberlein, *From the Rhine to the Susquehanna*.

34. The evolution of a national spoken and written language replacing both regional dialects and Latin was central to the development of German literature in the seventeenth century. The battle for Low German as a fully equivalent language remained joined throughout the eighteenth century, although by the nineteenth century it was increasingly fought on literary terrain.

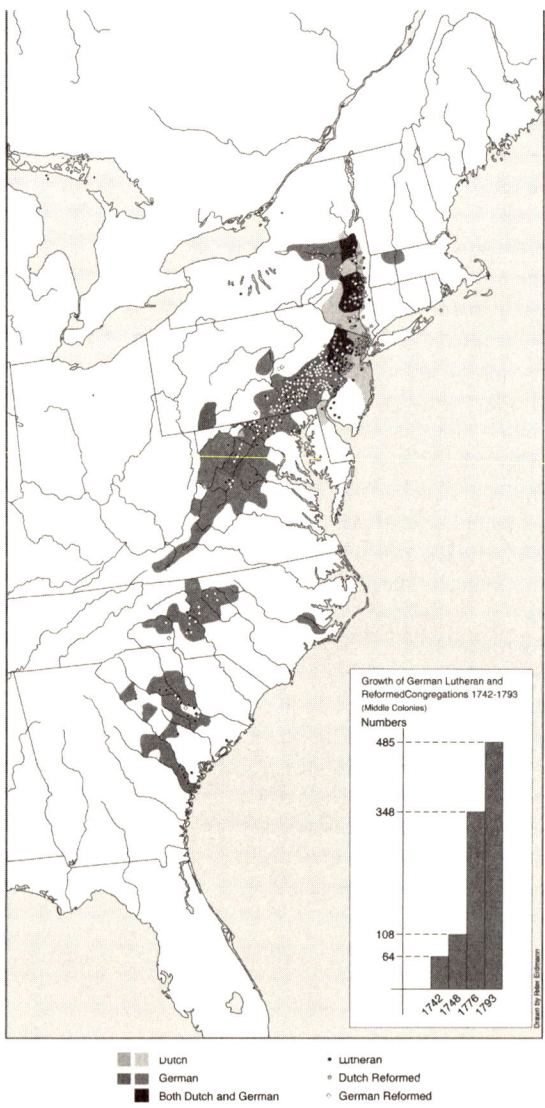

Growth of German Lutheran and
ReformedCongregations 1742-1793
(Middle Colonies)
Numbers

485

348

108
64

1742 1748 1776 1793

Drawn by Peter Erdmann

Dutch
German
Both Dutch and German

• Lutheran
○ Dutch Reformed
◇ German Reformed

Fig. 4.1

A medical catchment area defined by language and religious denomination: Areas of German and Dutch language settlements in the thirteen colonies, 1775, and distribution of Lutheran and German and Dutch Reformed congregations, 1775, using data on population distribution, relative population density, and location of congregations from Lester J. Cappon, *Atlas of Early American History* and C. O. Paullin, *Atlas of Historical Geography* (used with the kind permission of Princeton University Press). Paullin's data on congregations are updated to 1790 from Glatfelter, *Pastors and People*, vol. 2. Other denominations not shown. Light shading indicates up to 16 percent of the European population as German and Dutch; dark shading indicates 16–40 percent. (Graphic design by Peter Erdmann, Berlin.)

this language quarrel, which broke into the open in the 1720s between local and often unordained incumbents like Bernard van Dieren and their class-conscious new pastors Wilhelm Christoph Berkenmeyer and Wilhelm Knoll from Hamburg. Although until the 1770s congregations in turn often rejected ministers because of their inability to preach in Low German, this point of friction eventually declined. In some communities, the conflict was resolved only by attrition, some Low German congregations apparently preferring to move into the English sphere rather than adapting to High German texts.[35]

In a letter of 23 October 1713, the then Lutheran pastor in New York, Justus Falckner, writing to an unidentified correspondent in Amsterdam, expressed thanks for a large book shipment in Dutch and published by Amsterdam houses. Thirty years later, Heinrich Melchior Mühlenberg, who was the first pastor from Halle in the middle colonies and who spoke and wrote Low German, used the quarrel between speakers of Low German dialects and their Hamburg pastors to draw the New York–New Jersey congregations into his own sphere. He continued to confer with the Raritan congregation in Low German, in a series of legal wrangles over a legacy in the 1750s.[36] But by 1770, when his American-born son Gotthilf Heinrich Ernst assumed this congregation, the persistence of Low German is rarely if ever mentioned. There is no mention of medical texts or pharmaceuticals ordered from Amsterdam through the orthodox Lutheran clergy under the Hamburg synod. Speakers of Low German or Dutch wishing to use the Halle Orphanage medications, of course,

35. Hart and Kreider, eds., *Lutheran Church in New York and New Jersey.* In a letter by J. Friedrich Riess (KM 1:423, of 17 July 1751), concerning the New York congregation, the closeness of Dutch and Low German is reflected in the statement "an evangelical Dutch and Low Saxon congregation." Both the correspondence and the protocols of the Saint Matthew's congregation in New York, which include the period of Justus Falckner's incumbency, are either in Dutch or in Latin, although Falckner spoke and wrote High German. The transitions are well documented in *Records Relating to the Lutheran Church in Colonial New York, 1649–1772,* including minutes of the Consistory at Amsterdam, correspondence of the Consistory with Lutherans in New York, and petitions from New York to the Consistory, Hamburg, and the Dutch West Indies Company. Originals at the Archives of the Lutheran Church, Amsterdam; photocopies and transcripts at the New York Public Library. (Excerpts transcribed and published by Kreider, "Lutheran Church in New York," and Hart and Kreider, eds., *Evangelisch Luthersche Kerk [Netherlands]* [Protokolle der St. Matthäus Gemeinde].) Correspondence with Lutheran bodies in Amsterdam, Hamburg, London, and Skara, Manuscripts and Archives Section, New York Public Library.

36. Evangelisch Luthersche Kerk, Netherlands, 1703–83. Microfilm at Rutgers University Libraries, New Brunswick. The fact that Heinrich Melchior Mühlenberg came from one of the bastions of Low German, Einbeck in Lower Saxony, has not been noted by his biographers, whether German or English.

could purchase them and Dutch versions of the accompanying text from Amsterdam and Rotterdam.[37]

The number of Lutheran congregations grew substantially over the course of the century, both in the center of German settlement and at the periphery. In Pennsylvania, New York, New Jersey, Maryland, and Virginia, they numbered about 50 by 1748; by 1776, there were roughly 180; and by 1793, about 250.[38] Among the German Reformed, many congregations—roughly equal in number and growth rates to the Lutheran ones—shared churches with the Lutherans and thus almost doubled the potential points of contact for Halle influence, not least in terms of the sale of books and medicines.[39]

The central role of congregation and church for eighteenth-century North American community life and commercial activity need hardly be stressed. Of interest is the fact that after the relative prominence of radical Pietist sects early in the century, and despite Moravian incursions by mid-century,[40] there was a sixfold growth in Lutheran and Reformed congregations between 1740 and 1790, which almost matches the sevenfold growth in the German population over the same period[41] (see Fig. 4.1).

From the 1720s to the 1740s, many German settlements had been without regular pastoral attention, but by the late 1760s, basic needs seem to have been met, if at the cost of constant travel by ministers to outlying congregations. Continued complaints about the scarcity of preachers may have reflected clerical perceptions of need and placeholding concerns rather than

37. A Dutch translation of the *Short Account* by D. S. Madai was published as *Kort bericht* as early as 1734. Book imports in Dutch in general seem to have ceased by the 1720s (Roeber, "German and Dutch Books and Printing"), and North American Dutch imprints between 1700 and 1800 were few, running at most to five a year (in 1755) but usually not more than two to three titles. I thank Antje Matthäus for compiling this information.

38. As in much of the following, this account is indebted to the pioneering work of Charles Glatfelter, *Pastors and People*.

39. After mid-century, the substantial book imports from Halle began to include the Heidelberg catechism and Reformed Bible editions in increasing number; see Chapter 7, and Roeber, "German and Dutch Books and Printing."

40. See, most recently, Fogleman, *Hopeful Journeys*.

41. Numbers calculated after Glatfelter, *Pastors and People*, vol. 2, and Fogleman, *Hopeful Journeys*. The dechurching of the American population claimed by Butler, *Awash in a Sea of Faith*, does not fit this growth well, at least for the German population. It seems that Roeber's assumption (underlying *Palatines, Liberty, and Property*) of organized religious community, although perhaps overly reliant on professions of faith, may have a better fit with the congregation as a central social institution throughout much of American history.

actual need.[42] Many congregations were fractured by social strife, clerical inter-lopers persisted, and there was considerable variation in size and economic sta-tus. But in the end, the desire to maintain cultural and linguistic cohesion and internal order buttressed by church discipline overcame the resistance of many German congregations unaccustomed to the strict demands of the Pietist Lutheran clergy.[43] The story of the slow but sure takeover by Halle Pietists of many of these Lutheran congregations has been told many times and from many perspectives. It need not concern us here in detail other than to show that after mid-century, few areas of contiguous German settlement in the middle colonies had not been touched by the Pietist presence.[44]

Also, and this is important for the growth of a medical market, not all con-gregations were and remained full of the poor. Lutheran and Reformed congre-gations took in all baptized members of their European mother churches and thus had a wider range of members and probably more need for charity than the sects, which were more exclusive and often well financed from Europe or had brought capital with them.[45] But many Lutheran parishes soon became well-off, as reflected in donations and subscription and vestry lists from New York to Pennsyl-vania. In particular, the New York congregations were well connected to outside sources of funds from the beginning of the eighteenth century and well-off from the 1720s onward, as indicated by contribution lists for 1700–1740 in the Protocols of the Saint Matthew's congregation. The New Jersey congregations in the Raritan Valley made substantial contributions to the parish and established

42. With all due respect to these efforts, it should not go unnoticed that the highly regarded senior Mühlenberg placed his extremely young sons Friedrich August and Heinrich Gotthilf Ernst at the head of contested congregations. Neither was over twenty years old, and both were eventually ordained by the American Lutheran Ministerium, without any apparent objection by the new co-direc-tor of the Francke Foundations, J. G. Knapp. (See KM 4: Letter 538–39 of 16 and 21 February 1771, 253ff., and Letter 553, reply by Knapp of 26 April 1771.) See also Glatfelter, *Pastors and People,* vol. 1.

43. The dominance of language in conditions of relative religious freedom is obvious. The German Reformed shared with the English and Scottish Presbyterians many points of doctrine and church history. *Gemeinschaftliche* ("common") churches and church administration occurred not across these two confessions, however, but within the German Protestant congregations, despite initial dif-ficulties (Glatfelter, *Pastors and People,* 2:161ff.).

44. Tappert and Doberstein, *Journals of Henry Melchior Muhlenberg;* Glatfelter, *Pastors and People;* Müller, *Kirche zwischen zwei Welten;* Splitter, "A Free People in the American Air."

45. For example, this is true for both Schwenkfelders and Moravians and well known also for Mennonites. The Schwenkfelders, expelled from Silesia in the 1720s, came to North America after many years of exile but were neither redemptioners nor landless (Ward, *Protestant Evangelical Awakening,* 88; Berky, *Practitioner in Physick*). The extraordinary financing of the Moravian missions, which went well beyond the funds available from Halle, is well known. See de Schweinitz, "Financial History of the Province," as cited by Fogleman, *Hopeful Journeys,* and Smaby, *Moravian Bethlehem.*

legacies in support of a minister beginning in 1740.[46] Collections came from as far away as Saint Thomas and reflected relations with the sugar trade in the Dutch Virgin Islands and the processing centers in New York and Philadelphia.[47] Despite widespread poverty among urban and rural immigrant populations, particularly in the first generation, economic stability throughout the Pennsylvania field grew with demographic size and offered not just a charity but a paying public for the Halle trade in books and medications. As congregations prospered, they attracted the German medical diaspora other than the Halle clergy.

A Profile of German Medical Providers

The prospects of serving this growing market became most obvious to both German and English medical providers and others during the peak period of German immigration around mid-century. But a separate if seldom-recognized German medical culture had in fact existed since the first German settlements were founded by groups of religious immigrants in the early part of the century. In part, this was due to the traditional linkage between ministry and medicine of the period; also, as for the Spanish and French Canadian domains, planned settlements were usually equipped with medical staff.[48] In the German case, this was true for many of the radical and dissenting groups that arrived between 1690 and 1740. Least well documented but intriguing is Daniel Falkner, born in 1666, who came to Pennsylvania in the 1690s and returned to Germany and then to the colonies as an agent of the Frankfurt Company, an enterprise closely connected to the nascent Pietist movement.[49] He practiced medicine and served New Jersey and Pennsylvania congregations until his death in 1741. He corresponded with the elder Francke in Halle, and, as late as 1730, was referred to as a veritable "Galen" by the head of the Albany congregations, a man not known for his generous temperament.[50]

The Salzburger settlement in Georgia founded in 1733 always had at least one and for most of the time two medical providers sent from Germany, although

46. Hart and Kreider, *Lutheran Church in New York and New Jersey.*
47. For the rewards of the sugar trade in Philadelphia, see Doerflinger, *Vigorous Spirit of Enterprise,* 179.
48. Duffy, *Rudolf Matas History of Medicine,* vol. 1, chap. 1; Risse, Numbers, and Leavitt, *Medicine in the New World.*
49. Wallmann, *Philipp Jakob Spener;* Glatfelter, *Pastors and People,* 2:517; Sachse, *History of the German Role.*
50. Sachse, *The German Pietists in Pennsylvania.*

they were not salaried but were expected to make their living by selling Halle medications and providing charity or community care to the settlers in return for housing, firewood, and in-kind payments.[51] There were a good number of medical providers among the Moravian groups and the Schwenkfelders, the former mostly but not always serving as part of their community obligations, the latter practicing freely. Many of these practitioners took up practice in the 1730s and 1740s and were clustered in the eastern Pennsylvania and western New Jersey counties.

Secular and clerical medical providers of European origin serving the colonial population can be documented only in part; it is obvious from scattered and usually critical comments in the contemporary literature, such as the journals and correspondence of Heinrich Melchior Mühlenberg, that the range of their training was just about as large as that found in Europe. There were among all nationalities a few "legitimate" physicians, whether academically trained or apprenticed, who have been the major focus of American medical historians until quite recently[52] (see Table 4.1). There were some extraordinarily gifted men (and apparently a few women).[53] In the middle colonies, they included Abraham Wagner and George de Benneville, whose training, judging from their reputation and their writings, seems to have been intensive. Among the Moravians were Bishop Johann Ettwein and Johann Adolph Meyer, the latter a son of a pharmacist from Halberstadt, who came to the colonies in 1742. In midlife, Meyer practiced outside the closed Moravian communities but within the eastern Pennsylvania medical area. By the time of the Revolutionary War, he returned to the Moravian community at Lititz, where he died in 1781. Johann Friedrich Otto from Meiningen, who had studied at the Universities of Jena and Halle, was another Moravian who arrived with the first large wave in 1743, practicing in Bethlehem for most of his life, as did his brother.[54]

51. Wilson, "Die Halleschen Waisenhausmedikamente"; Wilson and Poeckern, "A Continental System of Medical Care."

52. Bell, *Colonial Physician*; Cowen, *Medicine in New Jersey.*

53. Both Bell, op. cit., and Meier, *Early Pennsylvania Medicine*, mention one or two practicing female physicians but could not document them. In one of his reports of medical provider surplus, Mühlenberg mentions "apothecaries, surgeons, physicians, . . . masculini et foemina, etc. generis" (KM 2:429, Letter of 9 October 1760 to Francke and Ziegenhagen).

54. For Benneville, see Savacool, "Illness and Therapy"; for Wagner, see Berky, *Practitioner in Physick*. Meier, *Early Pennsylvania Medicine*, gives a name-by-name account of many of the others, who also appear in diaries and letters. As for many eighteenth-century colonial practitioners, there is much medical filiopiety in particular with regard to European social antecedents and education. As noted

Table 4.1   Medical practitioners (including Moravian Brethren) from Central Europe known to have practiced medicine and pharmacy in the middle colonies (Pennsylvania, New Jersey, Maryland, and New York), 1700–1810 (in chronological order of known start of practice)

Names and Approximate Periods of Practice	Location of Practice	Training/Origin/Religious Affiliation
Daniel Falckner, 1690(?)–1740	Falkner's Swamp, New York Low German congregations	Saxony, Lutheran
Andreas Zwifler, 1737–50(?)	Georgia/Philadelphia	Apothecary, Hungary, Imperial Army/Lutheran, subsequently Moravian
Melchior Heebner, 1734–38	Falkner's Swamp	Silesia/apprentice training/Schwenkfelder
Abraham Wagner, 1738–63	Falkner's Swamp/Worcester	Silesia, apprentice Heebner, Schwenkfelder
Bodo Otto, 1740–80	Cohenzy, New Jersey, Delaware peninsula, Philadelphia, Revolutionary Army	Army surgeon, Germany, Lutheran
Johann Adolph Meyer, 1742–81	Bethlehem, Nazareth, Skippack, Lititz	Halberstadt, apprenticed to father, Moravian but practiced outside Moravian community in midlife
Johann Friedrich Otto, 1743–89	Bethlehem, Nazareth	Meiningen, University Jena/Halle (?), Moravian
George de Benneville, 1740–93	Oley, Philadelphia	London (Huguenot diaspora), Siegen (?), Church of Brethren

Adam Simon Kuhn, 1740–80	Lancaster	Not known
Johann Mathäus Otto, 1752–86	Bethlehem	Previous practice, Meiningen, Physician/surgeon, Moravian
Christian Friedrich Martin, 1755?–82	West Indies, Providence, Macungie, Lehigh County, Revolutionary War surgeon	Berlin, Collegium medicum chirurgicum, Lutheran
John Ettwein, 1758–77	Bethlehem, North Carolina	Origin and training unknown, Moravian bishop
Christian Friedrich Kampmann, 1786–90 (1808?)	Bethlehem (previously Hope, N.J.)	Niesky and Barby schools, Moravian
Johann Eberhard Freytag, 1790–1839	Bethlehem	Physician and apothecary, Moravian (?)
Godfrey Henry Thumhardt, 1791	West Indies, Bethlehem, Lititz (1794)	Not known
Joseph Dixon, 1792 (?)	Bethlehem, Emmaus	Not known
John Frederick Rudolph, 1795	Bethlehem, Lititz, Reading	Not known

SOURCES: Berki, "Practitioner in Physic"; Meier, *Early Pennsylvania Medicine*; Gibson, *Bodo Otto*; Savacool, *Illness and Therapy*; KM vols. 1–3.

NOTES: This table does not attempt to provide a complete listing of all German practitioners in the middle colonies. It is a selective listing from sources indicating some formal training or, in the case of the Moravians, selection by an official body probably using some criteria of German qualification. Attribution of medical training in Halle for some of the Moravians suggests merely similar exposure to clinical practice, as that noted for H. M. Mühlenberg and other Halle clergy. Academic medical faculty excluded (e.g., the younger Adam Kuhn, J. Eberle).

A troupe of former imperial army surgeons and apothecaries, who for some reason did not go east, as did most German emigrants of the early modern period, including medical providers,[55] drifted across the Atlantic, often attracted by medical opportunities in the West Indies. Andreas Zwifler was a Hungarian apothecary who came with the Salzburgers to Georgia in 1733. Christian Friedrich Martin apparently trained at the army medical-surgical college in Berlin and on his return from the West Indies practiced in Pennsylvania. Then there were countless quacks, some of them known from their newspaper advertisements, who like their counterparts in Europe may or may not have been competent herbalists, repairers of hernias, or cutters of the stone. There also was the generally unsung body of midwives, often the wives or widows of clergy.

The Lure of the Halle Pharmaceutical Trade

Most if not all American physicians regardless of national background and training prepared and dispensed their own medications, because fee bills and custom usually provided fees for the medication and not the visit, unless surgery or delivery was involved.[56] Even in the 1760s, when a younger cohort of physicians returned from Europe and John Morgan attempted to decommercialize the medical profession, most of the reputable and even famous among the American *medici* ran their own pharmaceutical business, including Morgan himself, the elder Shippen, Thomas Say, Adam Simon Kuhn (the father of Adam Kuhn in Lancaster), and the compiler of the first American pharmacopoeia, William Brown.[57]

---

on Tables 4.1 and 4.2, most of the material on these men comes from a few local histories that have tried hard to fill the gaps in the vitae of their subjects. The major and most reliable source for our group is Glatfelter, but the purpose of his work was to document clergy, not medical practitioners. In this study, I have relied for verification on the diaries and above all the letters of Heinrich Melchior Mühlenberg, who was not only the Lutheran patriarch of Pennsylvania but may well be called its Boswell. As expected, he made no mention of any Moravian medical practitioners despite geographical proximity in a tightly knit learned community and despite the very detailed comment on Moravian incursions into Lutheran and Reformed congregations. The only other well-known practitioner honored by his silence is the Unitarian George de Benneville, whose medical background is accessible through his formulary at the College of Physicians in Philadelphia.

55. Fertig, "German Migration."

56. Cowen, *Medicine and Health in New Jersey*, 10–11; Waring, *Medicine in South Carolina*.

57. For Shippen and Morgan, see Bell, *John Morgan, Continental Doctor*. For the attempt to specialize in medicine only, see Gelfand, "Origin of a Modern Concept of Medical Specialization." For Brown's work at Moravian Lititz, see Kremers, in the *Badger Pharmacist*, 27–30. More recently on Brown, see Cowen, "The Letters of Dr. William Brown to Andrew Craigie."

It should not come as a surprise, therefore, that the leader of these clergy, Heinrich Melchior Mühlenberg, included two major Halle institutions, a printing press and a small pharmaceutical manufacture, in his repeated efforts to set up a permanent Lutheran and Pietist establishment in the middle colonies. In a long report to his superiors in London and Halle in June 1751, Mühlenberg took up his perennial concern for the well-being of Halle American clergy who were ill or no longer able to serve and thus without a stipend unless they had acquired property or married well. He proposed erecting on his own land in the Pennsylvania parish of New Providence (Trappe) a small replication of the Halle bookstore and pharmacy, to be run by his even more poorly paid schoolmasters "seeing that the blessed Halle medications were most effective in this country and could be obtained at reasonable prices. . . . But as soon as Saur learned that we had received medications from Halle, and that everyone praised their use and effect, he advertised in his journal that he himself could reproduce the genuine Halle articles, and in fact he did imitate them and sold them at a high price."[58]

Like Christopher Sauer, the founder of German printing houses in the colonies, who had also tried to obtain German printing fonts from Halle,[59] Mühlenberg was successful in neither attempt. Halle saw no reason to delegate the profit and financial leverage of these enterprises to the American periphery, even after it had relaxed its cautious response to Mühlenberg's first and early request for medications to be distributed and sold in German communities. Eventually, and after clearing this trade with Court Preacher Ziegenhagen in London,[60] the Orphanage followed its usual mission policy of channeling bequests and legacies, one of the major sources of charitable income, through its own pharmaceutical manufacture and sent its medicinals to selected clergy in the middle colonies, not only for the customary charity distribution but for resale.

As noted in Chapter 3, the linkage of straight charity and commercial activity for a charitable cause had proved successful in Germany and in the missions in the Baltics and Russia. Halle medications were much in demand in

58. KM 1:406–15; the quotation is from 412ff. Mühlenberg insisted on the close linkage between a print shop and the pharmaceutical trade, the former to permit him to print his own weekly and to advertise his products. This proposal was repeated many times over the next twenty years. See also KM 2: Letter 146, 16 March 1754.

59. Schrader, *Literaturproduktion und Büchermarkt des radikalen Pietismus*.

60. Letter from G. A. Francke to Mühlenberg, KM 1:114, 29 September 1743.

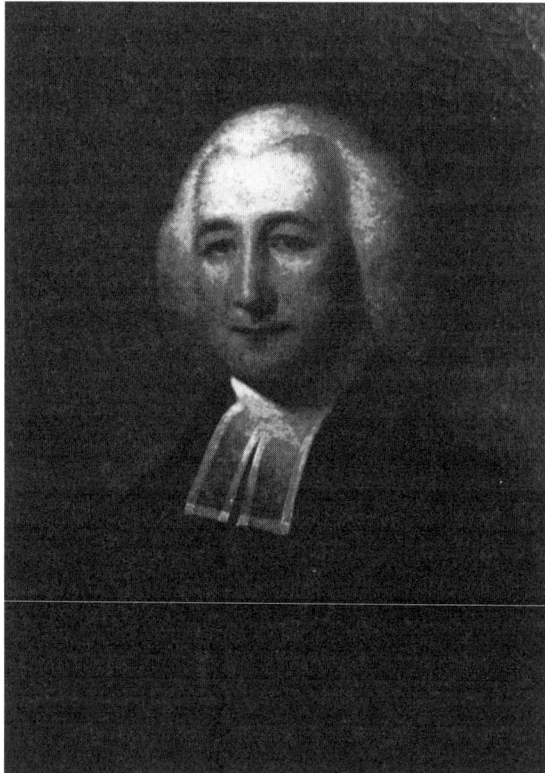

Fig. 4.2

Heinrich Melchior
Mühlenberg (b. 1711
Einbeck near Hanover,
Germany, d. 1787
Providence, Pennsylvania),
the first Lutheran minister
from the Halle Orphanage in
Pennsylvania. (Courtesy,
Pastor Frederick S. Weiser.)

Holland and England, where Friedrich Michael Ziegenhagen received regular shipments.[61] In North America as well, the merchant community in the Lutheran areas was eager to capitalize on a prestigious medical product. Heinrich Keppele, for instance, a well-known Philadelphia merchant with close trading and family connections to Holland and a close ally of Mühlenberg in his struggles for congregational control,[62] was willing and eager to provide financial backing for the import and manufacture of the Halle medications either through the Halle mission channels or his own connections in London and Rotterdam. On several occasions, he suggested appropriate candidates, including young Peter Mühlenberg on his return from Germany in 1768.[63]

61. The major primary sources for this and the following chapters are MAFSt, Series 4 C, D, and G, Series 5 E. Citations are documented separately and in context.
62. Best captured in Roeber, *Palatines, Liberty, and Property*.
63. KM 2:517, 607ff.

Almost fifteen years earlier, Heinrich Schleydorn, a sugar factor formerly from Saint Thomas and the New York congregation, had sent his son to Halle to study at the Orphanage, but then ran into difficulties in his trade in Philadelphia. He proposed that the son work in the Orphanage pharmacy, but Mühlenberg, in transmitting this request, insisted that young Schleydorn receive training that would make him useful in the English colonies.

> Method, theory, and practice [Mühlenberg wrote] are different among the English [that is, in the colonies] than among the Germans. Those who wish to practice as a doctor of medicine among the English must, first, be experienced in the English manner of surgery, second, must be sufficiently advanced in the apothecaries, art or in chemistry that he can prepare medicinals for internal and external injuries; and third be sufficiently knowledgeable in medicine and its constituent disciplines that he can practice on his own. In this manner, a real English doctor is at one and the same time a phlebotomist, surgeon, apothecary, chemist, and *medicum proprie sic dictum*. A young fellow who also has some Latin can learn the whole cursum in this country—*ex omnibus nempe aliquid*—in about three years, for a fee of about 100 pounds current. Then he can settle here and practice his art without any further examinations or license being necessary. Given that M. Schleydorn and we all seriously desire that this American plant might become a useful instrument of *the right kind of medicine* [emphasis added] for America, but as he lacks in the *sumtus ad aedificandam turrim*, we address to your Reverend Excellency the question if: (1) it is practicable for him to be placed under a reputable surgeon; (2) afterwards be trained for some time in the pharmacy of the blessed Halle Institutions; and (3) finally be admitted to the medical collegiis—both practical and theoretical.[64]

Mühlenberg, who had left Halle almost fifteen years earlier, probably still referred to a medical curriculum that did not yet feature surgery but was restricted to the classical course (physiology, materia medica, natural philosophy, dietetics, and anatomy),[65] but in most other respects, this was an astute judgment of necessary qualifications and reflects consideration of American needs beyond empirical training or apprenticeship.

64. H. M. Mühlenberg to G. A. Francke, KM 2:Letters 145, 153, 14 March and 26 July 1754.
65. Seils, *Friedrich Albrecht Carl Gren*; Bonner, *Becoming a Physician*.

European training for American-born protégés also seems to have been among the priorities of the London interest guiding Halle immigration to North America, although it is not clear whether there were diverging agendas in Halle and London. In the case of young Henry Schleydorn, this interest was pronounced (and therefore is documented) because his father was a longtime supporter of Halle clergy and one of his sisters had married the Reformed preacher Michael Schlatter, head of the Reformed Coetus since 1747 and one of the great clerical movers and proponents of union between Lutherans and the German Reformed in the middle colonies. Samuel Theodor Albinus in London, who by the 1750s supported the aging Court Preacher Ziegenhagen in running the Halle missions in India and North America, offered his own views on the appropriate practical medical training of the first German-American generation to return to Europe. Not unreasonably, he stressed the advantages of English apothecary practice, which included dispensing of medications and house calls, because London physicians made calls rarely and at high cost, while the dispensing chemists charged only for their medications, as in the colonies.[66] He or Ziegenhagen nonetheless wished to ensure that Schleydorn remained within the German sphere, suggesting that he be apprenticed, at the usual period of seven years and for roughly 200 pounds sterling, to a German apothecary in London who

> would teach him not only chemistry and the art of pharmacy but instruct him in surgery, both of which are required from an apothecary. . . . [H]e also will have the opportunity to learn from the many prescriptions sent in by English, German, Dutch, etc. *Doctoris,* [and] the different cures that are proposed by different doctors, who see their patients rarely. That is the business of the apothecary, who reports back to the medici on a daily basis, who then adjust their consilium and their prescriptions accordingly. . . . It is well known that several industrious apothecaries are considered more skillful and more desirable than the doctors, who ask for 2 guineas for every visit and 1 guinea for a prescription . . . and cannot be dissuaded from this practice.[67]

But G. A. Francke had made different plans more in keeping with the agenda of the Foundations. Replying directly to the elder Schleydorn and

66. For instance, Holmes, *Augustan England,* 206ff.
67. Secretary Albinus, Reply to Heinrich Melchior Mühlenberg, 20 October 1754, MAFSt 4 C 7, *Stück* 18, fols. 121–22.

offering his son in effect a scholarship in the Orphanage Foundations, he proposed to have training take place in the Orphanage pharmacy under the supervision of Inspector Schulenberg, who then headed Orphanage pharmaceutical manufacture and shipping. The latter also supervised and authorized most shipments to North America. Apprenticeship tenure was for six years, Francke noted, "which is a necessary period if the apprentice is to be well trained. The training here is considerably better than in other pharmacies. . . . And if your dear son should afterwards wish to study medicine proper, he will have excellent opportunity with our dear Professor Juncker, who may also be able to teach him the elements of surgery. He may well be needed in one of the wards of the Orphanage hospital and thus gain practical clinical experience for a future career in North America."[68]

Plans for training and dispatching medical personnel to the middle colonies continued. Reacting to a letter by Mühlenberg in March 1759, which set out plans to send his own three sons to Europe and discussing, as on a number of previous occasions, the medical situation in the colonies and the possible potential of the sale of the Orphanage medications, Inspector Schulenberg at Halle suggested the following:

1. Whether we should not offer Mr. Mühlenberg's sons to provide for their sustenance and schooling here at Halle if he can arrange for their travel.

2. His arguments concerning the need for a medicus [according to Halle principles] are not unjustified since young Schleydorn did not work out. We would not incur much in the way of cost unless we were to advance travel, which Mr. M. would have to undertake to repay. [insert on margin: If we could persuade someone from here to bear their own costs, it would be even better, although that person would then be less dependent on us.] Once there, he probably would not have to worry about his income, since conditions are not like in Ebenezer. And if he were to rely mainly on our medications, we might ensure considerable

68. MAFSt 4 C 8, *Stück* 14, Francke to Schleydorn, 16 September 1755. A similar request was made by another recently arrived and well-married cleric, Friedrich Handschuh, who in a letter of 28 May 1754 (ibid., 4 C 7, fols. 123–26) requested admission to Halle for the twelve-year-old son of his brother-in-law, Church Elder Hubele, at Lancaster, for want of appropriate educational opportunities. Hubele would prefer, Handschuh wrote, the study of theology, but if the boy lacked the requisite intellectual gifts, the father would be content if the boy acquired an education in pharmacy and be apprenticed in medicine.

sales which would more than cover interest on any advance we would have to make to provide initial stocks. If Dr. Schiffel were so inclined it would be a good proposal, since he is interested in chemistry and thus could help setting up a pharmaceutical institution (*Apothekenanstalt*). And if [young] Mühlenberg were to join him, he could find a living and be of use.[69]

In the event, the strict apothecary's or druggist's apprenticeship envisioned in Halle both for young Schleydorn and Peter Mühlenberg did not work out too well. It imposed on the American apprentices returned to Europe stifling and demeaning conditions of personal servitude delegated to lower social strata in their homeland. Schleydorn joined the Prussian army, and Peter absconded to return to North America.[70] But Peter and his father kept attempting to establish a commercial channel for the Halle pharmaceutical trade until the Revolutionary War and beyond. They eventually succeeded, but under very different conditions than originally envisioned at the motherhouse.

The Structure of the Colonial Medical Clergy

The medical markets of the late colonial period thus offered the Pietist clergy both opportunities and risk. The practice of medicine by academically trained and self-declared ministers of all Protestant denominations was generally accepted and not infrequent, although some congregations objected to their ministers' doubling of burdens.[71] Among Lutheran and Reformed pastors, the clergy known to have practiced medicine amounted to 8 percent of the total of 250 ministers listed by Glatfelter for the entire eighteenth century;[72] this is a conservative estimate because it relies on probate and inventory evidence at the end of life (medical, surgical, or pharmaceutical equipment as part of estates and

69. The letter to Halle is KM 2: Letter 186, 3 March 1759. The unsigned memorandum in response is apparently from Inspector Schulenberg to Francke, 19 November 1759, MAFSt 4 C 10, Stück 4, fols. 56–60.

70. Like H. M. Mühlenberg, Schleydorn and later his widow had much trouble discharging the not inconsiderable tuition and maintenance bills their son had run up at Halle (KM 2:419). School and board charges for Student Schleydorn were—for five quarters from Summer 1752 to Winter 1753—Rth 85 or 17 pounds sterling. To this was added a prior balance of Rth 320; MAFSt 4 G 2, fol. 149, 30 January 1754.

71. Duffy, *The Healers*, 34ff.; Bell, "A Portrait of the Colonial Physician," 13f.

72. Glatfelter, *Pastors and People*, 2:429–32. Glatfelter was apparently not aware of the scope of the Halle pharmaceutical trade.

a medical library or books). If the roughly twenty Halle clergy who had both some medical training at the Orphanage and access to and knowledge of Halle medications are included, this share goes up to 14 percent (see Tables 4.2 and 4.3). This proportion of German clergy among accepted medical providers before the Revolution was not much different from the one for the Anglican clergy in New Jersey in the 1760s.[73]

Several patterns were involved in this turn to medicine. A minority of both Reformed and Lutheran clergy were rejected as pastors by their congregations and fell back on the practice of medicine. This minority included some Halle disciples, such as Friedrich Schultz in New Jersey.[74] Some, such as Johann Martin Schaefer in Maine and Lucas Raus, who practiced in New Jersey and New York, combined what were probably poor or insufficient clerical livings with a very profitable medical practice. Raus definitely had some university education, but he was without medical training according to his own account of his education.[75] Two Pennsylvania Reformed ministers had formal medical training in addition to the ministry, Johann Bartholomeus Rieger even going back to enroll at Leiden in 1744 and returning in 1745 to North America, where he practiced until his death in 1769. William Stoy, who had degrees from Herborn University, is better and more widely remembered for his antirabies medicine and his treatment of Washington's servant than for his ministry.[76] There is no instance in Glatfelter's or other accounts of physicians turning into ministers, to the exclusion of their practice, but there may have been reluctant or failed physicians among the clerics coming over, such as Johann Friedrich Ries, who had apparently studied medicine in Jena before turning to theology in Halle.[77] And the final cohort of medical clerics coming over after 1765 included men choosing or wandering

73. Cowen, *Medicine and Health in New Jersey,* reports six clergy out of thirty-six members of the New Jersey Medical Society for the period 1766–76. This share had dropped to less than 10 percent by 1796.

74. MAFSt 4 C 9, Stück 13, Letter by Handschuh to Francke of 30 September 1757, fols. 113–23, mentions that Schultz had been given Halle medications. Schultz, although rejected in favor of the senior Mühlenberg by the fractious Raritan congregation, insisted that he remain as their physician.

75. Lucas Raus, who incurred the wrath of H. M. Mühlenberg for matters unconnected to medicine, had been born in Kronstadt and had studied in Pressburg, then a center of the Counter-Reformation. Glatfelter describes him as having studied in Jena, but in a long and rambling letter to G. A. F. Francke in MAFSt 4 C 3, Stück 34, of 12 March 1750, he stated that he had no medical training other than having lived in the house of a famous German physician in Hungary. He nonetheless was a successful practitioner and left a considerable estate.

76. Cowen, "Zum Dienst des Gemeinen Mannes."

77. KM 1:349, note 26.

Table 4.2 Lutheran and Reformed clergy (other than Halle Pietists from Central Europe) known to have practiced medicine and pharmacy in the middle colonies, 1700–1825 (in chronological order of approximate start of practice)

Names and Periods of Practice	Location of Practice	Training/Origin/Religious Affiliation
Lucas Raus, 1750–88	New Jersey congregations	Cronstadt (Hungary), University of Jena, no medical training, Lutheran.
Johann Bartholomäus Rieger, 1745–69	Lancaster and Pennsylvania congregations	Reformed, Leiden Univiversity. Returned to Europe in 1744, took medical degree from Leiden.
Heinrich Wilhelm Stoy, 1750–1801	Pennsylvania	Nassau Dillenberg, Reformed, Herborn University.
Casper Michael Stapel, 1760–66	New Jersey	Rostock-Mecklenburg Schwerin, Rostock University. Ph.D., Herborn University. Lutheran, converted to Reformed.
Johann Georg Schmidt, 1736–46	Philadelphia, New Hanover	"Empiric," irregular, Lutheran.
Gotthilf Traugott Illing, 1772–1800	Juniata Valley, Middletown, Lancaster County	Switzerland, Anglican, and sent by SPG, dropped affiliation and served Lutheran congregation.
Johann Conrad Andreae, 1748–54	Germantown	Zweibrücken, ordained clergy, Lutheran.
Frederick Miller, 1769–1827	Lebanon, and Windsor, Berks County	Place of birth and training unknown; Lutheran.

Johann Peter Ahl, 1772–1827	Baltimore, Virginia, North Carolina	Irregular minister, Lutheran, surgeon's mate and surgeon in Revolutionary Army.
Johann Martin Schaeffer, 1760–94	New Jersey, New York, Maine	Unknown education and origin, Lutheran.
Friedrich Valentin Melsheimer, 1779–1814	Pennsylvania	Helmstedt University; Lutheran; military chaplain of Brunswick dragoons in North America.
Carl Benjamin Danapfel, 1785–91	Bucks County, Northampton	Lutheran, irregular, Danzig (?), training unknown.
Anton Ulrich Luetge, 1785–96	New Jersey, Pennsylvania, d. Chambersburg	Origin and training unknown, Lutheran.
Johann Georg Jung, 1770–93	Maryland and Virginia	Lutheran, recommended by Pastor Anton Wachsel in London, origin and education unknown.

SOURCES: Glatfelter, *Pastors and People*, vol. 1; Berki, *Practitioner in Physic*; Meier, *Early Pennsylvania Medicine*; Gibson, *Bodo Otto*; Savacool, "Illness and Therapy"; KM vols. 1–3.

NOTES: Academic medical faculty excluded (e.g., Adam Kuhn, J. Eberle). Many of these men are not well known, although some left considerable estates, including Lucas Raus, C. B. Danapfel, and A. U. Luetge. Jung (Young) married into the Streit family. Best known is Heinrich Wilhelm Stoy, who invented and sold a famous rabies cure and is said to have saved the life of George Washington's servant.

Table 4.3   Halle Pietist or Lutheran Ministerium clergy distributing or ordering
Halle medicines in the middle colonies, 1742–1820

Heinrich Melchior Mühlenberg	1742–1780
Peter Brunnholz	1745–1757
Johann Nicholas Kurtz	1745–1790
Johann Helferich Schaum	1747–1775
Friedrich Handschuh	1748–1764
Johann Friedrich Ries	1749–1799
Johann Dietrich Mathias Heinzelmann	1751–1756
Johann Wilhelm Kurtz	1755–1799
Friedrich Schultz	1759–1780
Wilhelm Anton Graaf	1760–1805
Karl Wildbahn	1762–1802
Andreas Krug	1764–1796
Johann Ludwig Voigt	1764–1800
Christoph Emmanuel Schulze	1765–1805
Peter Gabriel Mühlenberg	1770–1776
Friedrich August Mühlenberg	1770–1776
Gotthilf Heinrich Ernst Mühlenberg	1770–1805
Johann Christoph Kunze	1770–1807
Johann Friedrich Schmidt	1770–1812
Justus Heinrich Christian Helmuth	1770–1820

NOTE: Dates are dates of arrival or documented start of medication sales and other practice to year
of death. All men on this list were clergy associated with Halle Orphanage through training,
position in Orphanage schools, direct dispatch, or patronage in North America. They were 8
percent of a total of 250 Lutheran and Reformed clergy, 1717–93 (according to Glatfelter, *Pastors
and People*), and one-third of the 55 clergy of both denominations who were ordained and called or
sent through London or Amsterdam. Listing does not consider continuous good standing with the
Pennsylvania Ministerium. For these core clergy, inclusion is based on direct evidence from the
Mühlenberg correspondence or on direct mention or orders in the Halle ledgers and archival correspondence. See Mission Archives 4 (Pennsylvania), Series C, D, G.

among the confessions, such as Gotthilf Traugott Illing, a Swiss who had been sent over by the Anglican Society for Promoting the Gospel in Foreign Parts but later served Lutheran congregations until 1800. As I show in Chapters 5 and 6, he became a regular if contentious purchaser of Halle medications.

As in rural areas of Europe, this clerical medical practice occupied a special niche, its practitioners being closer to their fully trained medical colleagues in classical background and social status than to their commercial counterparts in the surgical and druggist trades. They had access to a common reservoir of materia medica and shared comparable, occasionally overlapping medical traditions with their denominational allies in the medical profession. Even when fully trained American-born practitioners came back from Europe by the 1760s and attempted to set up an exclusive professional shop and a medical academe, practice continued among German clergy. It remained profitable in a few cases, as for Johann Peter Ahl, Benjamin Danapfel, and Anton Luetge, who according to Glatfelter left comfortable estates. It persisted among highly regarded men who were among the fathers of American botany, mathematics, and entomology, such as Heinrich Gotthilf Ernst Mühlenberg and Johann Christoph Kunze and the Streits and Melsheimers of the second generation of German immigrant clergy.

Medical historians have paid much attention to the Philadelphia academic physicians and their interminable quarrels in the last decades of the eighteenth century.[78] What is more amazing in our perspective, however, is that there is very little contemporary acknowledgment of the Germans among the medical clergy despite their presence in many fields and the esteem in which they were held as ministers and educators. It would be most satisfying, of course, to attribute this silence to the intent to medicalize the profession, or to Anglicize the clergy, or to use the German element for political reasons,[79] but there is no unambiguous evidence for any of these motives. It might well be, however, that by the end of the century, the Halle disciples in the medical field offended the academic establishment on two fronts. They continued to trade—and trade successfully— in what to many of their medical colleagues may have seemed an old-fashioned

---

78. This observation was made as early as 1969 by Bell, *Colonial Physician*, 6.

79. As was true for Benjamin Rush in his encomium on German virtues. See Butterfield, *A Letter by Dr. Benjamin Rush* (1787). One might add that the focus on medicine in Edinburgh and London and an antiloyalist tradition have led to the scholarly neglect of German physicians and teachers in Pennsylvania. Adam Kuhn and Casper Wistar still await a modern treatment. They are not central to this study, however, and are mentioned only in context.

or competing set of proprietary medication. And some of this clergy, if by no means all or even the majority, persisted in the use of German in both preaching and prescribing. This in fact may have been as serious an offense—and competitive advantage—as medical practice pure and simple. The strange persistence by immigrant clergy entirely capable of speaking English, such as the learned Johann Christoph Kunze and Justus Heinrich Helmuth, or by native speakers like Gotthilf Heinrich Ernst Mühlenberg, was indeed one factor that relegated Pietist medicine to the shadows of eighteenth-century Anglophone North American medicine.

But in many ways, this persistence was part and parcel of their calling. The elder Mühlenberg had never been shy about his medical practice and certainly considered the Halle medicine of his student days superior to most in effectiveness and medical ethics.[80] But he always insisted that clerical medical practice had to be secondary and not primary; the Halle clergy were with few exceptions fully committed to their German-speaking flocks, even if some had taken Anglican orders to be able to practice in Virginia, Maryland, and South Carolina. And their flocks were at one and the same time the now much enlarged German medical market, a good segment of which, notwithstanding adaptation to new and English-language legal and political norms, continued to use, among many other medical services, familiar medicines, familiar books, and familiar providers.

80. For example, in his letter to Francke and Ziegenhagen, of 3 March 1759, KM 2: Letter 186.

Building a

Transatlantic

Exchange

5

A network of transatlantic trading and exchange mechanisms was instrumental in creating a North American market niche for the Halle Orphanage medications. With some exceptions, pharmaceutical transatlantic sales during the eighteenth century are difficult to reconstruct because of the lack of much in the way of comparable documentation, particularly with regard to proprietary medicines. We do have some serial data over time for some traders and their business practices, mainly in London and its Quaker community, which supplied North American pharmacies as a profitable part of the dry goods trade, and some orders and invoices for the period after 1783, when American pharmacists had to restock.[1] There was no large-scale drug

1. For a detailed account of one exporter from England, see Steele, *Atlantic Merchant Apothecary,* for the beginning of the eighteenth century; for the famous Corbyn trade after mid-century, see Porter and Porter, "The Rise of the English Drugs Industry," and Palmer, "Thomas Corbyn, Quaker Merchant." Kremers has reproduced and commented on two orders from Philadelphia in 1785 ("Two Invoices of 1785") to the pharmacies of the brothers Marshall and the house of Moses Bartram. Interestingly, neither of the two substantial orders contains proprietary medicines. Cowen's work is the most comprehensive account of the development of North American colonial pharmacy, but in the main lacks financial data. However, see his recent "The Letters of Dr. William Brown." A very full account of the history of the pharmaceutical trade into the Dutch West Indies, an important market poorly

manufacture on the American side of the Atlantic before the 1820s. Compounding of imported simples and other materia medica by individual pharmacists remained the rule and was often practiced by physicians. Indian remedies were widely praised but not actually part of the standard armamentarium.[2] South American botanicals, such as Jesuit's bark or cinchona, were either smuggled into the colonies or had to be reimported through England. On the other hand, the range of items available in simple and compounded form was probably as large as in Europe, although supplies may have been spottier. Available English shipping and order sheets are lengthy and similar to European inventories, and we have a few local dispensatories and formularies from German practitioners in the middle colonies that are not notable for their parsimony.[3] For a fuller picture, we still lack an overview of price structures and profit margins, of their trends over time, and of the extent to which proprietary medications came from sources outside England over the course of the eighteenth century.

The Francke Foundations being a philanthropic organization heavily dependent on commercial income, their financial transactions with their missionaries and other dependencies abroad are minutely recorded. They therefore offer a rare opportunity to examine almost a century's worth of information on the structure and pathways of a small and circumscribed part of the colonial drug traffic, largely in proprietary medicines. On the German side, we have considerable and redundant detail about how Halle determined financial access by extending or denying credit to persons or groups; how specific accounts were kept and, when needed, creatively manipulated to keep the books in reasonable balance; how specific legacy incomes were applied effectively and without violating the donor's intent; and, at least until the 1780s, how the Pietist dependencies in Georgia and Pennsylvania compared with each other and with their more prestigious and politically important colleagues in East India. On the American side, we can document the type and business practices of specific clergy and their interaction with American merchants and congregations and with the larger world outside the German communities. Because there is a fair

---

developed in the English literature on the subject (Rutten, "Slavenhandel, ziekten en mortaliteit") is based on the archives of the Dutch West India Company, which was probably a monopoly carrier. I thank Dr. Steven Behrends for bringing Dr. Rutten's work to my attention and Dr. Rutten for generously sharing this and other work with me.

2. Cowen, "Impact of the Materia Medica of the North American Indians."

3. Savacool, "Illness and Therapy"; Berky, *Practitioner in Physick*; Estes, "Patterns of Drug Usage in Colonial America," idem, "Therapeutic Practice in New England"; Cowen, "The Letters of Dr. William Brown."

amount of detailed information on individual orders, we can also assess preferences for specific medications within and outside the Halle armamentarium by providers and consumers, both male and female, lay and learned.

A chronological account of this modest but durable traffic is important beyond its contribution to a comparative framework of the economics of the North American drug trade. It yields in addition a larger perspective and permits us to place the Halle clergy in North America and their trade in medicines into a wider and transatlantic context. The rise and fall of this trade was not in lockstep but reflected very different economic and political developments on both sides of the Atlantic. A period of American prosperity and a search for wider markets beginning at the end of the 1760s were reflected in increased orders. But this period ran parallel to serious financial difficulties at the Foundations after the death of the younger Francke, Gotthilf August, in 1769. These difficulties were in large part caused by a devastating property levy exacted by the Prussian state, itself in serious financial difficulties at the end of the Seven Years' War in 1763. Although the net profits from the pharmaceutical trade continued to flow into the coffers of the Foundations, they no longer matched expenses, and the new directors apparently were forced to mingle sources of income from legacies to keep afloat. In turn, Halle was barred by the American Revolution from using a number of new and considerable bequests on behalf of the American colonies to produce much-needed income.[4]

Pharmaceutical and book imports from Halle resumed after 1783 and at a fast pace, again under very different personal and financial constellations in America and Europe and beset by trade and currency difficulties.[5] Evidence also

4. One concern was the rate of interest for investment purposes stipulated in many of the Halle bequests. For example (MAFSt 4 D 2 fol. 1, letter of 12 November 1790), Inspector Stoppelberg complained of difficulties in placing the Streit capital at reasonable interest. Other concerns, as noted by Roeber in *Palatines, Liberty, and Property*, related to the difficulty of obtaining corporate charters and matching the conditions of German bequests and legacies to the legal practices governing the American markets; see the correspondence on the Solms-Rödelsheim legacy before the revolution (KM 4). For trade during the Revolution, there is reference to correspondence through Nantes, probably through Halle's Dutch and French connections and those of the Keppele family. For the continuing Amsterdam connection through the Dutch branch of this family, see memorandum by S. A. Fabricius, MAFSt 4 C 20, fols. 116–18, 2 November 1784, from Halle, both with regard to medicines and advertising of learned books in North America, in competition with the Frankfurt book trade. But by this time, and as noted by Fabricius, monetary exchanges through the enclave of Altona near Hamburg were as advantageous as through Holland (Letter to J. H. Helmuth, 24 December 1784, MAFSt 4 C 20, Stück 46/47, fols. 119–22).

5. For this period, demand for goods from Halle as a direct or intermediate supplier fits closely into the general pattern described by Doerflinger, *Vigorous Spirit of Enterprise*, III. McCusker, *Money*

suggests that the Foundations now looked to America for favorable opportunities to place their returns on capital as conditions in Europe continued to deteriorate.[6] Neither the French Revolution and the Austrian-French wars of the 1790s, nor the occupation of large parts of the German Empire by Napoleon's troops and the subsequent continental blockade by England, entirely interrupted their trade with North America until 1815; these events were devastating, however, to the independence of the Halle Foundations and to their trade in Europe. Both the marketing concerns at Halle and the persistence of a German-speaking public are therefore reflected in this North American trade under very new auspices.

Creating a Market Niche, 1745–1776

In the 1730s, when the ministers from the Halle Orphanage began to come to North America to assume the stewardship of Lutheran congregations, they had a twofold mission: to ensure that as many Lutheran Germans as possible would come under and remain under the guidance of Pietist moral and social tenets, church discipline, and evangelical forms of worship, and to extend across the North Atlantic the network of Halle philanthropy. In both objectives, they had until the War of Independence the support of the Bishop of London through the Society for Promoting Christian Knowledge and the Lutheran establishment in London. By the end of the war, at least in the former middle colonies, their hold over their congregations was no longer dependent on European patronage. By virtue of their community service, a strong and continuous pastoral leadership and church organization, and a growing network of marital and personal relationships, they had become a social and political force to be reckoned with.

Well implanted in most men trained in or sent out by the Halle institutions was a strong spirit of enterprise, tempered by an extraordinary and often tormented willingness to listen closely to an inner voice that could serve as reassurance of the divine will.[7] This spirit, which characterizes many evangelicals

---

and Exchange in Europe and America, 370, and Rappaport, *Stability and Change,* describe the colonial and postcolonial centers and channels of financial exchange.

    6. Roeber, "J. H. C. Helmuth"; Wilson, "Development of Eighteenth-Century Voluntary Institutions."

    7. Intense self-inspection is a generic and well-known trademark of the evangelical movements of the eighteenth century, but it has rarely been discussed as a generic trait also in relation to commercial ventures, although it was obvious in the case of George Whitefield (*Pedlar in Divinity*). For a Halle example in North America, Johann Martin Boltzius, see his *Detailed Reports,* ed. Jones et al., and Wilson, "Public Works and Piety."

of the time, was one of the legendary sources of the Foundations' success under August Herman Francke, starting in 1696, and it carried over into the trade in edification literature, Bibles, and pharmaceuticals in the early 1700s. Joined to the practice of Pietist medicine inculcated into most of the Halle clergy sent abroad, these ministers were fully aware that in their clerical and medical practice, they would use the Halle Orphanage medications to attract patients, to increase their stipends, and to assure the motherhouse of a reliable return on its American investment.

As with many colonial plans, things were not to run as smoothly as both the motherhouse and the clergy in the diaspora would have liked. The attempt to introduce not just Halle medicines but Halle medical practice while profiting from the reputation of the Halle motherhouse had existed from the arrival of the first Georgia ministers in 1733. The Georgia model envisioned the provision of medical care in a closed community where secular and church governance was in the hands of Pietist clergy paid from Europe. This model succeeded only in part. The story of the senior physician in Ebenezer, Georgia, Georg Ernst Thilo, is an instructive exercise in physician independence gained on the basis of both medical conviction and financial considerations, although Halle never fully stopped supplying its recalcitrant emissary.[8]

In Pennsylvania, Halle interests had to rely on the personal initiative and needs of the clergy, whose ministerial stipends were in turn dependent on the financial ability of their parishes and their willingness to support their ministers. In both cases, however, the original Halle emphasis remained. Charity care was joined to evangelical reform and church discipline, and the reputation of the Orphanage books and medications was carried over to a paying public attracted by the juncture of godly medicine and German tradition. The middle path chosen by Pietism as an evangelical movement, which by the 1740s had firmly rejected chiliasm, millenarianism, and other schismatic beliefs, ensured a favorable reception among the more traditional social strata. It also ensured to the leaders and the enterprising of the Halle clergy access to German-American merchant interests.

This access was buttressed by shrewd choices in marriage partners both on the part of the marrying clergy and of the families of the brides. These marriages were part of the personal and familial web that enabled German ministers not

---

8. Wilson, "Die Halleschen Waisenhausmedikamente"; Wilson and Poeckern, "A Continental System of Medical Care."

only to survive but to gain social ascendancy within and to some degree outside their congregations. They included not only Heinrich Melchior Mühlenberg's own marriage to Anna Maria Weiser, daughter of the famous Konrad Weiser, a "friend of colonist and Mohawk"[9] and a major force in the Philadelphia political community. Johann Dietrich Heinzelmann, one of Mühlenberg's vicars, married into the Weiser family three years after his arrival in 1751; he died in 1756. Johann Helferich Schaum, who had come in 1747, married into the well-off Pickele family of Raritan, but his wife soon died. Justus Heinrich Christian Helmuth, a man of driving ambition and much talent who would succeed Mühlenberg as head of the Lutheran Ministerium in the 1780s, married one of the Keppele daughters fourteen months after arriving in Pennsylvania in 1769. This marriage in particular ensured that the second generation of Halle clergy had a continued link to the tight web of Pennsylvania German and Dutch trading interests. Christian Emmanuel Schulze, who arrived in 1765, and the learned Johann Christoph Kunze, who arrived in the company of Helmuth and the two younger Mühlenbergs, both married Mühlenberg daughters, although the father of the bride modestly disclaimed any rank and status for the new Mrs. Kunze.[10] Even Friedrich August and Peter Mühlenberg, for all their Anglican and later patriot connections, married into German Lutheran families. On both sides, at least in the American setting, these marriages were entirely appropriate. They strengthened bonds among language and confessional groups whose members tended to both intermarry and deal largely with their own kind,[11] and they produced a network that supported the sales of Halle medicines and helped to create and maintain their market niche.

As noted in Chapter 4, Heinrich Melchior Mühlenberg had almost from the outset suggested opening a small pharmacy and bookstore on the model of

9. To quote the astute epitaph of one of Weiser's biographers, Paul A. Wallace.
10. Letter 561, to J. W. Pasche, 5 July 1771, KM 4:338. For a full account of this network, see *The Weiser Families in North America*, ed. Weiser et al.
11. The Pietist ministers' correspondence with Europe leans heavily toward complaints about clergy marrying or consorting below their status. There is less open emphasis on the more successful matches. The marriage of Johann Friedrich Handschuh to a servant, Susanna Barbara Belzner, is typical of the disapproval, by colleagues and above all by congregations, of marriages beneath the clergy's station. The widowed Mrs. Handschuh, however, turned out to be fully capable of pursuing her own interests after her husband's death in 1763. Clergy could aspire, even in Europe, to the status of gentlemen, and the Pietist clergy were no exception. August Hermann Francke, for instance, was married to a noblewoman in his first not altogether blessed marriage (his first wife was a von Wurm; see Zaepernick, "Johann Georg Gichtels und seiner Nachfolger Briefwechsel"), and the second wife of his son Gotthilf August was Eva Wilhelmine, née von Gersdorf.

the Halle institutions to support needy co-pastors and their dependents. His argument was a relatively favorable price structure compared with other imported and local proprietary medications and competition from at least one denominational adversary, Christopher Sauer, whom he accused of having sold cheap imitations of the Halle products once he knew of Mühlenberg's own dispensing. We know too little about actual profit margins and import costs in the colonial market in pharmaceuticals to confirm or negate this claim, which may well have been self-serving, but there is no question that in relative terms, the Halle products, like other proprietary medications imported from Europe, were expensive. Some advantages of purchasing through the Foundations were discounts of 10 to 15 percent (20 percent in rare instances)[12] and shipment through protected channels in London, rather than through travelers and immigrants carrying items aboard ship as personal baggage.[13] These advantages, however, must be set off against restrictive conditions of credit at Halle, at least as far as the trade through the Orphanage Foundations before the postrevolutionary period is concerned.[14] Credit was advanced for orders that were to be set off against future charity collections on behalf of the Pennsylvania congregations, not only in Germany but also in the middle colonies.[15]

By the 1750s, H. M. Mühlenberg was no longer the sole dispenser of Halle medications and medical advice. Although his proposal to set up a pharmaceutical dispensary was barred for lack of a suitable candidate with sufficient capital to establish an account at the *Medikamentenexpedition* in Halle, he shared the continuing shipments from home with his junior colleagues. To them he delegated much responsibility, and they in turn tended to be overly optimistic, accumulating considerable trading debts at the motherhouse. Over time, not all these debts could be fully repaid. There was a considerable negative balance against Pastor Brunnholz at the time of his death in 1757, and advances against future income usually exceeded reimbursements. Because the moneys for the medications had

12. MAFSt 4 G 3, 1774, fols. 82–84: "Für die Frau Pastor Mühlenbergin in Philadelphia werden gesendet aus der Waisenhausapotheke zu Halle den 5. Martius 1774."

13. See Beiler, "From the Rhine to the Delaware Valley."

14. Comparative study is needed to show whether Halle freight and insurance for shipment through Hamburg and London were higher than for the trade through Amsterdam.

15. MAFSt 4 G 6, fols. 58–59, final note to an unsigned and undated *pro memoria*, probably from the years 1751–55: "Nota: The [Pennsylvania] collection accounts here owe 1. To the bookstore Rth 110/2/3; to the pharmacy shipping account, 127/8/7 . . . Which must be paid off slowly from donations received. Where the Lord does not see fit to direct such donations to Germany we shall take the moneys from the Pennsylvania collection account, from which in that case the balance must be made over by draft. This has been agreed from the outset."

to be paid to Counselor Madai as head of the *Medikamentenexpedition*, losses from unpaid debits on the mission accounts would in principle have to be made up by the Foundations unless other means became available. Negative balances by Brunnholz's successor in the trade, Friedrich Handschuh, for instance, were set off against a German inheritance benefiting his American widow.

Owing to the Foundations' double status as a domestic philanthropy and a supplier of clergy and printed material to foreign missions and transatlantic German congregations, the arrangements for accounting, disbursing, and rolling over debt and credit demanded a considerable degree of sophistication and knowledge of the multiple eighteenth-century financial markets and the range of currency transactions. In their domestic accounts, it had taken the Foundations almost three decades to introduce a coherent system of accounting, and the reforms instituted by Counselor Cellarius, a well-known cameralist, had to wait until the interregnum between the death of the older Francke in 1727, and of his close collaborators Elers and Neubauer soon after, and the assumption of full control by his son Gotthilf August Francke in the mid-1730s.[16] East Indian and North American mission accounts were complicated by the involvement of Denmark and England, the exigencies of confessional politics, and the need to involve numerous agents and points of transaction.

The Mechanisms of Trade in Philanthropy

As shown in Chapter 3, business reform and expansion had come at the same time for the pharmaceutical trade at Halle. By the late 1730s, the pharmaceutical mail order business, while retaining the prestigious label of the Orphanage medications, had been separated from the Foundations proper under an agreement providing for the transfer of net profits from any sales plus a generous stipend of free medications dispensed in the Orphanage dispensary and hospital. However, legal separation of the strictly commercial components of the Halle enterprise from the Foundations proper did not rein in the spirit and practice of profitable commingling of moneys and effort that had been the wellspring of Halle's appeal and success from the beginning.

The eventual divisions of labor and commerce at the Foundations, coupled with some opaqueness in eighteenth-century bookkeeping and reasoning, have

16. Welsch, "Die Franckeschen Stiftungen als wirtschaftliches Grossunternehmen." I base these statements on recent work with the ledgers of the *Hauptkassen* of the Orphanage in VAFSt, Repertorium i and ii, from 1710 to 1800.

contributed to the difficulty of disentangling the financial transactions between Halle and North America over the course of the century. It is therefore worth quoting the following exchange, in which the long-term inspector of the Orphanage accounts, Sebastian Andreas Fabricius, submitted to the Orphanage director, G. A. Francke, a long set of "deliberanda wegen Pennsylvanien." In these deliberations, he commented on a letter by Heinrich Melchior Mühlenberg of 27 February 1759 to his patrons, Francke and Court Preacher Ziegenhagen in London, and suggested the following procedures, which as usual imposed a heavy bookkeeping and copying burden on the American emissaries:[17]

> Would it not be best to instruct him [Mühlenberg] as follows in this regard: [1] Please keep two item accounts for books and medications. (a) To the extent to which you keep accounts with the Orphanage, your are to consider as *your own debt* the amount of the books and medicines sent according to the specifications enclosed in each packet. From these we will discharge to the credit of the bookstore and the medication business as much as God shall move our benefactors to contribute. On the other hand, *that which was given as a gift in the form of medications, books, and bibles will be at the disposition of the ministers* [in Pennsylvania] so that they may dispose of those articles they do not need for their own houses, either as charity among the poor or, if that should not be useful in the circumstances, sell it, with the proceeds to go to the church box to be used for the glory of the Lord and the best of the congregations. (b) Those monies paid from our own collections [in Germany] in discharge of the above debts you should consider as payment in lieu of cash, and *these amounts will constitute the American collection box.*
>
> Your Excellency [G. A. Francke] will be in charge of these monies and decide what should go to this or that American congregation or church and for this or that of our emissaries to America if these are in need or for the benefit of our entire Pennsylvania congregations. But in view of the distances involved, these *decisions are to be left to the discretion, after due consultation with each other, of the two senior ministers in such a manner that they could use specific sums where there is evident need or a good purpose, always pending your*

---

17. These burdens, although entirely customary in the commercial practice of the period, are evident throughout the correspondence with the Halle colonial stations and indicate considerable disregard of the realities of labor available to their clergy. See the Mühlenberg journals and correspondence and the journals from Ebenezer (Jones et al., eds., *Detailed Reports*).

final approval. If, however, the incoming collections should not suffice to discharge [American] debts with the Orphanage [note on margin: in particular if there are large orders for bibles and medications] outstanding payments should be made on your directions from the book account [*aus der Büchercassa anhero zu remedieren*], before further monies are credited to the collections account. Against this, we must take into account freight and transport charges and any costs incurred in North America, plus some measure of profit. The latter are to recover any losses arising from their transactions, unsold books, for instance, or a bad loan. Also, Mr. Handschuh might in this way to be able to recover some additional monies in excess of the current 63 £ Penn. cour. for his trouble, in particular if he is in straightened circumstances.[18]

This multilevel arrangement seems to have been the matrix for financial exchanges and trade with North America at least during the period up to 1785. All four Halle clergy who arrived after the senior Mühlenberg but before 1755 (Brunnholz, Schaum, Heinzelmann, Handschuh; see Table 4.3) brought books and medications they had received as gifts; in addition, they soon placed substantial orders with the Halle motherhouse on their own account.[19] Peter Brunnholz quickly assumed control of most of this trade. Beginning in 1748, most orders were made by him, on his own behalf and that of Mühlenberg and a circle of lay and clerical associates. These soon included Michael Schlatter, a major figure among German and Swiss Reformed ministers and a close ally of Mühlenberg in the consolidation of the German congregations. Although Brunnholz's and Heinzelmann's careers were foreshortened by early deaths (in 1757 and 1756, respectively), Handschuh continued to trade until his own death in 1764, and his wife continued the trade as a widow. Johann Vigera, who had accompanied the third Salzburger transport to Georgia as commissioner and then drifted north to join Mühlenberg, also attempted to enter the trade, and we have a number of orders placed by merchants in Philadelphia and Lancaster and by associated clergy.

18. MAFSt 4 C 10, Stück 4, 3 March 1759, fols. 56–60. Emphasis added. Slashes denote marginal insertions and deletions in the original. The referenced letter from Mühlenberg is KM 2: Letter 184. The two senior ministers are Mühlenberg and his senior in American tenure, Johann Martin Boltzius in Georgia.

19. Throughout, the pharmaceutical trade of the Halle clergy in the middle colonies constituted about one-third to one-half of the value of their book trade with the motherhouse. However, in areas of distance from pharmaceutical markets, such as Georgia, materia medica was imported at levels well in excess of the book trade. See Wilson, "Die Halleschen Waisenhausmedikamente," and MAFSt 5 E.

Commercial orders through the Dutch ports were facilitated by the wider network that since the late 1740s had begun to supplement the transatlantic charity shipments through Friedrich Michael Ziegenhagen in London.[20] Pastor Brunnholz's instructions in an early letter of 20 November 1748[21] were for shipment of his order either through the London correspondents of Mr. Koch, a Pennsylvania merchant, or through the merchants in Amsterdam who handled the Madai business, and who should send them "with next year's ships carrying German immigrants to Philadelphia. This would almost be more convenient." Concerning payment, he added that "since I do not believe that there will be any surplus in the local [North American] collections, costs and shipping fees to Amsterdam should be debited to my account until there is occasion to remit a draft to Halle." In case of loss, however, each person placing an order was to be responsible for his or her share.[22] In this case, the shipments arrived, and payments were made within the year. In 1768, the senior Mühlenberg reported on correspondence and bills of lading from David Samuel von Madai, forwarded through his contacts in London and advising him of a shipment worth 405 Reichsthaler (Rth), which J. H. Keppele was to pay through his own London contacts, the famous house of Mildred and Roberts.[23]

Until the 1760s, documented orders were fairly evenly divided between medicine chests and separate lists of the preferred Halle medications. Selectivity in filling these orders is apparent mainly with regard to their fit into the distribution of tasks and sales privileges set up in Halle. A 1752 order with prices recorded in the dispatch ledger includes medications on the charity for all Halle ministers, items for sale on account, and a considerable number of the Richter and Madai treatises. By contrast, a Rth 200 medication order placed by the former Salzburg commissioner Vigera on top of a large book order was refused.

20. See MAFSt 4 G 6, fol. 27; 4 G 2, fol. 234: "I hereby certify that The Reverend Francke has paid to me by order and for account of M. George Moses Weinberger in Amsterdam 50 Dutch fl courant. . . . Halle, 7 January 1764, Dav. Sa. Madai."

21. MAFSt 4 G 2, fols. 51 ff. "Rth 64 from Pastor Brunnholz for medication which he ordered for himself and other friends under 10 November 1748, according to receipt sub a."

22. MAFSt 4 G 6, fol. 79, following an order of 28 August 1753 by the newly arrived Mathias Heinzelmann and a Captain Budden. A letter to Paul List (4 G 6, fol. 91, 27 April 1754), an agent in Amsterdam who handled pharmacy shipments for Madai to the East Indies and Philadelphia, indicates that three boxes were in fact lost at sea.

23. We do not know who sold these medications, but they probably went through the Keppele establishment. KM 2: Letter 430, to Francke and Ziegenhagen, of 8 June 1768, 607. See also Letters 398, 408, 423 n. 7, 424 passim. Ziegenhagen himself seems to have distributed or sold Halle medications in London; several of his orders appear in the mission accounts for India and Georgia.

That this was not a question of insufficient funds overall but of allocation of credit is suggested by the fact that the total of this order, which was sent in three carefully wrapped boxes to Brunnholz in Philadelphia, ran to Rth 319 for medications and Rth 450 in books and Bibles.[24] Similar orders were sent annually throughout the 1750s, with Brunnholz ordering on average Rth 300 worth of medications per year. His death in 1757 deprived the Pennsylvania team of an enterprising mind and, as noted, eventually caused fairly large and uncollectible debt overhangs, which dogged the Pennsylvania accounts even after Friedrich Handschuh took over the Halle accounting from Pennsylvania.[25] But although personal trading accounts may have been short, the early 1750s still witnessed a constant flow of donations specifically for Pennsylvania.

These donations still came from all over Europe and reflected the network of donors—and often simultaneous clients of the Halle pharmaceutical and book business—who had supported the Francke Foundations over the first half of the century. To give some examples: In 1754, at the height of Halle prosperity and pharmaceutical sales, a Finnish donor, Mr. Siliard, sent a draft for the equivalent of Rth 177; the court chaplain in Copenhagen contributed Rth 5 for Pennsylvania as part of a larger regular donation for India; an unnamed lady donor offered Rth 66; a Pastor Hoppe in Louvain forwarded on behalf of an M. Caspary in Besançon Rth 66 for the use of the "Pennsylvania Foundations." A sum of Rth 40 came through Inspector Wedel at the Salzwedel orphanage as a gift from a retired general; the poor box at the orphanage yielded Rth 25 from an unknown donor for the salary fund of the ministers in Pennsylvania.[26] Court Preacher Ziegenhagen in London decided to divert to the benefit of the Pennsylvania ministers £ 10 sterling, to be drawn from the funds yielded by pharmaceutical sales in Pennsylvania; this was credited as Rth 57 to the Pennsylvania debt in Halle. By the end of 1755, European collections

24. Some of these were never sold. See MAFSt 4 G 6, Lit A, fols. 47–50.
25. MAFSt 4 G 6, 1756, fols. 113–14: "Für Pennsylvanien Mens Jun 1756," with attachments. After the death of Handschuh in 1765 (see ibid., fols. 163–66), Mühlenberg was forced to handle the remaining debts until the end of the Revolutionary War. Reflecting his growing impatience with Halle's mercantile prudence and parsimony in the handling of these transactions, he did not hesitate to declare these amounts lost: "That hated word, bad debt," and suggested that the local charity fund be used to pay off Handschuh's remaining debt of Pa. £ 63. Handschuh and others sent into the Pennsylvania field were in fact closely tied to the Foundations by family and friends. His brother apparently worked as an accountant at the Foundations (MAFSt F 6 and 9, Streit legacy papers).
26. The assumption by Pennsylvania Lutheran ministers outside the Halle circle that there was a salary fund for the Halle ministers seems to have been shared by European donors (see Glatfelter, *Pastors and People*, 2:239ff.).

from that year and 1754 had yielded a total of Rth 401, almost enough to cover debits of Rth 491.[27]

The use of many of these donations for the construction of Lutheran houses of worship is well known from the Mühlenberg journals and letters.[28] The largest donation in the period 1748–55 came from the so-called Darmstädter Collecte, recorded in the amount of 579 florins (fl). But an equal sum went for credit, subsequently reimbursed, to fill a Brunnholz order for books and medications, sent through Hamburg in 1749. During the Seven Years' War of 1757–63, which pitted Prussia against Austria in Europe and England against France in North America, most shipments from Halle ceased, and the Pennsylvania accounts were left to regenerate themselves.[29] After the end of the war in 1763, they had been restored by a number of large interest-yielding bequests. Among these was a long-expected donation from Venice, the so-called Streit legacy, whose surviving annuitant had finally died; sums paid through Frankfurt on behalf of anonymous persons of rank; and a quite substantial legacy, the so-called Solms-Rödelsheim bequest of 1770, made largely to relieve Heinrich Melchior Mühlenberg of personal liability for the costs of church construction.[30] The income from these sources permitted a rapid expansion of credit to the Pennsylvania accounts, shown, for instance, in several large orders by Mrs. Mühlenberg.

Current account balances were rapidly eaten into by this book and pharmacy trade, for which long-term credit was extended,[31] with most of the proceeds of American sales going into congregational work and education. In 1763

27. MAFSt 4 G 2 fol. 151, annual account for 1754, dated 24 January 1755. Amounts and currencies are as stated in the original.

28. For church construction during this period, see Müller, *Obrigkeitsproblematik*; Roeber, *Palatines, Liberty, and Property*; KM 1.

29. MAFSt 4 G 2, 15 March 1759, fol. 818: "Final account (*Schlussrechnung*): All income for the last four years: Rth 809/16/9; expenses (as above), Rth 735/11/8; current account balance, Rth 74/5/1."

30. The full story of these and other North American bequests remains to be told. In 1762 (MAFSt G 2 fol. 219), a typical and large anonymous bequest of 500 fl, converted to Rth 327/4, was recorded on behalf of "a person of rank." The legacy by Count Solms-Rödelsheim (15,000 florin or £ sterling 1250: MAFSt 4 F 4 and elsewhere) was intended to free Mühlenberg and his associates from the personal liability for church construction in Philadelphia. Its income supported much of the trade and educational undertakings of the Halle clergy at the end of the century. See Roeber, "J. H. C. Helmuth." For the Streit legacy, which ran eventually to £ 3000 sterling, see KM, vols. 2 and 3, passim, and FAFSt 4 F 6. In 4 D 2, fol. 1, a letter by Inspector Stoppelberg of 12 November 1790, complains of difficulties in placing this capital at reasonable interest.

31. A Rth 205 bill for pharmaceuticals purchased by Brunnholz in 1756 was paid off to Madai in 1763 (MAFSt 4 G 2, fols. 230–31); a 1767 bill of Rth 320 was paid in 1769 (MAFSt 4 G3, fol. 9).

and on subsequent occasions, major sums went into fitting out and providing travel costs for the second generation of Halle preachers. Johann Ludwig Voigt and Andreas Krug arrived in 1764, and a year later came Christoph Emmanuel Schulze, who married into the Mühlenberg family and went on to become a major member of Halle's inner circle in North America. Although the Pennsylvania clergy were rarely paid more than £50 sterling per annum by their congregations, a sum similar to that of their SPCK-supported colleagues in Georgia, their outfits, furnishings, and travel costs were in the range of Rth 600 per person. They usually received a good amount of expense money for use in England until they boarded ship, the balance of which they were bound to return to their London patron and taskmaster, Court Preacher Ziegenhagen. The substantial outfits in clothing and travel money suggest the need perceived by the Pietist German fathers in Halle to impress Anglican supporters in London, but were clearly at considerable variance from the professions of humble status that pervade letters to Europe.[32] Clerical libraries and other equipment and a beginning stock of medications, books, and various editions of North American and East Indian mission news traveled along as well.[33]

Given the growth in Halle clergy and their increasing importance among the Lutheran and other German congregations in the middle colonies, the pace of orders from North America tended to be on the increase in the decade before the Revolution. This trend may have been encouraged by shipping opportunities and demand resulting from North American attempts to circumvent trade with the British metropolis.[34]

32. Of total Pennsylvania mission expenditures for 1763 (Rth 1,137/14/6 or well over £ sterling 200), two-thirds went for the travel and outfitting of two new American recruits, Pastors Krug and Voigt. Outfits consisted of gowns and underwear, fur boots, two hats per person at Rth 2/18 each, a fur cap at Rth 1/12, and fur gloves at Rth 1/12 a pair. The charge in London for room and board was Rth 4/10 or just under £ sterling 1, plus 2 shillings each for service and hot water for tea (4 G 2, fols. 2, 228, 237ff.). See fol. 297 for Pastor Schulze.

33. The role of this print network in securing funds has been noted by Ward (*Protestant Evangelical Awakening*) and Roeber ("J. C. H. Helmuth") and cannot be overestimated. Donors were inspired to make multiple bequests to H. M. Mühlenberg and his own congregation through this network; see MAFSt 4 G 3, fols. 13–14, for specially designated bequests for 1769–71, for example, a fund transmitted through Pastor Darnemann at Brandenburg, for a total of Rth 258/18. For this reason, and also for efficiency of bookkeeping, the Pennsylvania pastors were still subsumed under the term "missionaries" until well into the 1760s, although the German congregations clearly were not missions in our current understanding of the term.

34. The fit of the commerce in medicines and books with overall shipping and mercantile trends in the period 1769–76 requires more careful study. See Doerflinger, *Vigorous Spirit*, 173ff., table 1.3, and his figs. 1, 2, and 4, for trends during the prerevolutionary decade.

Moreover, the pharmaceutical trade financed from philanthropic accounts and church collections both in Germany and North America apparently ran parallel and often overlapped with the commerce proper conducted by the Madai *Medikamentenexpedition*, and there are good reasons to believe that well-placed Halle ministers acted also as agents or middlemen in this larger trans-atlantic trade. This commercial trade, however, is only partly and occasionally documented in the Francke archives. Shipments went through Hamburg or Altona and thence to Amsterdam, Rotterdam, and London.[35]

In Prussian Halle, the domestic situation of the Foundations deteriorated sharply after the death in 1769 of the founder's son, G. A. Francke, and overall net profits from the pharmaceutical business decreased for the first time since the 1740s. In view of these findings, the assumption that the American market may indeed have become an attractive alternative to stagnant pharmaceutical sales in Europe is not unreasonable, although it is qualified by the fact that trade through clerical channels was based on the stream of dedicated mission income. In 1771, books and medications worth Thaler courant 628 were debited to the Solms-Rödelsheim legacy on the call of Ziegenhagen in London, who raised them as £ 104/16 sterling through the firm of Thornton. Terms of payment in transit in England were handled through Ziegenhagen and his London connections.[36]

H. M. Mühlenberg in Pennsylvania and the new codirectors in Halle seem to have agreed to let some of the Halle trade be handled through another enter-prising minister, J. H. C. Helmuth, who used local merchants, including his father-in-law J. H. (Henry) Keppele, as his network for distribution. In a 1774 letter to one of G. A. Francke's successors, G. A. Freylinghausen, Helmuth pro-vided an overview of a well-established trade in books and medications and at the same time offered some insight into its agents, both male and female, within

35. Although London was doubtless the center of colonial trade and financial exchange to North America if only in terms of volume, trade by Dutch agents cannot be ignored. For their role in immi-grant transports, see Wokeck, *Trade in Strangers*; Brink, *Die deutsche Auswanderungwelle in die britischen Kolonien Nordamerikas*.

36. MAFSt 4 G 3 contains a summary of accounts for "die vereinigten evangelisch Lutherischen Gemeinen in Pennylvanien, von den Jahren 1769 bis 1771, 1772, 1773, 1774, 1775." The five-year account of income and expenditures, which involved cross-credits and debits through London and to the Solms-Rödelsheim account, was explained in an attached unsigned note, dated 4 September 1772 (4 G 3, fols. 15–18, 19–22). Individual receipts are in 4 G 7. Although the rate of exchange in London was 6 Rth/£ sterling at the time, yields in Pennsylvania currency were close to 15 percent above the exchange rates in 1770. See McCusker, *Money and Exchange in Europe and America*, table 3.7. Note that this exchange is denominated in Reichsthaler, as the money of account. See also Denzel, "Der Aufstieg und die Einbindung der Vereinigten Staaten von Amerika in die Weltwirtschaft."

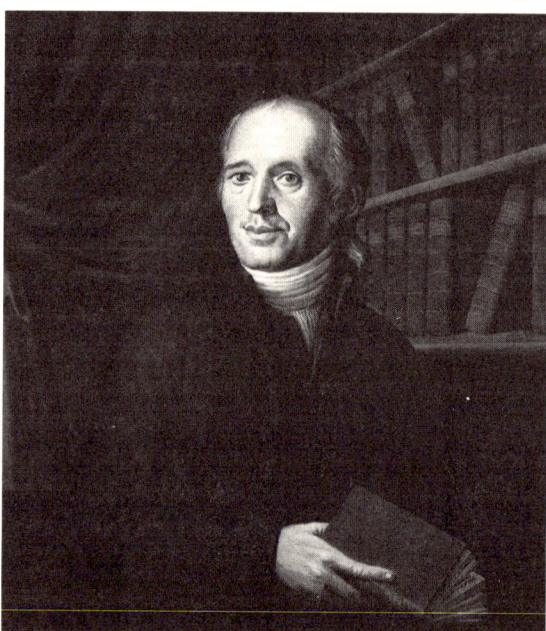

Fig. 5.1

Justus Heinrich Christian
Helmuth (b. 1745
Helmstedt, d. 1825
Philadelphia), former
instructor at the Halle
Orphanage Foundations;
Lutheran minister in
Pennsylvania from 1770 and
founder of the Mosheim
Society. (Courtesy,
Smithsonian National
Portrait Gallery.)

the clergy and without. "Both books and medications have arrived and been distributed. As soon as we learn about the detailed charges from Cowes, all items will be paid for immediately. If twice the amounts ordered had been sent, we would have sold them all, since the previous shipment order was received a good time hence."

Helmuth attributed this success to hunger for the word of the Lord and praised the opportunity to join the spoken to the written word, which Halle provided through its printed products. Thus, and having some moneys available for this purpose, he placed a further order on his own account. However, the sum mentioned (£150 Pennsylvania currency) was to go both into books and medications, "so that we can channel them to the poor at a lower than customary price. I do not intend to trade in these myself, for I have neither time nor skill for such matters, but to turn affairs over to a person who will accept my conditions and not charge more than a reasonable profit. I do not think that there is a better way of investing one's money. If God wills, I shall make payment as soon as the books will have arrived."[37]

37. Both quotations in MAFSt 4 C 17, Helmuth in Lancaster to Freylinghausen, 13 November 1774, starting fol. 298, with enclosures.

A bit more restrained but in the same vein, J. C. Kunze wrote to Ziegenhagen's assistant in London at the same time and with the same concerns.[38] All books and medicines ordered had arrived and were being sold at a fast pace. Medications were being handled by Kunze's wife, Margarete, in the absence of her mother, the elder Mrs. Mühlenberg. The books were placed with Laumann and Wirz, two merchants in Lancaster commissioned by one of the Mühlenberg sons. The political troubles with England besetting the colonies seem to have made little difference in commercial planning, with the senior Mühlenberg advising Halle that if current problems prevented ships from leaving England for the northern colonies, shipments might be made through the previous route, that is, "through the new ministers expected to travel via Holland. . . . With regard to the enclosed catalogue for books and medications, I note that my wife intends to continue the sale of the Halle medications, and although she has not yet used up her entire supply, she would like at all times to have a stock on hand. The books are ordered by my son Henry [Gotthilf Heinrich Ernst], who is a good housefather and manager, frugal but not stingy. I will guarantee their orders, if that is acceptable to you" (fol. 330).

Commercial agents were not to be given the favorable terms of payment through the Halle mission accounts, with debts set off from eventual charitable bequests, but placed on a cash and commission basis.[39] Only Mrs. Mühlenberg was permitted to charge her fairly large orders for medications directly to the Pennsylvania accounts.[40]

In terms of merchant interest, the recurrent strictures on trade with Great Britain, first after the Stamp Act and then after the nonimportation or boycott movement precipitated by the Townshend Acts, may well have caused German merchants with connections to the Dutch trading community to look for alternative sources of imports to North America, among them Halle medications.[41]

38. MAFSt 4 C 17, Stück 25, fol. 30, Kunze to Pasche in London, Philadelphia, 3 December 1774, copy received in Halle, 18 January 1775. At this time, Kunze owed the Halle accounts Rth 152/17 gr or close to £30 sterling.

39. KM 3: Letter 324 of 16 March 1765.

40. For example, 4 G 3, fols. 33, 34, several orders for books and medicines for herself and others, in the total amount of Rth 159 in 1774, and again in the same year, a shipment for Rth 377/11, of which Rth 131 was for medications. Her discount was 20 percent (fol. 84: "Für die Frau Pastor Mühlenberg in Philadelphia werden gesendet aus der Waisenhausapotheke zu Halle den 5. Martius 1774"). Whether these were Solms-Rödelsheim moneys is not clear, but likely in view of the sudden spurt of credit.

41. Although pharmaceuticals were often sold as part of the dry goods trade in North America, they were not a major part of this trade by value and certainly not by volume. For the general trend

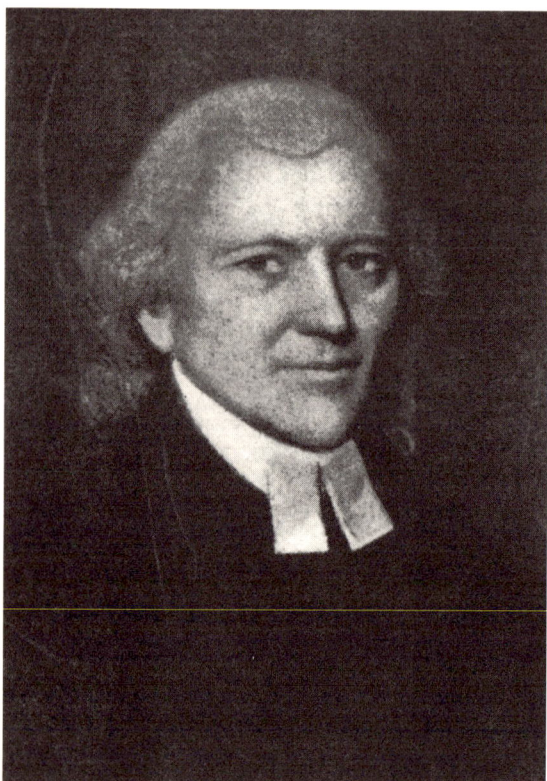

Fig. 5.2

Johann Christoph Kunze (b. 1744 Saxony, d. 1707 New York), taught at Leipzig University; Lutheran minister in Pennsylvania and New Jersey from 1770 and afterward in New York; governor of New York Hospital and professor at King's College. (Courtesy, Columbia University Archives.)

In addition to the Germantown merchants Reinhold, Leibert, and Billmeyer and Becker, and Laumann and Wirz in Lancaster, the major and best-connected merchant in this group was Johann Heinrich Keppele, who, as noted, seems to have placed his first direct orders through the Orphanage network at the time of Peter Mühlenberg's return, in 1768. Several later transactions both through England and, after the Revolution, directly through Holland and Hamburg, are recorded in the Halle ledgers.[42]

in dry goods imports and credit during this period and in this region, see Doerflinger, *Vigorous Spirit*, 168–80. There is insufficient information on trends in American pharmaceutical imports for this period to permit comparison with the Halle orders, which were for proprietary medicines only. For Europe, the financial value of the Corbyn trade as described by Porter and Porter (284–90) offers a base of comparison with the value of the total trade of the *Medikamentenexpedition* and seems to have covered pretty much the same markets, Russia being an exception.

42. The elder Keppele was an associate of the Weiser family and godfather to Peter Mühlenberg. His son Henry was trained in London in the 1760s. He traded with Halle first on his own and later

Increasingly, as portions of the North American trade shifted to Holland, the Keppele contacts and networks became indispensable. A large 1774 shipment from Halle, for instance, went directly to him via Altona and Rotterdam, in boxes labeled with his signature. The Halle factor informed the Hamburg agent, the firm of van Smissen, of total costs, insurance values, and freight costs and indicated that both freight and insurance moneys were to be paid by the designee on arrival in Philadelphia.[43] The total 1774 shipment was the equivalent of approximately £270 sterling.[44] Of this, two-thirds went for books and Bibles, and one-third for Orphanage medications, leaving a small balance in favor of the Pennsylvania missions on the eve of the Revolution.[45]

Trading in the New Republic, 1785–1815

By the mid-1780s, the Lutheran communities and their clerical leaders had, at least in the middle colonies, overcome the shoals of faction between patriots and loyalists. Although the Halle clergy in particular, with the exception of Peter and Friedrich August Mühlenberg, had not embraced the Republican patriotism of their new compatriots with overt enthusiasm, their attitude was not so much one of divided loyalties as of a well-tempered distrust of worldly faction and strife. If they suffered from disapprobation, they bore it silently like their distant if not affectionate cousins, the Quakers.[46]

---

through his son and his son-in-law J. H. C. Helmuth. Keppele and his family have not yet found an American biographer, and his trading interests are less familiar to the colonial historian than is his role as a trustee of Saint Michael's in Philadelphia and his support of the German Society.

43. MAFSt 4 G 3, fols. 63, 88, 98–100, the last item to the Altona agent van Smissen Sons, 9 June 1774. Insurance rates were 5.5 percent from Altona to Holland and Holland to Philadelphia. Freight and Dutch fees were to be paid in Philadelphia. On fol. 100, it was noted that extra books and medications were added, which the esteemed Mr. Keppele would surely be able to place, with moneys from these sales to go to the widow Handschuh for setoff from the German estate of her husband. The value of unsolicited orders was Rth 228, out of a total order of Rth 1,662. The practice of sending unsolicited goods to introduce one's wares may have been standard business practice; see Porter and Porter, "Rise of the English Drugs Industry," 291.

44. This shipment is particularly well documented in MAFSt 4 G 3, fols. 63, 101–2.

45. MAFSt 4 G 3, fol. 110, "Ausgaben, 1775." The debit balance from 1774 was Rth 196/4; expenses included items such as Rth 20 for Frau Schulze; Rth 392/8/4 to the bookstore; Rth 302 for the *Richtersche Medicamentenexpedition*; Rth 216 for the *Cansteinsche Bibelanstalt*; or a total expense, including advances, of Rth 1,126/22/4. Against these stood income of Rth 1,259/4/8, leaving a balance of Rth 132/6/4 on 2 January 1776. Roeber's reading (*Palatines, Liberty, and Property*, 256) of the relative decrease in income for North America was apparently based on the final annual balance, not on total transactions.

46. Several pronounced loyalists, including B. M. Houseal from New York, went to Canada and Nova Scotia, or like the unfortunate C. Friedrich Triebner from Georgia, returned to London to work

At least in terms of European trading opportunities, there seems to have been no political discord among the political factions. Conditions on the American side of the Atlantic fluctuated but over the course of the 1780s appeared as favorable if not more so than before the war for trade from continental Europe. By 1785, trade with Europe picked up again, whereas the former Halle trading position had been further eroded. Disbursements in Germany from the Halle accounts went mainly for remittances to the living relatives of clergy. Current income from church and institutional collections, which had been the backbone of Halle income to 1755, had almost ceased. But the old legacies accumulated throughout the century and continued to bear interest. Moneys for 1787–88 assigned to Pennsylvania came from this accumulated interest and from principal repayments for secured loans of legacy and similar capital.[47]

There is only anecdotal information on the financial course of the Francke Foundations to the end of the century, and a satisfactory and fully documented account of the details and modalities of transfer of some of these funds to North America is not possible at the current stage of research.[48] That some transfers from Germany were invested in Pennsylvania real estate cannot be doubted, because some of the debtors and their bonds are listed repeatedly in the Pennsylvania ledgers at Halle. But again, it appears that much if not all of this involved trading with Halle, with proceeds reinvested in North America, rather than straight capital transfers.[49] In a 1784 letter, Helmuth had inquired into the

for the SPCK. See Glatfelter, *Pastors and People*, vol. 1, for men like Houseal. For Quaker detachment but undiluted business purpose, see Doerflinger, *Vigorous Spirit*, 300, quoting Chaloner on the occasion of the founding of the Bank of Pennsylvania in 1784. See also Rappaport, *Stability and Change*, chap. 7.

47. MAFSt 4 G 4, fols. 10ff. The Streit legacy, for instance, yielded roughly Rth 400–450 per year over its forty years of documented investment. According to documents in MAFSt 4 F 6, payments from this legacy to North America continued until 1825 and probably beyond.

48. The work by Welsch, "Die Franckeschen Stiftungen als wirtschaftliches Grossunternehmen," takes us only to 1730; my own work with the sources in the Wirtschaftsarchiv is tentative and has so far permitted only a summary of aggregate income and expenses. The only American researcher who has tried to brave this thorny complex of questions for our period of interest is Roeber, who details some of it in his work on Helmuth. The major North American legacy files are in MAFSt 4 F 1–10 and are matched for Pennsylvania by detailed but incomplete accounts at the Lutheran Seminary Archives in Germantown.

49. 4 G 8, fol. 30(?), a 1787 letter from Helmuth and Schmidt reports that a total of £ [sic] 1,573 in income from the Solms-Rödelsheim legacy had been placed in the Philadelphia real estate market and with several firms, including David Schaefer heirs, Philips Edeborn, Herbst und Lex, Heinrich Keppele (Jr.), and Laumann and Daum. This and most other transactions with Halle during the next decades are still denominated in pounds, probably in Pennsylvania currency, which was still being used in merchant circles for most financial exchanges; see Denzel, "Der Aufstieg und die Einbindung der

conditions of the Streit legacy, its beneficiary and exact purpose, and indeed suggested that it might be more profitable, and less burdensome for the Halle administrators, to invest the capital in Philadelphia. His stated concern was to relieve the Pennsylvania Ministerium and its members of the onus of accounting for this money, shifting this task instead to an intermediary who would post bond. Another concern was to discharge the debt still extant from previous church construction and related expenses, although these affected mainly the Mühlenberg family and its standing.

At this time, Helmuth correctly pointed out, the balance of payments was heavily in favor of Europe, although he correctly predicted an eventual upsurge in American conditions. But he and his business associates knew full well that although the capital from Halle might be welcome, there was little marketing opportunity for any American exports to Halle; on the other leg of the trade, customs and freight charges would continue to eat into the profit from trade in books and medications.[50] In the end, the Fabricius scheme proposed in 1759 and involving setoffs and transfers through Halle products was adapted to the very different circumstances of the 1780s and beyond, although the scheme put Halle in the position of offering more goods than the market might be able to bear. For some time, however, actual demand exceeded expected demand, and the trade with Halle did not succumb.

In North America, a new division of labor among the leading clergy had become apparent even before the death of H. M. Mühlenberg in 1787. His two older sons—Peter and Friedrich August—had retired from the clergy and entered politics. Gotthilf Heinrich Ernst practiced his ministry and medicine and tried to run Franklin College in Lancaster. In his diaries, he commented with some distance on the goings-on in Philadelphia.[51] Under the terms of the Pennsylvania legacies, however, he remained part of the core group concerning financial dispositions and continued to order substantial quantities of medicine and books from Halle for his own and other accounts. His brother-in-law, J. C. Kunze, and some of his disciples went to New York in 1785 and apparently

---

Vereinigten Staaten," 157ff. In Georgia as well, legacy capital remained in Europe. A hundred years later, a letter from the minister of the Evangelical Lutheran Church of the Ascension, Reverend W. S. Bowman, to the chairman of the Board of Trustees, E. G. Weitman, of 15 March 1887, refers to income continuously received from the Degenfeld legacy established in the 1740s.

50. MAFSt 4 C 16, fol. 245. For the postrevolutionary boom and the subsequent drop in imports, see Rappaport, *Stability and Change*, 159ff.

51. Mühlenberg papers, American Philosophical Society, M 892, vol. 2.

ceased to play an active role in the Pennsylvania Ministerium. Kunze, as university professor and senior Lutheran minister, was to become prominent both as a professor of King's College and a governor of New York Hospital. In Philadelphia, Justus Heinrich Helmuth and Johann Friedrich Schmidt assumed the leadership of the Lutheran Ministerium, of the movement for the maintenance of German teaching and academic instruction,[52] and, last but not least, of the accounts with Halle.

By the end of the 1780s, regular shipments of books and medications had resumed and for a while proceeded on an unprecedented scale. This was despite the fact that transatlantic accounting, which even before 1776 had often caused friction because of varying rates of exchange and the cost of credit, now was mired in the chaotic conditions of the money market in North America in its transition to relative financial independence. As senior minister in Philadelphia and head of the Lutheran Ministerium during much of the last two decades of the century, Helmuth was now at the center of the German network in Philadelphia and well placed by opportunity, family connections, and temperament to take the lead in restoring commerce with Halle and expanding it to fit the new and boisterous if risky opportunities of the period. In a letter to Fabricius of 14 April 1785, he suggested rerouting shipments through Hamburg, Bremen, or Ostende to save freight charges, this time circumventing not only the English but the Dutch as well. As the head of a growing German educational establishment and in close contact with the University of Pennsylvania, Helmuth ventured into new imports, such as compasses and rules and scientific equipment.[53]

Reimbursement by drafts, the route previously taken, had become impractical; Helmuth noted that £2,000 in drafts on Holland had been returned to his aging father-in-law in view of the absence of American creditworthiness.[54] As a result, moneys taken in from the sale of German products had accumulated and now had been lent out against bond to various members of Saint Michael's corporation. Helmuth was urged by the borrowers to initiate repayment, because

52. More fully described in Roeber, "The Mosheim Society"; idem, "J. H. C. Helmuth."
53. First pushed against the wall by a vendor of English instruments and forced to give away one set as a courtesy, he subsequently ordered two dozen sets, to be sold by an English printer, Francis Bailey, who also sold Halle medications and books (Letter to Fabricius, 14 April 1785, MAFSt 4 C 20, Stück 46, fols. 202–5): "I have passed on the medications to Francis Bailey and the printer Billmeyer in Germantown."
54. MAFSt 4 C 20, Stück 58, fols. 244–47, Helmuth and Schmidt to Fabricius, 30 August 1785. Most of this material is in 4 MAFSt C 20.

this would favor their position at a time of galloping inflation.[55] Both Helmuth and the Mühlenberg sons were concerned to avoid the appearance of nepotism in the use of these moneys, and Helmuth suggested reinvestment with a secure firm or, his own preference, purchasing stock in one of the new banks.[56] Despite these difficulties, the wish to rush into the European trade was difficult to resist if it could be joined to the good cause of supporting the Foundations in their decline. Inspector Fabricius was urged to send a large contingent of books and medications intended for the prosperous Germantown firm of Leibert and Billmeyer, whose credit Helmuth was willing to vouch for. A substantial order from Baltimore worth several hundred pounds was in the offing if the merchant proved creditworthy. And the medications, Helmuth wrote with a fine disregard for the trade of his predecessors from 1750 to 1775 or for the institutional memory of the Halle leadership, were beginning to be well known and to acquire a measure of fame. He himself intended to translate the instructions for use into English,[57] all with the goal of letting the "beloved Orphanage benefit from all possible advantages accruing from North America."

He was above all convinced of the prospects of supplying a German market with specifically German products—books and medications—and hoped to find an agent to conduct this trade, even advertising in the American German newspapers to push the product, in yet another reversal of conservative Halle practice. Although German immigration during the next two decades was to slow to a trickle,[58] he saw great promise in the arrival, within the span of a few days in 1784, of three boats carrying German immigrants, one from Germany and two from Holland. Like his contemporary Benjamin Rush, he shared the view that Germans were highly popular arrivals because of their willingness to settle toward

55. The amount involved in this instance was £660 current in income from the Streit legacy. The borrowers asked for return of their bonds from Halle as a condition of repayment. Another £ 300 were held by the father-in-law of Friedrich August Mühlenberg, the merchant Schaefer.

56. It is unclear whether he referred to the Bank of North America founded by Robert Morris or the planned but short-lived Bank of Pennsylvania, which seems to have been envisaged by the merchant community excluded from the Morris circle but then was absorbed by the Bank of North America; see Doerflinger, *Vigorous Spirit*, 296ff.; Rappaport, *Stability and Change*, 160ff. Unfortunately, neither Doerflinger nor Rappaport pays much attention to the Dutch and German commercial element, whether for lack of sources or lack of linguistic access. Forthcoming work by Rosalind Beiler on the Wistar family should open up research into this commercial sector, which was clearly of some importance.

57. The 1784 English version of Madai, *A Brief Account*, contains a detailed conversion table for florins and pounds sterling but apparently was not meant for the American market; see Table 3.3.

58. Grabbe, "Besonderheiten der europäischen Einwanderung in die USA."

the west of the new republic. His appreciation of the common working folk did not, however, extend to possible competition by learned immigrants, in particular lawyers and clergy arriving without a call.[59]

The death of Inspector Fabricius in 1790 caused yet another collapse in Halle financial stewardship,[60] and Helmuth urged the restoration of some kind of order, pointing out that "Mssrs. Becker urgently await the books ordered [for Helmuth's German academy]. We hope that their and my drafts on London, as those of Dr. Mühlenberg and Mr. Laumann, can be safely settled through London. We could also resume the sale of medications, but I must see a full account first."[61]

This trade with Halle now included dry goods not previously obtained through the motherhouse.[62] It was carried by the familiar range of merchants and by a new generation of enterprising young men. Helmuth's orders during the next twenty years concentrated largely, but not exclusively, on books, for which orders ran to about Rth 1,000 per year and for which he and his co-assignee Schmidt held their own account with the Bible Institute.[63] His medication orders, although containing the usual Orphanage medications, were directed at efficiency of dispensing, whether by himself or for resale. He requested the usual packing slips for individual medications, but asked that

59. There is no mention by Helmuth, in contrast to the previous preoccupation by H. M. Mühlenberg, of Philadelphia physicians or pharmacists, although the latter in particular were to constitute an interesting German immigrant stream throughout this period (Higby, *In Search of American Pharmacy*). A good number of Philadelphia pharmacies were in German hands by 1815 (Parrish, "Pharmacy in Philadelphia").

60. Sebastian Andreas Fabricius was the last of the old Halle functionaries and had befriended the Mühlenberg boys during their stay in the 1760s. On inspection, his books, as at previous occasions of institutional turnover at the Orphanage, were found to be in disorder, but the new accountants did not last long enough in their positions to manage a smooth transition. Fabricius maintained an extensive correspondence with Helmuth as American administrator of legacies on the new conditions of trade and on old debts and balances of the missions (MAFSt 4 C 20).

61. Letter by Helmuth, MAFSt 4 D 2, Stück 50, fol. 47, with book *pro memoria* on fol. 51, dated 10 May 1790.

62. A much-ordered item was German lace; see MAFSt 4 G 4, fols. 10ff. Some of this lace was apparently manufactured in orphanages and *Stifte* close to the Foundations. In a letter in MAFSt 4 D 6, Stück 10, of 23 December 1809, John Baker (now using an English name) confirmed an order of spices and books and medications through Halle, and continued: "[I]n the event that the English should lift the blockade, make sure that you have both books and lace ready for shipment. . . . 400 Rth worth of white lace of specified widths."

63. MAFSt 4 G 4, 1789, paid on account of the "Herren Mandatarien," Rth 800 Streit legacy interest, from a total expense of Rth 862; fols. 24–25, 1791–93, "für Rechnung der Herren Mandatarien zu Philadelphia, Rth 550." On fols. 41–43, for instance, Inspector Stoppelberg explained that the Streit legacy set a mandatory rate of interest on capital of 5 percent, which at the time was not available in German markets but could be had in Philadelphia (see Rappaport, *Stability and Change*, 168).

printed instructions be included that not only discussed indications of use and anticipated effects but also a proportional dosage scale, so that "these could be used for future prescriptions."[64]

Thirty years after the failed attempt to set up Peter Mühlenberg in his own pharmaceutical trade, J. H. C. Helmuth wrote to Halle with the request to establish credit for his son Gamble, an aspiring merchant: "[M]y youngest son has established a storehouse . . . and wishes to inquire if in addition to his other business he can enter into the pharmaceutical trade with Halle, which is close to his heart for his father's sake. He is interested in establishing a mutually beneficial traffic."[65] One year later, this trade was apparently established, with Gamble ordering ten crates of goods, including, as Item 12, a crate of medications containing four small boxes.[66] Gamble Helmuth's enterprise ended in bankruptcy twenty years later, and he left no record of his preferences in the trade in pharmaceuticals, which by now was competing with an increasingly strong and stable domestic apothecary system, at least in Philadelphia.[67]

The size and range of the trade with Halle were still confined to a close circle of associates, although the clergy were by now no longer in the majority. Of the total of Rth 2,195 owed to the Canstein Bible Institute in 1789, the Orphanage bookstore, and the *Medikamentenexpedition* for shipments from 1787, half was owed by Helmuth himself, by Helmuth and Schmidt jointly as assignees and trustees of Halle income (*Mandatarien*), and by G. H. E. Mühlenberg; the rest of the debt reflected sales by the Philadelphia and Lancaster firms of Laumann, Becker, Leibert and Billmeyer, and Michael Billmeyer.[68]

In 1788–89, medication orders totaled the handsome sum of 457 Louis d'or, of which Pastor G. H. E. Mühlenberg in Lancaster took the lion's share, with

64. MAFSt 4 D 2, Stück 60, fol. 249, letter from Helmuth to Fabricius, 5 April 1784.

65. Letter from Helmuth of 13 September 1796, MAFSt 4 G 10, fol. 1.

66. MAFSt 4 G 10, fols. 143–44, detailed order from Gamble Helmuth of 3 December 1797. The order was for several Richter medications, but apparently at a trial level and was not comparable to the quantities and scope of the orders by G. H. E. Mühlenberg discussed in Chapter 7. See also the letter from G. H. E. Mühlenberg to van Smissen (MAFSt 4 D 3, Stück 9) of 10 September 1796.

67. Although German apothecaries had a large share in this market, we lack detailed inventories that could indicate whether their trade in proprietary medications, if any, favored German over British products. Personal communication, G. Higby, American College for the History of Pharmacy.

68. MAFSt 4 G 8, 1787, "Lieferungen nach Pennsylvanien [fol. 25] copia, N. S. an die Herren Mandatarien zu Philadelphia." The firm of Becker (later Baker) placed substantial orders between 1789 and 1794, including one for twelve Ludwig and twelve Bayley English dictionaries on one occasion and large orders of Bibles and religious literature. Orders are in 4 G 9, fols. 29–33, 35–36, 187, 195. These were no longer the same merchants but were in most cases the same firms with whom Halle had dealt in the 1750s. See Roeber, "German and Dutch Books and Printing."

Helmuth and the firm of Bergmann ranking next.[69] Mühlenberg placed similar and continuing orders throughout the decade and also handled orders for Pastor Traugott Illing, who had been practicing medicine and using the Halle medications in western Maryland since the 1760s. Smaller amounts were ordered by J. C. Kunze in New York and by his student and protégé, Friedrich David Schaefer, also in Maryland.[70] That this trade persisted under the very different economic conditions and medical markets of the 1780s and 1790 is remarkable; I discuss some of the likely reasons for the loyalty of providers and public in the next chapter. There is no doubt, though, that at this time both initiative and guidance came from North America, from a group of clergy closely related to the Halle motherhouse by tradition and sentiment, but no longer tied to its strictures. They no longer lacked their own funding and held a secure position in American society. In a 1795 letter to the Foundations, Helmuth mentioned the fire that destroyed the Zion Church in Philadelphia, for the reconstruction of which the congregation subscribed £10,000 [sic] in two weeks. He and Schmidt proposed that one-quarter of the annual income from the Streit legacy should benefit their old and beleaguered motherhouse, in consideration of the "concern and labor you have expended on our behalf now for many years."[71]

In 1796, H. G. E. Mühlenberg complained to the new Orphanage inspector of account discrepancies, estate matters, and inefficiencies, but at the same time requested continued use of the Halle shipping facilities for his far-ranging botanical correspondence, including books and instruments. He continued that "regarding medications and books and pending the arrival of outstanding shipments, I will continue my previous orders in the amounts stated, and probably will need more. . . . No doubt Mr. Laumann will also wish to place another

---

69. MAFSt 4 G 9, fols. 41, 185, 195.

70. MAFSt 4 G 4, fol. 25, 1793, which includes Rth 100 for medications for D. Mühlenberg, and fols. 26–27, 1794, "an die Medikamentenexpedition für Herrn D. Mühlenberg, Rth 180/21/8." Orders by Gotthilf Heinrich Ernst Mühlenberg are documented in Chapter 7. Orders by Reverend Illing for books and medications are ibid., fols. 28–29. In 4 D 4, Stück 36, Pastor Schaefer wrote to Inspector Nebe (18 January 1799) with a note on the envelope that the letter would be delivered at the North American Post Office in Hamburg, and that payment would be made to Pastor Schmidt in Philadelphia, that is, not remitted to Germany, because the cost of drafts during this period made both books and medications too expensive for sale. Schaefer clearly dispensed himself, because his order is in pharmaceutical quantities. The Mühlenberg order for medications in 1806 ran to Rth 238/9 for himself and others (MAFSt 4 G 4, fol. 53).

71. The fire is reported in MAFSt 4 G 10, fol. 11. The remainder of the annual Streit income was to be used to purchase a large order of the *Pennsylvanische Nachrichten*, which carried news from Pennsylvania and the middle colonies but was compiled and printed in Halle; MAFSt 4 G 10, fols. 11–14, 18 November 1795.

order."[72] In a postscript, Mühlenberg thanked the Orphanage pharmacy for a gift of medications apart from his order, which would enable him to dispense more medications on the charity.

Clearly, the notion of philanthropy from the metropolis to the colonial dependencies had undergone considerable change. But almost without exception, the descendants of the Halle pioneers proved well up to the new conditions of the market. In a 1797 letter to yet another crew of accountants at Halle, Mühlenberg insisted that the previous conditions of credit for twelve months after shipment should be maintained, with only balances remaining to bear interest. "This is the common practice here among the English merchants, and the Americans are accustomed to this generous practice." Freight and customs duties had again increased, but the ability to send books and medications directly through the Danish port of Altona and thence onboard American vessels remained an advantage. Mühlenberg as well thought that there was enough of a market in North America to maintain the size and composition of his previous orders. His brother Friedrich August, then a member of Congress and Postmaster General, used his connections to introduce business associates of his son-in-law Jacob Sperry to the Halle book and medications trade.[73] Sperry himself apparently had already been in touch with Halle, now dealing through the house of Kleinworth and Moeller in Hamburg.

The foregoing summarizes nearly seven decades of transatlantic trade under German philanthropic auspices, extending from 1730 to 1810. In this larger perspective, we find that during the colonial period, the Halle motherhouse used its English and Dutch network to support its dependencies through trade in medicines and books, which were carried across the Atlantic both as regular commercial and charity shipments and by means of the small-scale carrying trade on board immigrant ships. In North America, these imports helped the Halle ministers to gain a place in the merchant community that augmented their clerical influence. During the decline of the Francke Foundations and the poor economic and investment conditions in Germany at the end of the eighteenth century, this trade, which had been a small fraction of total Halle trade during

---

72. MAFSt 4 G 10, fols. 15–17, 20–22, of 6 April 1796, and 4 D 4, Stück 47, Mühlenberg to Inspector Nebe, 24 November 1797. The final separation of the Bible Institute and the Pharmacy business from the Orphanage proper had upset previous trading and setoff conveniences. Mr. Laumann did in fact die in 1798, but his widow took over the books and promised to pay for them.

73. MAFSt 4 D 4, Letter to Nebe, Stück 27, 22 September 1798. C. J. Vogel was traveling to Europe and to Halle on business for H. M. Mühlenberg's son-in-law, Jacob Sperry.

the years 1740–70, became relatively more important. To the established ministry in North America, this shift and the availability of funds for investment at relatively high rates of interest in the currency-poor American republic provided a source of economic influence at a time of shifting allegiances and competition among professional and language groups for social status. The European mother-house thus joined its newly independent sons in continuing its trade. This, I argue, was entirely in accordance with the spirit of enterprise that had prevailed in Halle at the beginning of the eighteenth century. Philanthropic stewardship then as now requires continuous placement of legacies and bequests at the best rates of return. In the case of the Halle Orphanage Foundations, the founder's development of a printing house and a pharmacy and the sale of products in Europe and across the ocean had proved a wise investment in the new philanthropy of the eighteenth century. Both trades made it possible to transfer the income from dedicated legacies and bequests to their intended beneficiaries, absent a developed banking system and transfer mechanisms. At the same time, the trade in medicinals introduced Pietist medicine and therapeutic opinions into this country and offered their users, both learned providers and lay patients practicing self-help, choices not otherwise available in the market for eighteenth-century medicinals.

German Lay Preferences

and Choices

6

The market for the Halle Orphanage medications in North America was defined by commercial trade under philanthropic auspices, clerical medical practice, and merchant and consumer demand. For patients and practitioners, the continued attraction of these medications lay in part in their identification with a pharmaceutical armamentarium sanctioned by charity practice at a famous medical institution. Another likely motive was patient unease at being confronted by a different medical nomenclature and a different system of care in times of illness.

The resulting preferences for familiar remedies and treatments not only related to illness behavior, but served larger purposes for different social actors: to preserve cultural identity among users and providers, to establish an economic advantage in a large and unregulated market, and to confer social distinctiveness. It assured the godly and conservative German element in North America, or at least the better-off among this element, that they too could draw on a mainstream culture in Europe that was as good as if not better than that of their American contemporaries. In addition to supply through the Pietist clergy, German merchants from Philadelphia and Baltimore to New York used their connections in Frankfurt, Leipzig, and Amsterdam to supply some of this demand. German agents traveling to Europe on legal and commercial errands availed themselves of the advantages of size and weight offered by the packaging of Halle medications and similar products, bringing them over in their personal luggage and reselling them in the middle colonies. An advertisement by Johann Adam Franck, in the *Wöchentliche Pennsylvanische Staatsbote* of 29 April 1765, repeated in May 1765, advertised both Halle and Thuringian medications arrived in the last ship from Holland. The Thuringian merchandise probably consisted of the traditional *Oleitäten*.[1] Thus, commercial factors were joined to social aspirations, brand loyalty, and faith in one's own traditions to maintain Halle medicines as a factor in the domestic and medical culture in German settlements.

Language played a large part in this, and the Halle armamentarium was a felicitous combination of medical incentives offered through a common reading medium. The traffic in German-language self-help texts is best known for the period after the Revolutionary War and the early nineteenth century.[2] In addition, as German-language groups in North America stratified and became more prosperous, there was some demand for current German textbooks in natural philosophy, chemistry, and other learned works by the medical and scholarly community who had access to German lists.[3]

Pharmaceutical orders from the middle colonies that went through the Halle mission accounts came from a variety of people: the Halle clergy, merchants and other commercial agents, male and female providers of medical care in or connected to the Halle network, and educated laity who bought specific items for self-medication. Both providers and users exercised considerable

1. For the commercial carrying trade, see Beiler, "From the Rhine to the Delaware Valley." I thank Christine Hucho for bringing this advertisement to my attention. For the continuing eighteenth-century popularity of *Oleitäten*, a series of early modern arcana, see Peickert, *Geheimmittel im deutschen Arzneiverkehr*, and more recently Beisswanger, *Arzneimittelversorgung im 18. Jahrhundert*. Franck's purchases, which he used to attract patients for his uroscopy practice, were clearly outside the mission supply route, although he lived close to the Lutheran Church and knew the elder Mühlenberg.

2. Cowen, "Zum Dienste des Gemeinen Mannes"; Cowen and Wilson, "Traffic in Medical Ideas," have more recently integrated the major Halle offerings, treatises, and sales brochures by C. Friedrich Richter and Samuel von Madai into this corpus.

3. See Cazden, *Social History of the German Book Trade*; and Roeber, "German and Dutch Books and Printing." For an interesting medical consumer who did not, for all we know, purchase Halle medications through the channels described in this book, see MFSt 4 G 7, fols. 45–46, 1771: "Pay from the Pennsylvania accounts: 1. For Dr. Kuhn, to the bookstore, Rth 62/14, to the Canstein Bible Press, Rth 9/6/3." Adam Kuhn, professor of medicine and botany at the University of Pennsylvania Medical School, had studied medicine in Leiden and Upsala and was well known in the Mühlenberg circle; he paid a visit to the elder Mühlenberg before his departure to Europe.

discrimination in selecting from the Halle armamentarium, particularly after first purchases of a medicine chest and its accompanying medical literature. Often, the chest was considered an investment by many of the direct users (the medical laity) that was then replenished with preferred substances. Merchants reflected their customers' preferences and stocked in expectation of proven demand. Medical providers ordered both according to the preferences of their paying patients and, as we see in one well-documented case, made some substitutions based on considerations of medical efficiency, obtaining similar effects at a lower price.

We can examine some of these preferences and choices at the level of the lay public, both men and women; in Chapter 7, I turn to the learned practitioner, including the clergy, and to some instances of trained medical providers, to determine whether patient and provider preferences coincided and what we can learn from differences and similarities. Not surprisingly, practitioners' selections were more diverse and contained greater quantities of individual Halle items. Practitioners served a larger clientele, saw a wider range of symptoms, and probably were more discriminating in their dispensing.

In all cases, it is reasonable to assume that none of the users, whether providers or patients, restricted themselves entirely to the Halle prefabricated medications, whether for reasons of medical choice, price, or availability. This is as true for the relative therapeutic frugality of physicians like Ernst Thilo in Georgia as for Heinrich Melchior Mühlenberg and his medically far less frugal son, Gotthilf Heinrich Ernst.

The German Lay Public

Preferences were expressed in specific instructions to Halle from the first recorded orders of Halle pharmaceuticals sent from North America in the 1740s. These, both in terms of merchant orders and direct patient orders passed along in letters to Halle, concentrated on a limited number of items from both Halle lists, but not only those in the chests advertised in the self-help texts. (See Table 6.1 for the product names, classified in the following as belonging to the A or B list, and Table 6.2 for approximate weight equivalents. For information on product composition, clinical indications, and prices, see Tables 3.1–4 above.) Here we face the first test of interpreting choices: Why did consumers choose one medication over the other, given that the medications on both lists originated from the same manufacturer and that they did not know the composition of the items offered? What they did know—either from hearsay or from previous experience—were the likely effects of the medications. They could also infer uses by their names, which in general stuck to traditional nomenclature, such as the *pulvis bezoardicus* and the *essentia antihypochondriaca*. Orders therefore reflected the expectation of reliable production of specific effects. The manufacturers retained familiar names despite occasional changes in composition over the course of the eighteenth century and beyond. This attitude of trust had in fact been anticipated by the author of the *Höchst-nöthige Erkenntnis* in the early eighteenth century.[4]

On the other hand, from the beginning of the long-distance merchandising of Halle medicine chests, it had proved difficult to make the public conform fully to the medical choices made by their developers, however carefully they explained these choices in the Richter manuals. Orders from Russia at the beginning of the eighteenth century had concentrated heavily on the *essentia dulcis* and *e. amara*, on *pulvis vitalis* and *balsamus cephalicus*, and the *elixir polychrestum*, for instance, but omitted bezoard powder and laxatives containing mercury;[5] orders from military camps in Hungary showed similar preferences. North American choices proved to be equally pronounced.

As early as 1744, two years after his arrival, Heinrich Melchior Mühlenberg ordered what already seem to have been among American favorites: polychrest pills, pills for purging and against obstructions, *pulvis vitalis*, and the *essentia dulcis*. Although most orders placed in 1748 follow the A list for the chest, a Mrs. Koch already restricted her order to *essentia dulcis*, *Milzessenz* (*essentia hypochondriaca*), *pilulae polychrestae* and *purgantes*, and *pulvis vitalis*, suggesting familiarity with the Halle offerings.[6] Heinrich Melchior Mühlenberg himself ordered fully Reichthaler (Rth) 10 worth of *essentia dulcis concentrata* and *pulvis vitalis*. Requests for omission of the chest and for the full Richter manual suggest parsimonious purchasers and refills.[7]

---

4. According to Poeckern's ongoing study of various formularies in the Halle archives, substitutions occurred in Galenic or botanical compounds, like the *essentia amara* or the *pilulae polychrestae*, where bitter substances or their extracts were exchanged; more important, the constituents of the chemiatric medications changed slowly by the substitution of *cinnabaris factitia* or iron filings for crude antimony, as in the *pulvis bezoardicus* (Poeckern, personal communication).

5. See, for example, the order by Pastor Roloff in Moscow, December 1712, VAFSt Repertorium ii/296.

6. For instance, Pastor Brunnholz, MAFSt 4 G 2, Item 4.

7. MAFSt 4 G 2, "[O]nly that I would like these in a simple box and without a bound text [here the 1746 *Short Instruction*]."

Table 6.1   Halle Orphanage medications, as advertised for sale in standard chests (A list) and additional medications (B list)

A List	B List
Essentia dulcis, or sweet essence	*Pulvis solaris*, or golden powder
Essentia amara, or bitter essence	*Pulvis laxans*, or softening powder
Essentia antihypochondriaca (*Milz-öffnende Essenz*), or spleen-opening essence	*Pulvis niger*, or black powder
Pilulae polychrestae, or pills of many virtues	*Pulvis polychrestus*, or powder of many virtues
Pilulae contra obstructiones, or antiobstructive pills	*Pulvis stomachicus* (*Resolvierendes Magenpulver*), or stomach powder
Pilulae purgantes, or cathartic pills	*Pulvis uterinus griseus*, or *nigricans*, or gray or black uterine powder
Pulvis contra acredinem, or powder against acrimony	*Elixir polychreston*, or elixir of many virtues
Pulvis antispasmodicus, or antispasmodic powder	*Magisterium diaphoreticum*, or sweat-inducing powder
Pulvis bezoardicus, or bezoar powder	*Balsamus mineralis*, or mineral balm
Pulvis vitalis, or life-giving powder	*Electuarium antiphtisicum*, or lozenge for phtisis
Balsamus cephalicus, or balsamic nerve strengthener	*Tinctura salina*, or saline mixture
	Tinctura corallina, or coral tincture

NOTE: Latin names are according to Richter, *Höchst-nöthige Erkenntnis*, 1715 ed., and Madai, *Brief Account*, 1784, with English translations per Madai. See also Tables 3.1 and 3.2.

Table 6.2   Pharmaceutical and commercial weights used, and gram equivalents

1 grain	0.06 g
1 drachm	3.8 g
1 lot	15.5 g
1 lb	372.1 g
1 oz troy	31.0 g
1 quentchen	3.8 g

NOTE: The values given approximate those of Beisswanger, *Arzneimittelversorgung im 18. Jahrhundert.* Most orders listing shipments to North America were in commercial quantities, including lot and quentchen. Orders from North America reflected differences in persons ordering and over time, and included a large range of unit sizes and weights, from doses, packets, and glasses of varying weights and volumes to pounds.

But for the more prestigious substances, in particular the tonics and forti-fiers, price does not seem to have been an obstacle. In the early 1750s, Conrad Weiser ordered half of the contents of a Rth 10 chest in *pulvis vitalis*, or an expen-sive 120 doses of four grains each. His son-in-law H. M. Mühlenberg ordered a Rth 20 chest filled half with *pulvis vitalis*, the rest with *essentia hypochondriaca* and polychrest pills; the packing room in Halle added yet another sixteen packets (or 192 doses) of *pulvis vitalis*.[8] A large if unfilled order by Schoolmaster Vigera[9] also concentrated heavily on *essentia dulcis, pulvis vitalis*, and *pil. polychresta*.

These individual orders for small quantities seem to have ceased in the decade after the Revolution. That this must be attributed more to the scarcity of foreign currency and similar obstacles to renewed European trade than to reduced demand is reflected in the larger orders by the direct contributors in the Halle trade, mainly Gotthilf Heinrich Ernst Mühlenberg, Justus Heinrich Helmuth, and some of the German and English merchants in the trading net-work. Only after 1805 do problems of decreasing demand surface in comments by merchants stocking the medications.

Compared with the large and competitive medical market in Pennsylvania, there was a relatively small but stable and tightly linked patient reservoir in Georgia after the 1750s, when the German settlements increasingly became an enclave outside the Georgia economic mainstream.[10] A large influx of settlers around mid-century had provided a resilient German population. Not all were servants and poor marginal farmers but added to an interesting German-Swiss community of learned settlers on the Savannah, one of whom corresponded with Albrecht von Haller on local plant specimens.[11] Even after the death of their two regular medical providers in 1764, the German settlers did not become part of the dominant but distant medical culture in Charleston.[12]

8. MAFSt 4 G 6, fol. 31, no date.

9. MAFSt 4 G 6 and lit. A. "Nach Pennsylvanien, 1752" (fol. 39). For the full order sent that year, with prices, see lit. E e.

10. The population of Ebenezer and its satellites was around 1,500 adults and children of European descent by the beginning of the 1760s and increased only slowly thereafter as a result of nat-ural growth balanced by outmigration. The German-Swiss settlements on either side of the Savannah River counted roughly another 3,000 people, but were less homogeneous and contained substantial slave populations. The German contingent in Savannah ran to a few hundred people during this period and included notables like Joachim Zubli and Johann Treutlen, Georgia's first governor (Jones, *Salzburger Saga, Georgia Dutch*; Wilson, "Land, Population, and Labor").

11. Jones, "Savannah River Intelligentsia."

12. Waring, *Medicine in South Carolina*, 62ff., describes a fairly standard practice of medicine, with much bleeding and forced excretion, but a lively medical culture that went far beyond the rudiments

Medicine in the German and Swiss settlements was practiced not only by the few German and French surgeons who had found their way to and remained in Georgia, but again by clergy—both the Lutherans of Ebenezer sent by Halle and several Swiss Reformed, some converted to the Anglican Church. From the 1750s onward, in addition to regular charity shipments for Ebenezer, orders for the Richter medications came from the Reverends Joachim Zuebli and J. Zouberbuhler in Savannah, from the Georgia-born son of the second Ebenezer vicar, Timothy Lemcke, from several merchants in the community, and from the Reverend Christoph Triebner, the last Halle-trained successor to the position of the senior minister of Ebenezer. Neighboring notables, including the almanac maker Johannes Tobler, ordered large and small medicine chests and individual items for their home practices.[13] Interestingly, the most economically active member of the Halle clergy in Georgia, and its first plantation and slave owner, Christian Rabenhorst, apparently did not practice medicine or trade in the motherhouse medications. The name of one of the most learned Georgians of the prerevolutionary period, the surveyor and Augsburg emissary Gerard de Brahm, is likewise absent from the Halle records.[14]

A comparison of orders by Timothy Lemcke and the Reverend Triebner from 1771 and by Reverend Joachim Zuebli in 1761[15] with the standard order sent annually to Ebenezer from Halle as charity offers a good basis for examining relative preferences for the proven Halle armamentarium. As in the orders from Pennsylvania, additions to this eleven-item list indicate direct familiarity

of neighboring Savannah, Georgia, and already showed signs of an excess of providers (87). There was apparently little contact with the Germans across the Carolina border, and we note an insistence on noble or at least professional English backgrounds for Charleston practitioners, for example, p. 251. A reference to the "médicine expectante" practiced at the end of the century by a French refugee from Saint Domingue is of interest (253–54) in view of comparable attitudes in the French territory of Louisiana (Duffy, *Medicine in Louisiana*, vol. 1).

13. All in MAFSt 5 E 4, as lit. added to the ledgers, and more or less adhering to the standard orders from the A list. Orders by merchants Flerl and Wertsch preceded the arrival of Triebner in 1770; the last order filled for the physician E. Thilo is dated 30 August 1764, in the amount of Rth 92/23 (lit. D). For the later history of the settlement, see Jones, *Georgia Dutch*, chap. 7; Wilson, "Halle Pietists in Georgia."

14. De Brahm (de Vorsey, *De Brahm's Report*) included a lengthy and not very original treatise on disease prevalence and causation in his survey of the southern colonies. He clearly belonged to a very different medical tradition and never mentioned the Halle University or the Richter medications by name.

15. All orders are in MAFSt 5 E 4: Lemke and Triebner ordering in 1771, Zubli in 1761. The annual charity shipments from Halle are in Wilson, "Die Halleschen Waisenhausmedikamente," table 1, and ran to about Rth 150 per year.

with older Halle medications and/or with the full Richter text, several dozen copies of which had been shipped to Georgia in the period to 1765. As part of the Ebenezer clergy, Triebner probably could draw on the continuing annual orders placed at the disposal of the Halle ministers. Additionally, he placed a small order in drachms and other prepackaged dose units for *essentia dulcis* and some of the "old" Halle medications (the B list); these were chemiatric powders like *pulvis solaris* and *p. niger* and *p. stomachica*.

The orders by Timothy Lemcke and Reverend Zuebli were quite large but dissimilar. Zuebli was at this time in Savannah as the head of a large congregation, but Lemcke's interest is less clear. He may have taken over the practice of the deceased physician Thilo or may merely have sold the medications to other lay practitioners or patients. He ordered an assortment of seventeen items, in most cases about half the volume of the standing charity shipments from Halle, but still not a trivial amount. One-third was in prepackaged multiple doses, and again we find a small amount of B-list items. Apart from the popular chest electuaries compounded from traditional botanicals, these, like Triebner's orders, were remedies of the chemiatric school; the *pulvis laxans* in particular was a calomel preparation no longer on the standard or A list. Zuebli's orders from Savannah were somewhat smaller but still too large for personal use. On all orders, the *essentia amara*, a mixture of bitter herbs, and *pulvis contra acredinem*, which mixed crushed oyster shells with red currant juice, were matched by the *pulvis bezoardicus* and *antispasmodicus;* both were diaphoretics containing antimony and mercury, respectively. Small amounts of two other chemiatric preparations, *pulvis vitalis* and *p. niger*—two strong and expensive tonics also popular in the Pennsylvania orders—were ordered in unit packaging.

Lay orders other than those by clergy and the few merchants with established credit were rare in Georgia for the period up to and following the War of Independence, when internal dissent and alternating occupation by the British and regular and irregular revolutionary forces severely damaged the cohesion and economic health of the settlement and its surviving German settlers.[16] The situation stabilized during the 1790s, however, and as in Pennsylvania, money from old bequests continued to accumulate in the Georgia accounts at the Foundations. The request from Halle to reduce some of this surplus by renewed book and medication orders led to a few large-scale lay imports of the Halle medicines into the new environment of the plantation South. It is in these orders that the

16. Wilson, "Halle Pietists in Georgia."

persistence of lay medical traditions again becomes obvious. The volume of the orders suggests that most were intended to supplement existing domestic or other remedies in a climate marked by endemic malaria and other southern diseases.[17]

There is no record in Georgia of indigenous or newly arrived German practitioners during the postrevolutionary period, a surgeon from Prussia called Holzmann being one exception. Because of their poor fit with the slave-owning plantation society that made up most of early antebellum Georgia, the rural German settlements were probably not considered attractive places of practice. The link to the settlers' legendary past as religious refugees from Catholic Salzburg is clear from the continuity of the names on the order list,[18] as is their continued use of German for domestic, including medical, routines. Both males and females ordered for their own households.[19] Of twenty-five people ordering from Halle in 1892, four were women placing their own orders, of whom two ordered the abbreviated Madai-Richter manual in German and one also in English. Three orders for the manual by men (all asking for the German editions) were placed, as well as orders for a number of individual flysheets. The twenty-one men ordered a total of seventy-one items or 3.4 items on average; women ordered fifteen items or 4.7 items on average, all in unit packages. Here, by far the front-runner among all orders was *balsamus cephalicus*, an ointment containing balsam of Peru and numerous essential oils in a mixture of suet; one man ordered as many as eighteen jars. Next in rank was an unidentified red powder (possibly the *pulvis antispasmodicus*, which was similar in composition to Glauber salts and is described as a *pulvis ruber* in the Halle Orphanage formularies),[20] followed by the *essentia amara* and *e. dulcis*—the latter ordered twice as a remedy against headaches. The only item not from the Richter list was Schauer

17. Cinchona bark had been urged on the settlers against the wishes of the pastors and the local physician from Halle since the 1750s by new arrivals from Augsburg, including Captain de Brahm. For the southern disease environment, see Savitt and Young, *Disease and Distinctiveness in the American South*; Krafka, "Medicine in Colonial Georgia." See Wilson and Poeckern, "A Continental System of Medical Care," for the disease perceptions in the Salzburger community.

18. Jones, "German-Speaking Settlers in Georgia," lists all the names on these lists. Most were the children or indirect descendants of the original settlers. For the view that the decline of the first Pietist-sponsored settlement in North America should be attributed to the population's continued use of German, see Jones, *Georgia Dutch*. Roeber, *Palatines, Liberty, and Property*, has a somewhat more enlightened view of assimilation versus mutual acculturation. I argue (most recently in "Land, Population, and Labor") that the main reason for this decline and the ensuing marginality of the Georgia German group was not language but the inability to fit into the plantation economy of the South.

19. All orders are in MAFSt 5 B 4, 1802, "*ad* Item 23."

20. See Schneider, "Geheimmittel und Spezialitäten," 33–34.

balm, a famous ointment often sent as a gift and possibly for resale during the early years of the settlement by its Augsburg manufacturer, who had been a patron of the Salzburgers.[21]

The largest single order came from a Mrs. Johanna Lackner née Schubdrein, with a total of ten items from the standard list, some in multiple units. Christian Israel Heit asked for a German *Arzeneybüchlein* (most likely the Madai *Brief Account*), but preferred to build his own chest from local wood. A brother and sister of Salzburger descent asked for a "16-Dollar" chest and two manuals, apparently ranking the standard items from an old text for their own purposes: "[T]heir order is for items of particular popularity. Their preference is for bals. cephalicus (*Balsambüchsen*), ess. dulcis, ess. amara, pil. polychrestae, pulv. bezo-ardicus and antispasmodicus, as well as contra acredinem, and small amounts of pulvis vitalis and solaris."[22]

Overall, the preferences of this group of lay German users at the end of the century were not all that different from those observed for earlier lay orders from Pennsylvania, with the possible exception of the *balsamus cephalicus* and the popular red powder. Whether the ingredients of the *balsamus cephalicus* were effective in the relief of fever symptoms or whether the remedy was used for other purposes is difficult to judge. Of greater interest is the fact that these orders reflect a continuing tradition of the use of Halle medications beginning in the 1730s, although by 1802, the isolation of the German communities in Georgia and their economic dependence on Savannah were in sharp contrast to the large and still expanding German medical market in the middle colonies.

Pietist Women in the North American Medical Market

In all lay orders, the presence of women ordering directly and on their own account is noticeable. As noted in Chapter 5, correspondence with Halle frequently refers to the ministers' spouses and widows as engaged in the Halle pharmaceutical trade.[23] The Halle Orphanage medications specifically addressed

21. Beisswanger, *Arzneimittelversorgung im 18. Jahrhundert*, 158, describes Schaur balm as a well-known arcanum manufactured in Augsburg since the seventeenth century and sold as a panacea.

22. The person transmitting the order—probably the then minister of the congregation, Bergman—highly recommended for future contact another established Salzburger, a Captain Kogler, who ordered six boxes of *bals. cephalicus*, as a "homo varii ingenii" who already owned one of the Richter or Madai texts. Johann Kogler was the son of one of the original Salzburger settlers.

23. For New England, see Gevitz and Sullivan-Fowler, "Making Sense of Therapeutics"; also Duffy, *The Healers*; Murphy, *Enter the Physician*.

female complaints and were offered as specific and potent remedies. The access of Halle spouses and widows to these trusted and reputable female medications should have increased their standing among pregnant women and among those needing help in childbirth and its aftermath.

The linkage of philanthropy to medical care by and for women in the Pietist and other Lutheran settlements of North America thus deserves closer examination, even given the obvious limitations of the data. As throughout this volume, we must rely on the available record, in particular the diaries and correspondence of the German-American clergy, to gather information on the personal involvement of clerical spouses and their circle of women. This record exists at two levels, both produced by men: the journals recording the daily performance of the office of the minister, and the personal and business correspondence with Halle and England.[24] In the Georgia mission, made up of a small and relatively stable congregation, it was the minister's duty to trace every man and woman's road to salvation; in addition, the colonial patrons in Germany and England specifically and continually demanded a wide range of demographic and morbidity data relating to marriages, births, and deaths.[25] In populous Pennsylvania, the elder Mühlenberg's letters are more oriented to the larger set of political problems, although the ministerial mandate to report on deaths, births, marriages, and funerals is observed in his journals.[26]

In both sets of accounts, female leadership and agency are hidden behind a discourse reflecting gender and class hierarchies and overt lack of financial authority and accountability.[27] Until mid-century, the Georgia diaries are full, often to excess, of the minister's Pietist concern for women in terms of their state of salvation, physical and spiritual health, and church discipline and as Christian

24. To my knowledge, there is no comparative study of the reporting from Pennsylvania and Georgia over time. In Georgia, where the shift of reporting duties among the senior pastor and his vicars to 1765 is well known, a generational change becomes clear with the assumption by a new vicar, Christian Rabenhorst, of record keeping in the 1750s. The extant congregational journals of the younger Pennsylvania ministers, in particular the Mühlenberg sons and J. H. Helmuth and C. F. Kunze, have not been published or evaluated on a systematic basis.

25. For the interest in American mortality data recorded by Anglican and Congregational clergy, see Cassedy, "Church Record Keeping and Public Health in Early New England"; and Estes, "Therapeutic Practice in Colonial New England."

26. Tappert and Doberstein, *Journals of Henry Melchior Mühlenberg*. It is well known that all Halle mission diaries underwent rigorous edition and emendation before publication for the Pietist audiences in Europe and North America. See Tappert and Doberstein, op. cit., introduction; Jones and Wilson, *Detailed Reports*, vol. 18, introduction; Wilson, "Public Works and Piety."

27. For the layered Pietist rhetoric of female conduct on the American side of the Atlantic, see Wilson and Nolte, "Diary of a Country Parson."

agents of successful marriage and community life in the Lutheran tradition. The crucial but anonymous labor input by local women into agriculture and silk culture is given much attention, and the reliance on widows as independent labor is stressed in the tradition of the Francke institutions. The Georgia diaries thus provide a richer, if one-sided, picture of female roles than do the reports from Pennsylvania. The wives of the clergy and the local physicians were by virtue of their marriages of superior social status; their health, therefore, was presumed to be more fragile and consumed considerable attention in the medical correspondence with Europe.[28] Thus, we have accounts of ill health from North America, and diagnostic and treatment advice from Halle, concerning the female complaints of Mrs. Boltzius. But if it were not for the occasional revealing reference, we would have little idea that German silk culture in Georgia was led almost single-handedly by this minister's wife, a Salzburger refugee, and that she provided midwifery services in competition first with an Indian-French woman and later with a male accoucheur coming from Savannah.[29]

In Pennsylvania, the Pietist clergy from Halle had married women in German-American Lutheran communities to cement congregational relationships and to build networks. In many cases, these led to strong and lasting partnerships, and some led to the provision of medical care. Wives and widows of parsons and vicars were frequently mentioned as ordering medications and intending to conduct a pharmaceutical retail business. Two Mühlenberg daughters, Maria Katharina and Margareta Henrietta Kunze, both ordered medicines on behalf of their mother and on their own.[30] The wife of Friedrich August Mühlenberg came from a merchant family, ran a store in the country at Trappe (New Providence) in the 1780s, and counted on supporting herself and her husband by selling medicines and books from Halle. Before them, the widowed Mrs. Handschuh obtained support from Halle and the moneys owing from an inheritance through the vehicle of the Richter medications. But here again, silence reigns as to the specifics and scope of their involvement in medical practice, and

28. Wilson, "Die Halleschen Waisenhausmedikamente"; Wilson and Nolte, "Diary of a Country Parson."
29. For a summary of Mrs. Boltzius's silk culture as reported by a knowledgeable neighbor, see Wilson, "Public Works and Piety."
30. MAFSt 4 C 1 contains a letter by letter from J. C. Kunze in Philadelphia of 3 December 1774 (received in Halle 18 January 1775, fol. 309), confirming that recently arrived shipments were being sold rapidly, the medications through his wife in the absence of his mother-in-law, and the books commissioned to two merchants in Lancaster.

whether they ordered medications for resale only or offered them to women as part of domestic practice. As in Europe, this may have reflected discretion in view of competition from other healers. The German newspapers in the middle colonies carried a number of advertisements by female healers.[31] Because the Mühlenbergs were a tight-knit family and compendious letter writers and left behind a family clan of astonishing size, we find recurrent accounts of the same events, usually quite laudatory, in particular of the women involved. A good example in more ways than one is the famous story of the older Mrs. Mühlenberg's terrible burns, attributed to a fall during an epileptic seizure, which in turn was attributed to a female complaint.[32] She was nursed and restored to health by her daughter Maria Katharina Mühlenberg, who seems to have been an extremely competent caregiver.

Overall, however, we do not have much in the way of diaries and other correspondence for North American clerical spouses that would equal the diaries of Elizabeth Drinker and of Thatcher Ulrich's Maine midwife,[33] or the patient diaries and letters that recent writers in Europe have used to reconstruct some of the mental states of the eighteenth-century female patient.[34] There are numerous accounts by Moravian women in North America, but they relate to the settlement of new American communities and not specifically to the division of labor in medical care.[35] But as elsewhere in this study of transatlantic philanthropy, we can pick up the thread visible through the occasional half-sentence occasioned by the Halle business interest and follow it to its source. This interest, apparent in many of the specific orders summarized earlier, offers as well some access to the woman as patient exercising preferences and choices for medications during pregnancy, birthing, and postnatal care.

31. One is mentioned by Meier, *Early Pennsylvania Medicine* (136–37), and a Dr. Brandt is mentioned by Bell, *Colonial Physician*, but for neither is there any supporting material. That female healers and herbalists and midwives abounded is attested to by Mühlenberg, who lumped the potential Halle competition into "chymicis, galenicis, et foemina generis, etc."

32. Although not a scholarly work, one of the best sources for the Mühlenberg women is a family history by Wallace, *The Mühlenbergs of Pennsylvania*. See p. 265 for Mrs. Kunze. For Mrs. Mühlenberg's complaint and the professional care provided by her daughters, see ibid., 217ff. Mrs. Mühlenberg's epileptic fits were attributed to fury of the womb, a standard eighteenth-century diagnosis.

33. Forman Crane, *The Diary of Elizabeth Drinker*; Ulrich, *A Midwife's Tale*.

34. For European accounts of patient mentalities, see Lachmund und Stolberg, *Patientenwelten*; Duden, *Geschichte unter der Haut*; Lane, "The Doctor Scolds Me."

35. Some of them mined by Fogleman ("Herrnhuter Frauen and Moravian Women," in *Hopeful Journeys*) and Smaby (*Transformation of Moravian Bethlehem*). Christine Hucho is making a similar study of Schwenkfelder women.

First, the charity orders to North America and almost all the special orders specified the *pilulae polychresta*, usually in combination with fortifiers. None of the orders for a standard chest specifically excluded them. The materia medica orders from Georgia by the two resident medical men, Thilo and Mayer, both contained generic and specific orders for emmenagogues.[36] Thilo's orders do not name the *pilulae polychrestae*, although they came as part of the regular charity shipments. One early order by Heinrich Melchior Mühlenberg included a quantity of castoreum (*Bibergeil*) ordered for a male friend. In Georgia, however, there are a large number of small orders (a total of eighty-five) placed by laymen and -women in 1802, which contained only four requests for *pilulae polychrestae*.

The structure of the demand for the Richter medications by and for women in the middle colonies is illustrated by several orders that Anna Maria Mühlenberg placed beginning in 1774. The matriarch of the Mühlenberg family herself came from an enterprising family of some means, and it would be surprising if she had been less actively involved in her husband's business affairs than her European-born opposite number in Ebenezer or her English contemporaries in Pennsylvania. Her orders may have been placed through her husband, or on his return by her son Gotthilf Heinrich Ernst, or by her daughters. Her larger orders coincide with increases in credit from Halle and an apparently promising market, similar to the pattern observed for her youngest son after the Revolution.[37] Two orders placed in 1774 were in fact very substantial, the first running to almost 1,000 lot or 500 oz troy, the second to 636 lot or 318 oz troy, almost all in dispensing units sizes such as vials, packets, and individual doses. Both included the entire standard or A list of the Richter medications, but the second one included as well seven items from the older or B list (see Tables 6.3 and 6.4). In both orders, the *pilulae polychrestae* were actually ordered in relatively small quantities, while demand for the *pulvis vitalis* was extraordinarily high in view of its price (running to about 600 doses in one order and 360 in the next one, plus 144 doses of the *pulvis solaris* from the B list). The *essentia amara* and *e. antihypochondriaca* and the *pulvis antispasmodicus* ranked at the top in order of weight, while the *essentia dulcis* and the *pilulae contra obstructiones* ranked first and second, respectively, in order of total value. The total value in pounds

36. One of the orders from Georgia discussed in Chapter 7 requests $^1/_2$ lb *spc. emmenagogae* (MAFSt 5 E 2, fols. 129–30).

37. Reported first in Wilson, "Die Halleschen Waisenhausmedikamente." One Rth 1,000 order for books and medicines was crossfiled in MAFSt (Georgia) 5 E 7: 69–73. Orders by Gotthilf Heinrich Ernst Mühlenberg are reported also in Chapter 7 of the present study.

sterling for the A-list orders in 1774 was almost £ 100 sterling, or twice her husband's annual stipend. Mrs. Mühlenberg's last available order from the Halle records, placed in 1795—seven years after her husband's death—involved much smaller but still substantial quantities, possibly designed for her own use or that of her family other than her son Gotthilf Heinrich. In her 1795 order, the *essentia dulcis* outranked all other medications in terms of monetary value, followed by the *pilulae polychrestae* and *pilulae contra obstructiones*.

In view of the indications for use provided in the *Höchst-nöthige Erkenntnis* (and the Madai *Brief Account*), the emphasis in her orders and traditional practice reflect items intended for or demanded by women in labor and during and after pregnancy. The *essentia amara* served among other uses as a blood purifier to be taken together with the *pilulae polychrestae* once or twice weekly. The *essentia hypochondriaca* was recommended for fury of the womb and for women with hysteric passions, and the *pulvis antispasmodicus* to relieve excessive bleeding and menses. It should be noted, however, that a cathartic, the *pilulae contra obstructiones*, was ordered in amounts that were well above other laxatives and medications for intestinal distress. Interestingly, Mrs. Mühlenberg and later her son did order several antiseizure medications, among them the *pulvis niger*.

The Mühlenbergs were at that time resident in Philadelphia, where a large and competitive pharmaceutical and provider market existed. Absent specific mention of who functioned as a midwife in her circle, we have the choice of assuming that she or one of her daughters was present at lyings-in and there dispensed these fortifiers and aids to promote labor or attenuate labor, or sold medications to expectant mothers or one or more midwives in her circle. In terms of pain relief, we note again that substances containing opium, often prescribed by qualified physicians of the period, were not part of the armamentarium reflected in her orders, nor was the famous Hoffmann's anodyne (*sine* or *cum* opium).

Potent Medicines for Women

Recent work on the history of pharmaceuticals in reproductive health permits us to examine these questions in ways more appropriate to the eighteenth century than were the tender consciences of nineteenth-century medical historians.[38] Modern ethnographic approaches that focused on the marginal groups providing or using female medications and their stigmatization have been criticized

38. See Riddle, *Eve's Herbs*, chap. 8.

Table 6.3 Three orders for Halle Orphanage medications by Anna Maria Mühlenberg (A list)

Medication (Latin)	Medication (English)	1774 (Order 1) (drachms)	1774 (Order 2) (drachms)	1795 (drachms)	Total Weight, Each Substance (drachms)	Total Value, Each Substance (Reichsthalers)
Essentia dulcis[a]	Sweet essence	200	150	100	450	113
Essentia amara	Bitter essence	720	480	80	1,280	53
Essentia antihypochondriaca	Spleen-opening essence	840	560	80	1,480	62
Pilulae polychrestae	Pills of many virtues	188	100	80	368	46
Pilulae contra obstructiones	Antiobstructive pills	336	336	80	752	94
Pilulae purgantes	Cathartic pills	64	32	80	116	15
Pulvis contra acredinem	Powder against acrimony	128	64	—	192	6
Pulvis antispasmodicus	Antispasmodic powder	840	560	160	1,560	65
Pulvis bezoardicus	Bezoar powder	312	144	40	496	22
Pulvis vitalis[b]	Life-giving powder	36	22	—	58	40
Balsamus cephalicus	Balsamic nerve strengthener	84	40	40	164	41
Total value, each order, Rth		287	198	73		557

NOTE: Weights are standardized to drachms for purposes of comparison. The *pulvis vitalis* was ordered in packets of 12 doses per packet. See Table 3.3 for unit sizes and prices. The Reichsthaler at 24 groschen and rounded to the next Thaler. Rounding errors not corrected.
SOURCE: Missionsarchiv Franckesche Stiftungen (Abteilung 4, Pennsylvanien), 4 D and G.

[a] Both orders in 1774 also contained orders for 2.5 oz. *ess. dulcis concentrata* each, or a total of Rth 40.
[b] Ordered in packets of 12 doses, the dose at 4 grains or 0.24 gram.

Table 6.4 Three orders for Halle Orphanage medications by Anna Maria Mühlenberg (B list)

Medication (Latin)	Medication (English)	1774 (Order 1)	1774 (Order 2)	1795	Total Value, Each Substance (Reichsthalers/Groschens)
Pulvis solaris (doses)	Golden powder	—	144	144	12
Pulvis laxans (lot)	Softening powder	—	10	10	4
Pulvis niger (doses)	Black powder	—	6	12	6
Pulvis stomachicus (packet)[a]	Stomach powder	56	40	30	8
Pulvis uterinus griseus or nigricans (doses)	Gray or black uterine powder	—	—	20	10
Tinctura salina (lot)	Saline mixture	—	90	—	15
Tinctura corallina (lot)	Coral tincture	—	48	10	9
Electuarium antiphtisicum (lb)	Lozenges for phtisis	—	6	6	12
Total value, each order, Rth		4	42	31	77

SOURCE: Missionsarchiv Franckesche Stiftungen (Abteilung 4, Pennsylvanien), 4 D and G.
NOTES: Orders shown in original units. Weights not standardized because of the wide range in dose and unit sizes. See Table 3.4 for dose weights, prices, and unit sizes, in particular for the various powders, which were usually ordered in multidose packets of doses ranging from 1 grain (*pulvis niger*) to 4 grains (*pulvis solaris*). Reichsthaler at 24 groschen and rounded to the next Thaler. Rounding errors not corrected. Prices calculated from Madai, *Brief Account*, 1784, and Richter, *Kurzer und Deutlicher Unterricht*, 1705.

[a] Packet at 3 doses in these orders.

as insufficiently generalizable to everyday practice.[39] Attention has instead turned to the whole range of reproductive medicine as more relevant to social and medical history than are instances of draconic punishment or legal misogyny.[40] On the other hand, there are now occasional and intriguing attempts to identify the possible effectiveness of botanical and chemical agents in preventing conception or interrupting pregnancies.[41]

Depending on the locus and source of advice, the advocacy or use of many medicinals reflected not only the intent to forestall or terminate unwanted pregnancy but as well the physiological and therapeutic understanding of the era and the nonspecific action of many substances.[42] Midwives, surgeons, physicians, or herbalists were recognized and consulted for their knowledge of fertility problems and the dangers implicit in spontaneous abortion, delayed labor, and expulsion or extraction of a dead fetus or afterbirth.[43] In the early eighteenth century, when the medicalization of pregnancy was still of relatively recent origin, even the intrusion of demographic concerns eventually had some beneficial effects on the mother's life. These included a fuller and more general medical awareness of serious adverse effects, questionable outcomes, and the indiscriminate use of powerful drugs.[44] We have only limited work on this subject in North

39. See, for instance, Jütte, "Die Persistenz des Verhütungswissens."

40. Kinzelbach, *Gesundbleiben* (258), mentions the practice among registered midwives of administering "treibende Medizinen." The work of Adrian Wilson on English midwifery contains similar references for the seventeenth and eighteenth centuries, as does the work of Walzer Leavitt for the latter part of our period (A. Wilson, "Seventeenth Century Childbirth," 33–37; Leavitt, *Brought to Bed*, 38). I have not read Wilson's fuller treatment (*Childbirth*). For the active role taken by attending nonmidwives in the North American urban setting, see Murphy, *Enter the Physician*, 33–37.

41. Riddle, *Eve's Herbs*; Leibrock-Plehn, *Hexenkräuter*. The latter is particularly valuable for an index that examines, from a biochemical perspective, the possible levels of efficacy and untoward adverse effects of the trove of medications, usually of botanical composition, that persisted into the eighteenth century and beyond. The jury is out on rates of effectiveness, but Leibrock-Plehn's work, which owes much to Erika Hickel's pharmacological historical experiments, is proof, if such is needed, that adverse effects had to be common and often debilitating or lethal in view of the preparations used. See also Lindemann, *Health and Healing in Eighteenth-Century Germany*, 346. None of these concerns of course were new, and they are reflected in the relative openness of the classical authorities cited by Riddle, *Contraception and Abortion*, particularly chap. 8, and, for the early Middle Ages before the reception of Arab medicine, chap. 9.

42. See, for example, Estes, "Pharmacology of Nineteenth-Century Patent Medicines."

43. For the complex questions involved, see the review of Riddle, *Eve's Herbs*, by Monica Green, *Bulletin of the History of Medicine* 73, 2 (1999): 308–11.

44. Lindemann, *Health and Healing in Eighteenth-Century Germany*, chaps. 4 and 5; a similar picture evolves, if from a different perspective, from the analysis of Friedrich Hoffmann's materia medica by Lanz. As noted by most historians of the early modern period, pregnancies not carried to term and not resulting in an infant that survived to baptism are almost impossible to enumerate.

America before the end of the eighteenth century, but there can be little doubt that similar considerations applied.[45]

In the case of the Richter medications, we can investigate some assumptions beyond the dichotomy of positive law and presumed practice. It is difficult to imagine that the Halle Pietists, under intense scrutiny by orthodox Lutherans in positions of medical and religious authority, would have openly violated the Christian consensus against abortion of a live or quick fetus. And indeed, this issue is not raised in the manifold anti-Pietist polemics of the early eighteenth century, although by that time the entire set of Richter medications and their effects and uses had been fully developed and described. The 1710 edition of the *Höchst-nöthige Erkenntnis* insisted that the *pilulae polychrestae*, the most explicit offering in the medicine chest for opening the womb and restoring the menses, and for cleaning the womb in the case of spontaneous abortions, "are a highly desired and strong medicinal in particular for women: For they open the uterus [*die Mutter*] and restore the missed monthly cleansing, if use is resumed at the appropriate time and continued as long as necessary. For such a condition, once rooted in the organ [*eingewurzelt*], cannot or may not be resolved at once or even by excessive doses."[46]

In other words, the *pilulae polychrestae* were justified for a number of acknowledged gynecological problems, although the ingredients (lesser centaury, fumitory, black hellebore, gentian, pistacia lentix resin, hedera, aloe, myrrh) could have made them suitable for abortion, given large enough doses and other promoting circumstances. A prescribed dosage in the 1715 edition of the *Höchst-nöthige Erkenntnis* was eighteen to twenty *pilulae polychrestae* of one grain each. At least three medications offered as part of the Richter medicine chests can be classified as containing *drastica* promoting violent physiological reactions; to the knowledgeable, their ingredients, all botanicals, were recognizable as abortifacients.[47] This was the case in particular for the components of the *pilulae contra obstructiones*, a panchimagogue extract containing colocinth, agaric, and black hellebore, but also of the similarly constituted *pilulae purgantes* and the *elixir polychrestum*. The Richter text specifically recommended only the *pilulae polychrestae* and the *elixir polychrestum* for restoration of the menses and similar uses, and the elixir was not part of the standard offering. In the 1715 edition, even use of the

45. Riddle, *Eve's Herbs*, chaps. 7 and 8.
46. *Höchst-nöthige Erkenntnis* (1710 edition), 759.
47. Leibrock-Plehn, *Hexenkräuter*. chap. 7. I rely in the following on her work and testing procedures and on my own translation of her German nomenclature.

pilulae polychrestae was considered counterindicated if chronic menstrual problems and signs of internal bleeding were present.

However tempting it may be to unravel these implicit or even explicit practices, too much concentration on the presence of actual or presumed abortifacients in the Richter offerings would misinterpret their place in the medical literature.[48] The *Höchst-nöthige Erkenntnis* was not a seventeenth-century herbal transmitting classical and medieval botanical and other knowledge, nor was it a midwifery text. Rather, the second part of the text stood in the tradition of the pharmaceutical dispensatory (*Arzneibuchliteratur*), although adapted to a set of proprietary medications. Among many other topics, it contained suggestions, recipes, cautions, and recommendations that addressed specific morbid conditions in all potential patients, male, female, adult, and child.[49] In general, this literature made some mention of the need for medications promoting expulsion of a dead fetus, but these recommendations were a small percentage of overall advice. And in the Richter scheme, all medications, except for the *pilulae polychrestae*, were recommended for multiple purposes in males and females, some specifically for pediatric use, with cautions and specific doses provided for both children and adults.

Also, none of the botanic *drastica* were in fact new medications in terms of names or ingredients.[50] Their likely effects, if not their precise compositions, would have been well known by the persons ordering them. The often-noted caution that warnings against strong abortive effects should be read as reverse advice may apply here as well, but it would be difficult to argue that the Richter text was quite as matter of fact and abundant in contraceptive and abortifacient advice as many of the female herbals of the early modern period. Four of the

48. The term *abortefacient* does not appear either in the Richter text or in any of the orders, reflecting in all likelihood the legal distinction between restoration of the menses and abortion, which was well established since the time of Soranus. See Riddle, *Contraception and Abortion*; idem, *Eve's Herbs*, 37.

49. For the nosography or classification of diseases offered in the *Höchst-nöthige Erkenntnis*, see Savacool, "Illness and Therapy." For this genre and its gynecological advice and materia medica for female complaints, see Leibrock-Plehn, *Hexenkräuter*, chap. 2.4. In many ways, the *Pharmacopoia medica physica* by Johann Schroeder and its many editions and revisions is a good example of and precedent to the Richter manual, in particular because Schroeder's work had been available in the vernacular since 1685 and was not an official pharmacopoia. Schroeder described the expulsion of the dead fetus as a morbid condition and offered a large number of suitable substances to ensure proper termination; despite the author's chemiatric leanings, only four out of thirty were chemiatric preparations (Leibrock-Plehn, *Hexenkräuter*, 62).

50. See, for instance, Lanz, *Arzneimittel*, 151, for Friedrich Hoffmann's practice and its precedent. See also Riddle, *Eve's Herbs*, and Leibrock-Plehn, *Hexenkräuter*, chap. 2.

most prominent and original medications in the Richter armamentarium were recommended for use as tonics and fortifiers during and after labor. This ambivalence, I argue, suggests both the actual eighteenth-century practice and the scope of the intended audience. A few examples may serve to illustrate the range of implicit and explicit advice that the Richter text offered to the potential user or provider:[51]

Item 8. [Concerning the] essentia dulcis . . . a most potent medication and often exhibits a quick effect, but at the same time safe and entirely free of harm. It strengthens nature, increases vigor, etc., and is a general strengthener in all diseases. . . . [Item 12] It . . . exhibits a peculiar gift in suppressing and *ameliorating pain* [*Stillung und Linderung*] and to induce sleep, including *antispasmodic* action. . . . Item 15. It is good for pregnant women to reduce *premature strong motion of the fetus in the last 6 weeks,* and similarly for delivery and post partum problems, who receive the benefit [unspecified] quickly and safely. . . . To be taken or administered also in cases of spontaneous abortion, where it alleviates symptoms and after-effects such as hemorrhages, retained afterbirth, arthritis, all three cases of gout (chiragra, gonagra, podagra). . . . Even in cases of contractions, use should not be discontinued but interrupted if pain is excessive and later resumed.

(p. 756) The essentia antihypochondriaca is in particular recommended against melancholy emanating from the spleen, menstrual difficulties, maternal problems, Epilepsy uterina.

(p. 758) Pilulae polychrestae are . . . for women, opening the mother, and promoting return of menses if use is started at the appropriate time; however, the problem is difficult to resolve if loss of menses has become chronic. The medication is also recommended for symptoms after a stillbirth, and during delivery to stop excessive flow of blood. Daily use during confinement is recommended.

Item 73. Pulvis vitalis promotes motus vitales or natural movements and strengthens. Safe and without side effects, to be used by all. Promotes light sweat and strengthens. Good for fevers, small pox, scarlatina [*Frieseln*], red and white fluxes where it quietens cramps and promotes excretion of noxious stools. Also helps against scurvy, venereal diseases, and all putrid sores and boils and fistulae.

51. All extracts are from Richter, 1715. My translation.

Item 81. Balsamus cephalico-stomachico-nervinus. . . . Ointment serves for apoplexy, fainting spells, dizziness, against noise in the ears. Topical application, with heat where indicated. For colics and for women in labor as well.

Item 94 ff. Elixir polychrestum. Laxative to be taken for all fevers, and leading to diarrhea after 8 or ten hours. . . . Specificum for . . . *obstructiones mensum.*[52]

Table 6.5 summarizes these and other selected Richter medications for the whole range of female medications in terms of recommended use. Columns 2–4 show the range of indications based on the Richter text. There is in fact little if any overlap, suggesting some selectivity. Column 1 lists the same medications in terms of their content—that is, having ingredients recognized as emmenagogues in women's herbals and midwife manuals of the early modern period.[53] The two medications specifically recommended as emmenagogues in the Richter text qualify for this list, as does the *essentia hypochondriaca,* which was also considered a major remedy for afflictions of the spleen in males.

Orders from Halle between 1731 and 1802 suggest that demand encompassed the entire range of medications shown in Table 6.1, although there were shifts within the three groups. Whether these were due to preferences by the consumers or their providers (in one case, Gotthilf Heinrich Ernst Mühlenberg; for his orders, see Tables 7.1 and 7.2 below) cannot be stated with any certainty because we lack information on the relative demand for local over imported substances. However, in the following chapter, we can gain some insight into the dispensing rationale that evolves from the journals of the younger Mühlenberg and discern some factors of price and availability of substitutes in the former colonies. In his first attempts during the Revolutionary War to replicate the Halle armamentarium,[54] Gotthilf Heinrich Mühlenberg had mentioned the *elixir Hoffmani,* a Helmontian preparation "contr. haemorrh., fl. uteri et fluor album (Helmont)," and an unspecified "essentia emmenagoga Halensis." An entry in his journal as early as 1782 listed an emmenagogue ("Pillen für Frauenzimmer,

---

52. Emphases added.

53. Leibrock-Plehn, *Hexenkräuter.* Her scheme does not take into account chemiatric medications, which in contrast to the ancient botanical lore seem to be rarely mentioned in midwifery and similar texts.

54. Gotthilf Heinrich Ernst Mühlenberg, journals and diaries, M 892, vol. 2, American Philosophical Society.

Table 6.5 Halle Orphanage medications classified by their use in reproductive medicine

Containing Substances Recognized as Emmenagogues in Women's Herbals and Manuals		Recommended for Restoring Menstrual Flow and Related Problems in Richter Texts		Recommended as Fortifier During Labor, for Protection of Fetus, and During and After Labor in Richter Texts		Recommended in Cases of Female Complaints and Excessive Bleeding	
Latin	English	Latin	English	Latin	English	Latin	English
Pilulae contra obstructiones	Antiobstructive pills			*Essentia dulcis*	Sweet essence	*Essentia anti-hypochondriaca* (in particular, fury of the womb)	Spleen-opening essence
Pilulae polychrestae	Pills of many virtues	*Pilulae polychrestae*	Pills of many virtues	*Pulvis vitalis*	Life-giving powder	*Pulvis antispasmodicus*	Antispasmodic powder
Pilulae purgantes	Cathartic pills			*Pulvis solaris*	Golden powder	*Pulvis uterinus griseus or nigricans*	Gray or black uterine powder
Pulvis Laxans	Softening powder			*Balsamus cephalicus*	Balsamic nerve strengthener		
Elixir polychrestum	Elixir of many virtues	*Elixir polychrestum*	Elixir of many virtues				

SOURCE: Based on the composition of the Richter medications according to Poeckern, on their indications in the *Höchst-nöthige Erkenntnis*, 1715, and on the classifications in Leibrock-Plehn, *Hexenkräuter*.

wenn die menses verstopft sind") as one of twelve necessary items for a domestic medicine chest. When his own wife suffered from a pain in the right side in
1786, he described her as having missed her menses and as possibly pregnant
and prescribed daily doses of several mild Halle preparations for the relief of
gastric discomfort, an additional weekly dose of asafetida (*assa foetida*) or polychrest pills, together with physical exercise and a blood-cleansing diet to restore
circulation and lift the spirits. Similarly, in 1788, when reflecting on what medicines to prepare at home from local substances rather than order from Halle,
he led off his list with "pills which purify the stomach and the blood and have
a similar effect as the pilulae polychrestae."

In his orders from the last decade of the century, he at first maintained the
preferences suggested in his mother's orders by but changed them over time.
Among the medications for female complaints, the *essentia hypochondriaca* was
eventually eclipsed by the *pulvis antispasmodicus* by the end of the century. The
so-called fortifiers or tonics (*essentia dulcis ordinaria, pulvis vitalis, balsamus cephalicus*, and *pulvis solaris*) were present in his orders to the mid-1790s, but by the
end of the century, only the *essentia dulcis* remained a steady and, considering its
price, a large-volume item. The *pilulae polychrestae*, except for a particularly large
order in 1794, remained at a constant level throughout the decade 1790–1800,
although below the amounts ordered by his mother in the 1770s. Among the
other preparations containing substances recognized as emmenagogues, only the
pilulae contra obstructiones remained an important item ordered from Halle
throughout, and these may well have been used as laxatives pure and simple.

As for other illnesses and complaints, German women in North America
who used one or the other of the Richter medications for the problems of pregnancy could find in them accessible, familiar, and, so they might hope, safe and
reliable remedies. We do not know the hidden numbers behind this use and can
only speculate on the specific uses to which some of these medications were put.
The increased concern with bearing children to term, which is reflected in the
advice tendered in midwifery books and domestic medicine texts by the end of
the eighteenth century,[55] does not appear in the Richter text, which belonged
to an earlier and apparently more pragmatic tradition. That women providers
and patients in the German-speaking communities may have circumvented the
new medical trends is suggested by some of the German imprints in North

55. Many of these sources are cited in Murphy's detailed study of American domestic medicine,
Enter the Physician, chaps. 1–3 in particular for our period. She does not refer to any but English-speaking women, however.

America at the end of the eighteenth century.[56] Several of those titles figure prominently in the early modern secrets literature and herbals.[57] These may have offered a reservoir of recipes not previously available and outside the strictures (and possibly the reading comprehension) of English-language male physicians and accoucheurs in North America. Also, newer European midwifery texts published after the 1790s and a younger generation of European practitioners from Central Europe and England may have changed gynecological practice by the end of the century, although the presence of women at birthings remained an important feature of rural community life until well into the nineteenth century.

Again, for the lay public demanding medications from the Halle Orphanage, considerations of price seem not to have been decisive. The *pulvis vitalis*—but not the *essentia dulcis*—was replaced over time, but the equally expensive *pulvis solaris* was substituted instead. Given the general lack of explicit sources, it is difficult to decide whose preferences are expressed in the orders from North America. What is indisputable, however, is that to the extent that the German female patient in colonial and early republican North America knew of and could obtain Halle medications, she had little need to rely on unknown English proprietary medications but could order reputable and potent German medicines if she was willing to pay the price.

56. Cowen and Wilson, "Traffic in Medical Ideas."

57. Eamon, *Science and the Secrets of Nature*; Leibrock-Plehn, *Hexenkräuter oder Arznei*, both referring to Eucharius Rösslin and Jakob Rueff (Ryff), but also the apocryphal Albertus Magnus books of secrets. See Leibrock-Plehn, op. cit., chap. 5.1, 4, and p. 171. Emphasis on the magical and ethnographic aspects of these texts (see, for instance, Brendle and Unger, *Folk Medicine of the Pennsylvania Germans*) has until now prevented a closer look at this component of *secreta* advice coming across the Atlantic. See Cowen and Wilson, "Traffic in Medical Ideas," although again, we should not presume that information on birth control and abortion was the only material of interest they presented.

7

Men and women of European descent in North America in the eighteenth century still relied on and drew from the central traditions of Western medicine. Within this framework—deriving from humoral pathology and its explanatory schemes—medical practitioners used and mingled a range of therapies depending on their training, cultural origin, and religious bias and the expectations and financial ability of their patients. Among these, the practices of some Germans trained in the Halle way did indeed suggest some features of a gentler—if not necessarily more effective—medicine.[1] In pharmaceutical terms, a number of the Halle medications departed from seventeenth-century and early eighteenth-century practice in significant ways, despite their continued reliance on traditional botanicals and mineral compounds, including mercury and antimony derivatives. Most notably, opium and cinchona bark had been rejected by Stahl and his followers and remained excluded from

1. This proposition is above all advanced by Habrich, "Zur Ethik des pietistischen Arztes im 18. Jahrhundert," and idem, "Characteristic Features of Eighteenth-Century Therapeutics," and by Richard Töllner, who has recently devoted a symposium to this subject ("A Gentler Medicine," symposium on the occasion of the 200th anniversary of the founding of the Halle Orphanage pharmacy, Halle, April 1998).

the ingredients of the remedies making up the standard Halle medicine chests. The formula of the star of the Halle offering, the tincture of gold or *essentia dulcis*, seems not to have changed over the course of the eighteenth century, but by the 1740s, iron filings and less toxic chemicals had begun to replace crude antimony and mercurous chloride and other chemiatric byproducts of the early preparations. However, these substances did remain part of the medicinals sold individually, including the chemiatric byproducts of *essentia dulcis* manufacture, such as the *pulvis niger*.

On the other hand, many of the botanical components were both traditional and hardly gentle in effect. We must therefore rely on the choices and preferences of the providers of Halle medications for the claim that the major Halle medications—for the indications and in the dosages recommended—may have been among the safer remedies available in North America.

A Gentler Medicine and Some of Its North American Practitioners

In the first decades of the eighteenth century, some students of Stahl—in particular J. S. Carl and J. Juncker—had gone beyond their teacher in seeking a gentler medicine and proposed a selective use even of the Halle medications. Juncker's student in Georgia, Ernst Thilo, was in fact accused by his clerical superior of biting the hand that fed him and the settlement by refusing to dispense the Halle medications.

Although Thilo's medical frugality may have been based on a number of not entirely medical reasons, his extant orders for materia medica provide a fascinating illustration of selective pharmaceutical practice. Despite his frictions with the motherhouse, he benefited from his status in the Ebenezer community and from female patrons in the Francke family to order fairly large amounts of supplies directly from Halle, particularly after the arrival of several hundreds of new German settlers during the period 1749–52.[2] Both Thilo and his substitute and sometime competitor, Johann Ludwig Mayer, apparently a surgeon from Swabia, placed regular orders for materia medica with Halle in addition to the supplies of the Richter medications that were sent over, as in Pennsylvania, on the charity. These orders have no parallel in the Pennsylvania correspondence, because the network of drug outlets there would have counterbalanced any

2. Wilson, "Die Halleschen Waisenhausmedikamente"; Wilson and Poeckern, "A Continental System of Medical Care."

financial gain from shipment through Halle. They permit an interesting base on which to judge at least in part how claims for a gentler medicine carried over into daily practice.

We have four lists drawn from the Georgia accounts for 1749 to 1759, making up a total of roughly seventy-five items of materia medica, including items from the Halle list and those named for their therapeutic indications (general mixtures such as *spec. emmenagogae* and *ess. anthelminticae*).[3] The sixty-item order of 1749 filled by the then head of the Halle laboratory, Schulenburg, had a total value of Reichthaler (Rth) 54 and contained only ten items from the main Richter list. To provide a measure of size, orders for various materia medica, both vegetable simples and *composita*, ranged in quantity from two pounds (twenty-four oz troy) of *sal. tartari* and one pound of *tinctura antimonii* to one drachm (one-eighth oz) of *tartar emeticus*. The use of the materials for drug preparation in Thilo's own laboratory, for which he had previously ordered and obtained a portable Becher furnace and other materials,[4] is apparent from the orders for containers (100 each at one and one-half lot) and 200 cork stoppers.

The Richter medications in the 1749 order included *ess. dulcis concentrata* (two lot), *ess. dulcis ord.* (six lot), and *ad oculos* (two lot), two orders (one-quarter of a pound and one pound) of *ess. amara*, twelve lot of *ess. antihypochondriaca*, and three lot of *balsamus cephalicus*. A smaller but more expensive order filled in July 1751 (for a total of thirty-one items) contained eight proprietary products, but these included both Hoffmann's anodyne liquor (noted as *sine* opium) and two preparations by Thilo's teacher Juncker (balsamic pill mass and a stomach liquor). None of the items on the Thilo lists was unknown to the trade, but some interesting differences appear when his preferences are compared with a later and much larger order by volume and number of items. This order was sent by former Army Surgeon General William Brown to Apothecary General Craigie when Brown contemplated the establishment of a joint medical and pharmaceutical supply trade in the 1780s. The most intriguing fact about the Georgia lists is the general lack of opium, ipecac, iron, and cinchona and only one specification for mercury in four orders, compared with at least five different mercury preparations ordered by Brown.[5] Overall, the materia medica used

3. MAFSt 5 E 2, fols. 13, 115–16, 125, 129. Quantities are as stated in the orders.
4. MAFSt 5 E 7 (4), fols. 160–61.
5. Based on Cowen's comparison of the Georgia orders with Brown's much larger order (these are published in Cowen, "The Letters of William Brown to Andrew Craigie"). As elsewhere, I am much indebted to David L. Cowen for this information. The mercury order from Thilo is for *mercurius dulcis*

by this Halle disciple corresponds to Brown's armamentarium in less than 25 percent of items.[6]

The documented distaste of some of the Southern medical community for Halle preparations,[7] although most likely based on the desire for professional control rather than on the community's own more beneficial and effective practices, may in part reflect these differences in materia medica. The refusal to use cinchona bark in an environment endemic with malarial fevers may have contributed to the disdain for Halle practice. On the other hand, opposition to smallpox variolization, a tenet of Stahlian medicine, was medically well supported until the latter part of the century.[8] We have two additional examples of Thilo's tendency to rely on course of nature. He was opposed to bleeding, particularly in cases of physical depletion, and refused to bleed the vicar at Ebenezer in 1745 as he lay dying from consumption, much to the dying man's and the senior minister's chagrin. Ten years later, he refused to administer drastic remedies in a lengthy and recurring eye problem suffered by the senior minister. After a long period of impairment, the problem eventually resolved on its own, and sight was restored. Thilo was credited with having used the correct treatment, although in fact he had treated as little as possible.[9] However, relative benefit in outcomes, cost, and safety of the regimens followed in North American German communities would be difficult to demonstrate except in a few instances. Halle practitioners situated in a more densely populated medical market than rural Georgia tended to conform more closely to prevailing practice and to patient expectations.

In Pennsylvania, there was some indication of gentler tendencies at least with regard to sparse venesection in two practitioners from Central Europe,

---

or mercurous chloride, or calomel (Lanz, Arzneimittel, 197). One possible exception to the exclusion of opium is a theriac (specified on the list as *theriacus coelestis Junc.*). A similarly named electuary by Hoffmann, described as an arcanum by Lanz (206), did contain opium, which Hoffmann in contrast to Stahl used frequently.

6. Although some of the differences may be due to changes in the materia medica over the twenty years elapsed between these orders (for example, Lewis observed in his 1753 *Dispensatory* that both earthworms and ants were no longer used in English practice [13 and 155]). But there is no obvious wholesale shift away from traditional materia medica in either Brown's or the Georgia lists.

7. An order placed by the Ebenezer minister, Bergmann, in 1802 (MAFSt 5 B 4, fol. 77) noted that " the physicians in town [Savannah] refuse to tolerate the sale and use of Halle medications. [One] Christopher Gugel therefore asked for placement of an order for 18 boxes of balm [*balsamus cephalicus*] demanded by patients who had fared well with this medication in cases of rheumatism and gout."

8. Duffy, *Epidemics in Colonial America*, chap. 11; Waring, *Medicine in South Carolina*, 38ff. See also Geyer-Kordesch, "Fevers and Other Fundamentals."

9. See Jones and Wilson, eds., *Detailed Reports*, vol. 18; entries for January 1745; MAFSt 5 B 3, 4 C 8, 1754–55.

George de Benneville and the so-called Schwenkfelder doctor Abraham Wagner, who were both trained in radical Pietist communities. De Benneville, whose training in the circle around Samuel Carl and Gerhard Tersteegen can be considered proved, left an American medical testament, the *Medicina Pennsylvania*, which is still largely oriented to chemiatric practice.[10] It contained a large number of standard antimony, opium, and mercury preparations, although the author repeatedly advised extreme caution in the use of these remedies and careful observation of patients suffering from adverse effects such as salivation.

As reported by his biographer, Abraham Wagner's daybook and dispensatory, *Remediorum Specimina ex Praxi A. W.*, begun in 1740, was full of references to favorite Halle medications, including bezoard powder and polychrest pills, *balsamus* and *pulvis vitalis*, and even items long since dropped from the Halle lists, such as *spiritum discutiens*.[11] Wagner was not averse to crude antimony as an emetic and for dysentery and inflammatory enteric conditions prescribed small doses of laudanum (opium) and an older theriac (*theriac andromachus*). But mercury is indeed singularly absent from his list except as an external ointment for the "itch." His framework relies to a large degree on nosography and therapy derived from family precedent, including his great-grandfather, a Silesian apothecary and *medicus* named Georg Hauptmann, and his American patron, Georg Hubner. His preparations in many instances, such as the *Lebenspulver*, parallel the Halle medications, and Wagner seems to have been quite familiar with the Richter family before coming over in 1737.[12] We do not know whether he dispensed or obtained any of the Richter preparations at the often-quoted but apparently apocryphal "Halle storehouse" in Philadelphia. Because of his religious affiliation, he could not have been part of the Halle mission trading system. But Wagner was obviously a competent pharmacist and *medicus* and occasionally supplied small amounts of materia medica to the elder Mühlenberg.[13]

10. The manuscript is at the College of Physicians in Philadelphia. See Savacool, "Illness and Therapy."

11. The manuscript was used by Berky, *Practitioner in Physick*, but this author could not locate it at the Schwenkfelder Library, its original depository. Wagner's nomenclature, however, indicates that he was also familiar with the armamentarium used by Friedrich Hoffmann. See Lanz, *Arzneimittel in der Therapie Friedrich Hoffmanns*.

12. See Berky, *Practitioner in Physick*, 82ff., for Wagner's medical background and library. For Wagner's own account, see KM 2:69, Letter 137, Wagner to Mühlenberg. The similarity in medications and names observed in this instance supports the assumption by Wilson, "Traffic in Halle Orphanage Medications," that the Halle armamentarium in fact picked up older remedies with slight modifications.

13. KM 2: Letter 177, 22 June 1757. Unfortunately, Berky's material is poorly documented, and the translations are suspiciously modern in some instances. That Wagner was not generally considered

In terms of clinical practice and training, Wagner, Thilo, and de Benneville were the most highly trained of German colonial physicians. They were experienced practitioners with a known grounding in the materia medica and some of the pharmaceutical trends then current. Even the limited evidence we have of their therapeutics and prescribing suggests that American physicians trained at the end of the early modern era tried to combine their theoretical insights with changing paradigms and their ethical mandates with clinical decisions.[14] Wagner and de Benneville remained outside the framework of the Francke Foundations and had no financial incentives to sell the Richter medicines. Thilo very consciously, and in conflict with his patrons, was a reluctant provider at best. But for the clergy trained at the Halle motherhouse and confident of its reputation, demand for the Richter medications was difficult to ignore when Halle sent charity shipments, outsiders copied them, and trade offered financial rewards not otherwise available. We see these forces influencing therapeutic choices in several generations of Halle practitioners, from the unquestioning assumption of the superiority of Halle medicine and medicines by Heinrich Melchior Mühlenberg in the 1750s to the more complex and ambiguous pattern observed for his son G. H. E. Mühlenberg. His practice patterns were no longer in accord with the tendencies of the Juncker school. Apart from any influence of his training at Halle in the 1760s, that is well after Juncker's death, they illustrate the slow adaptation of an American practitioner to the exigencies of the colonial and postcolonial medical market.[15]

---

a mere druggist by his colleagues and in fact enjoyed a considerable medical and personal reputation is clear from his complex and detailed will, in which he left one-third of his considerable estate (well in excess of £1,000) to be distributed to the poor through a number of surviving associates. He died in 1763. The bequests included a donation of £20 to Pennsylvania Hospital, and he forgave his impecunious patients their book debts, incoming moneys to be added to the charity trust.

14. Admittedly, this is a small group owing to the absence of daybooks or similar material from contemporary German physicians in North America, but it yields some insight into the vexing question of actual practice decisions and may support some cross-cultural comparison in the American setting. See Estes, "Therapeutic Practice in Colonial New England."

15. For his practice, this study can draw on two parallel sources: his large and exceptionally well-documented orders placed with Halle during the 1790s and beyond, and a series of journals that are part of his large written legacy in the United States. The journals are in the Papers of Heinrich Gotthilf Ernst Mühlenberg, American Philosophical Society, in particular vol. 2 of signature M892. The excerpts here do not include material from his botanical journals seen by Maisch, "Mühlenberg als Botaniker," in the same depository. The journal is undated and unpaginated, and most dates, including years, given here were added by a different hand.

An American-Born Practitioner of Pietist Medicine

Gotthilf Heinrich Ernst Mühlenberg was the American-born and Halle-trained son of Heinrich Melchior Mühlenberg. Born in 1753, young Mühlenberg was sent to Halle for schooling in 1763, by which time the generation of Stahl and his students were gone. Both Juncker and Carl died in the 1750s, the Halle medical school underwent a serious period of decline,[16] and its links with the Orphanage had become frayed. G. H. E. Mühlenberg returned to North America in 1770 at the age of seventeen with his near contemporaries J. H. C. Helmuth (b. 1745) and J. C. Kunze (b. 1744). Although not receiving a call to North America through the usual Halle procedures, he was ordained by the Ministerium led by his father and almost immediately took over several New Jersey congregations. In an age when intellectual precociousness was not a rarity, he overcame whatever intellectual and personal obstacles his youth and lack of experience may have posed to his position and authority and started his research into American plants and their usefulness as materia medica even while in this first New Jersey call. His father recommended him to Halle as a good *oeconomus* and sober mind. And so he indeed proved to be. He was without doubt the most extraordinary, in terms of scholarship, of the Mühlenberg sons and an internationally known natural philosopher among his own German-American cohort, which included recognized scholars like Friedrich Melsheimer. American accounts of his medical practice have taken a backseat to those involving his father, both for reasons of accessible documentation and the general lack of work on the second generation of Pietist pastors.[17]

His journals and daybooks begin in 1777 and extend to the 1780s.[18] They show him immersed in the attempt—apparently with some, but limited, success— to reproduce Halle and other European medications, using available materia medica and local herbs and a large number of recipes and formularies he had

16. Seils, *Friedrich Albrecht Gren*, quoting Conrad, *Statistik der Universität Halle*.
17. The work of Glatfelter and Roeber cited in this volume being notable exceptions.
18. Volume 2, M 892, American Philosophical Society. I have tried to be as faithful as possible to Mühlenberg's terminology while translating German names into English. His nomenclature is mixed Latin and German, with American plants designated in Latin or English (for example, Carolina pinkroot). Some of the German names may be regional variants, such as "Gagrille." Where possible, I have used eighteenth-century translations as provided by Lewis in a 1768 edition of the Edinburgh dispensatory (see Cowen, "The Edinburgh Pharmacopoeia") and the following later sources: Brookes, *General Dispensatory* (1807); Dunglison, *A New Dictionary of Medical Science* (1839); J. Redman Coxe, *The American Dispensatory* (1806).

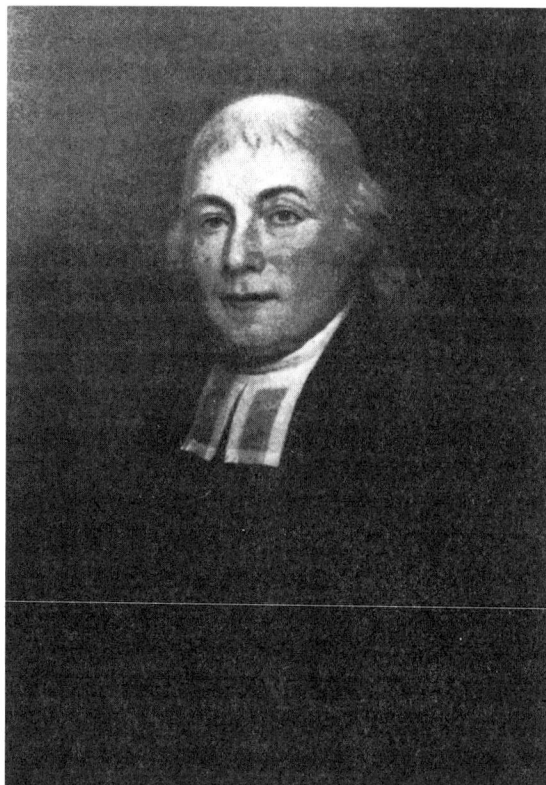

Fig. 7.1

Gotthilf Heinrich Ernst Mühlenberg (b. 1753 Trappe, Pennsylvania, d. 1815 Lancaster, Pennsylvania), youngest son of Heinrich Melchior Mühlenberg, student at the Halle Orphanage and the Friedrich University. From 1780, Lutheran minister in Pennsylvania and New Jersey, and eventually an eminent American botanist. (Courtesy, Pastor Frederick S. Weiser.)

brought back from Europe.[19] At the time, he served in New Hanover outside the British lines, separated from Philadelphia and its medical resources. In the last weeks of August 1777, he wrote down his own suggested list for a domestic medicine chest (*Vorschlag zu einer Hausapotheke*), which included twelve items not dissimilar from the Richter list, although using only a few of its names. Topped by a safe laxative and emetic, he listed a calming remedy against shock or rage (*niederschlagend Schreck oder Zorn Pulver*) and one to stop turbulence or the excessive flow of blood; a good stomach powder, especially for children; pills for women to restore the menses; a remedy against obstructions; a strengthener (he preferred an anodyne liquor); an antidiarrhetic or gastric sedative (he

19. A long recipe, apparently from memory and European sources, tries to recreate the *Pil. poly-chr.[esta] Halens.[is]*.

preferred the *tinctura salina*); a remedy against coughs and chest complaints; an *essentia amara*; and a remedy against the chills and cold fevers. His intent to include local herbs is suggested by comments on a plant used by Indians against dysentery, *sp. apulypia*, which could be given in powdered form or as a decoction.

Although we do not know the extent of his laboratory apparatus at the time and during his later tenure at Lancaster, it is clear that he was involved in some pharmaceutical experimentation and procedures. He attempted to extract salts (*sal fix. alcal.*) from herbs and noted his preference for neutral salts in putrid fevers because oyster shells, chalk, and so on promoted putrefaction. His recipes, in full pharmaceutical notation of the period, include in addition a *pulvis vermifugis laxans* and, notably in view of previous Stahlian practice, an antifever medicine containing ground Peruvian bark and tarwater. Like Friedrich Hoffmann, whose armamentarium he partly incorporated into his own, he considered *sal plantarum* an excellent remedy and speculated that it might be identical with the *sal tartari* of the Richter stomach powder.[20] For his own stomach powder, he noted that he was trying to replicate this medication (*arcanum duplicat.*), by using *tartar vitriolatus, nitrum depuratus*, conch shells, and three to four grains of high-quality cinnabar.[21] A similar process was followed for Richter's common fever powder (*pulvis bezoardicus*), a diaphoretic that had changed composition several times since its early inclusion in the standard offering from Halle.

Despite the strenuous efforts by the *Medikamentenexpedition* to safeguard the composition of its medications from reproduction or imitation, Mühlenberg's closeness to the Orphanage staff during his school days seems to have yielded a range of information. A whole page in his 1777 journal is taken up with generic recipes by the Halle greats, including "elixir Hoffmani, essentia asthmatica, and emmenagoga Hal., pil. contra obstructiones Hal. or aperinthes stahli, Pulvis contra accredinem Halens., . . . Pulvis laxans, and pectoralis Junckeri," and so forth. He thought he could infer the composition of Hoffmann's *balsamus pectoralis* and several of his electuaries, the *essentia dulcis*

20. "The stomach powder, I should think, consists of: Sal tartari or sal plantar—it can't be the former, for it does not dissolve when exposed to air—tartar vitriolatus, Nitr. depurat., Cinnab /or is it the nitrate that is responsible for the right color; del/."

21. Note the insistence on red as the most appropriate color, probably reflecting public expectations based on cinnabar medications. The same composition and nomenclature are attributed to a Hoffmann medication by Lanz, *Arzneimittel*, 188. It appears that the generally accepted division between Stahlian and Hoffmann's materia medica and their arcana in particular was not maintained in the practice at the Orphanage pharmacy by the latter part of the century.

and a *tinctura salina* after Teichmeyer, as well as the famous Richter *essentia amara*, from "among those Halle medications known to me, particularly from the Dispensatorium Brandenburgito."[22]

These fragmentary attempts of a European-trained rural clergyman practicing medicine indicate some of the problems of prescribing during a period of scarcity in pharmaceutical supplies caused by the Revolutionary War. Local medicinal herbs abounded, and many were known, but American botany and classification were still in the trial stage. Indian remedies passed on from the early colonial period, like *janaceto*, an herbal tea taken by G. H. E.'s wife on her own, were used but had unwelcome effects (excessive heat in this instance). Minerals like potash and tartar salts and other pharmaceutical supplies seem to have remained available locally, but imports of European medicines with reasonably predictable effects had as good as ceased. When they returned to North America in the 1780s, Mühlenberg reincorporated them into his practice, depending on availability and local preferences, but leading to a heady mix far removed from therapeutic abstinence. It seems that the Richter medications now regained an indispensable but by no means exclusive place in his armamentarium and that with few exceptions English patent medicines had not taken their place.

Botanicals remained Mühlenberg's overriding interest, both those available only in North America and species common to both continents. He continued experimenting, adding pennyroyal to the Richter *pulvis bezoardicus* for the alleviation of coughs and bronchial complaints in children. He laxated his child with rhubarb and tartar emetic in a case of unspecified eczema with fever, but used as well mint tea and millefolia to calm the system. When he used "Gagrillenthee" mixed with Carolina pinkroot as an anthelmintic, this caused a heavy and acid vomit, which he improved with "my own tinctura salina, restoring appetite and bowel movements." He used this tincture in other cases of excessive acid, particularly to restore appetite (giving one-half teaspoon as a gentle laxative for a small child). He treated his own eczema on lips and nose with an ointment of sugar of lead and sugared mercury (*mercurius sacharatus*), following laxation.

---

22. Whether this was in fact possible is difficult to ascertain. Poeckern, *Die Halleschen Waisenhausarzeneyen*, notes that when the recipe books were retransferred to the Orphanage Foundations in 1840, several entries were defaced, in particular the composition of the *essentia amara*. Mühlenberg's library is no longer extant, but if he had a copy of the Brandenburg dispensatory, it would be among the first copies in this country. I thank Glenn Sonnedecker for this information and other valuable and critical suggestions.

His recipes contained numerous traditional herbs like sage and Saint John's wort, but it is unclear whether he used extracts or how he prepared his botanical mixtures. His materia medica included much cinchona bark, which he like others at the time considered an excellent bitters or tonic against fevers, the fluxes, extreme heat, and epilepsy.[23] He mixed it with Hoffmann's *liquor mineralis* and Sydenham's liquor to produce an effective and mild diaphoretic, which acted both as fortifier and antispasmodicum similar to the common *essentia solis* (also an older Richter medication with similar indications). One remedy against toothaches was made of locally available botanical substances, here a *pursicaria* plaster.

More generally, and despite the inclusion of numerous new herbs, he did not ignore the traditional regimen of heavy medication combined with changes in diet. Finding himself with a painful stomach complaint and constant salivation, G. H. E. set about "restoring nature's balance by taking 12 pil. c. obstructiones in four doses with sweetened tea, afterwards a mixture of Cortex peruv. and roots and cortex aureum, with 2 glasses of table wine," adjusting his diet to consume more vegetables and less meat, and adding bitter herbs like chicory, dandelions, and *hierarium*, and proposing travel and a change of scene. During periods of seasonal fluxes (*Ruhr*), he collected *asclepias tuberosa* and *veronica spicat* "to prescribe this for people after proper evacuation." But he also prescribed initial doses of four grains of Ipecuhania [*sic*] and then ipecac and rhubarb, followed by dried root of *A. tuberosa* in a decoction to be taken three times daily.

In the case of a thirteen-year-old boy who had intestinal cramps and pains in the side and had already taken ipecac and rhubarb, he added three Richter *pilulae contra obstructiones*, followed on the next day by twenty grains of scurvy grass in a tea of yarrow (*millefolia*). When his son was sick with diarrhea from eating too many cherries and exhibited a lot of abdominal noise, he treated less actively, giving a mild emetic and fortifiers like mint and cinnamon. One dose of *pilulae polychresta* had no effect, as on previous occasions, nor did antidiarrheals (*stopfende Dinge*) such as *pulvis solaris* with Saint John's wort (*hypericus*). Suspecting hydrops or edema despite contrary symptoms ("no swelling of the head, but swollen glands"), he considered administering *tinctura hyperici* mixed with *Ciruviam* and some *sal tartar.*, as well as *pulvis niger, solaris*, and *vitalis*, and some stomach powder from the Halle repertory.

---

23. See Estes, *Dictionary of Protopharmacology.*

After trade with Halle had been restored in the 1780s, financial considerations (lack of species, difficulties in having drafts accepted in Europe) began to play a more prominent role in the choices exercised by what must have been one of Halle's best-informed clients in North America. Mühlenberg contemplated restricting his orders, noting that he had made a special observation about the polychrestum pills in a letter to Halle. In 1784, he considered his future and the steps to be taken to ensure a measure of financial security. These included much attention to agriculture on his own land, and the following medical component:[24]

> 1. Have a store of medications and dispense them. I will have, in addition to those for venereal diseases (*ausser den Gallischen*), tinctura salina, red powder, and liquor mineralis und tartar emeticum, and dispense these with the best herbs. A good bitters for the stomach is necessary, best made of gentian, orange peel, lavender, and several extracted oils. As it is, I hardly make enough use of my knowledge of herbs (*Kräuterkenntnis*). I also should *prepare* (emphasis added) some of the following: pulv. antispasm., bezoard., stomachalis, Tincturae amara, corallina, salina.

On 1 March 1788,[25] he even concluded that he should limit the medications ordered from Europe to those needed for himself and his family. By 1791, however, the date of his first large order, these doubts had proved short-lived. G. H. E. Mühlenberg now summarized the advantages for continual medical practice including the Richter medications as follows:

> 1. It yielded profit from the sale of medications bought in large quantities, in particular the *emetica* (unidentified but probably the *pulvis bezoardicus* and the *pulvis polychrestus*), the *pillulae contra obstructiones* and *polychresta*, the *essentia dulcis*, the *pillulae purgantes*, and so on.
> 2. Practice brought him into contact with the people in the vicinity and afforded the opportunity to make friends. However, a few changes in dispensing strategy were indicated:

24. These observations are in vol. 2 of M 892. We find no specific mention of the ongoing plans for Franklin College, but the changing scope of the author's medical dispensing may well have been affected by these plans, which brought their own difficulties. The College was founded in 1787 but suffered from a lack of funds from the outset, which was remedied only much later.

25. This passage is at the end of the second third in vol. 2, M 892.

"a. I should collect the best herbs I can find here, cut them into small pieces, and dispense them. This will also afford a good opportunity for my family and myself to get some exercise; I will prepare a register for the best plants: Trifolium fibro, Hypericum, millefolium, polygala senega, adranum, polypodium, cunida geranium, and oleum Ingl.

"b. Then purchase from local sources several items in quantity, including pinkroot, ipecacuhana, jalap, rhubarb, tartar emetic, forco stennes.

"c. Prepare several tinctures on my own for use in labor, stomach liquor, anodynes, and distribute the Halle medications singly rather than in bulk (*mehr einzeln austheilen*)."

This general plan was complemented by a more specific list of necessary items with separate indications for children and women:

1. Pills for cleaning the stomach and purifying the blood that resemble the pilulae polychresta in their effect.
2. A good stomach powder of the Halle kind for which I can use a good sal medicum;
3. A powder against the heat, antispasmodicus.
4. Pulvis bezoardicus for catharal fevers.
5. A good emetic and expectorant (*Auflösungspulver im Stickfluss*) after the Halle pulvis polychrestus (*ad mod pulv polychrest*).
6. A powder for children according to the pulvis contra acredinem (*Magn. albumantim*).
7. Drops against sore throat and cough in children: Learicoram, several herbs, geranium with mint oil.
8. Drops against uterine pains (*Mutterweh*) or hysterical attacks: Hoffmann's or Sydenham's anoydine liquors at 10 grains in oleum menthe.
9. Something to calm early labor and post partem pain (*wilde Wehen und Nachwehen*).

How these plans fared in practice is suggested in Tables 7.1 and 7.2. Amounting to an almost continuous ten-year series, the tables show standing and revised orders placed by G. H. E. Mühlenberg from 1791 to 1801 from both lists of the Richter medications and offer some insight into changes in demand.

Table 7.1   Selected orders for Halle Orphanage medications, by Gotthilf Heinrich Ernst Mühlenberg, 1791–1801 (A list)

| | Medication (English/Latin), in drachms | | | | | | | | | | | |
Year	Sweet Essence (Essentia dulcis)	Bitter Essence (Essentia amara)	Spleen-Opening Essence (Essentia anti-hypochondriaca)	Pills of Many Virtues (Pilulae polychrestae)	Antiobstructive Pills (Pilulae contra obstructiones)	Cathartic Pills (Pilulae purgantes)	Powder Against Acrimony (Pulvis contra acredinem)	Antispasmodic Powder (Pulvis antispasmodicus)	Bezoar powder (Pulvis bezoardicus)	Life-Giving Powder (Pulvis vitalis)	Balsamic Nerve Strengthener (Balsamus cephalicus)	Total Value Each Order (Reichsthalers)
1791 (Order 1)	100	120	160	120	100	40	40	240	120	15	24	102
1791 (Order 2)	80	—	—	100	50	—	—	200	120	8	—	60
1794	140	40	120	200	100	20	—	160	40	6	10	95
1795	100	80	80	80	80	20	—	160	40	—	40	72
1796	140	80	80	60	80	20	—	160	40	—	10	72
1798	200	120	—	60	40	—	—	240	40	—	—	77
1799 (Order 1)	200	120	80	80	80	20	—	160	40	—	10	92
1799 (Order 2)	200	120	—	80	80	—	—	320	40	—	20	96
1801	250	120	—	80	100	—	—	320	40	—	10	108
Total weight, each substance, in drachms	1,410	800	520	860	710	120	40	1,960	520	23	124	776
Total value, each substance, in Rth	353	33	22	108	89	15	2	82	22	18	31	

SOURCE: Missionsarchiv Franckesche Stiftungen (Abteilung 4, Pennsylvanien), 4 D 2, 3, 4, and 5.

NOTE: Weights are standardized to drachm (except for *pulvis vitalis* [doses]) for purposes of comparison. The *pulvis vitalis* was ordered in packets of 12 doses of 4 grains per packet. See Table 3.3 for unit sizes and prices. Reichsthaler at 24 groschen and rounded to the next Thaler. Rounding errors not corrected.

Table 7.2 Selected orders for Halle Orphanage medications, by Gotthilf Heinrich Ernst Mühlenberg, 1791–1801 (B list)

Year	Medication (English/Latin)										Total Value, Each Order, Rth
	Golden Powder (Pulvis solaris)	Softening Powder (Pulvis laxans)	Black Powder (Pulvis niger)	Powder of Many Virtues (Pulvis polychrestus)	Stomach Powder (Pulvis stomachicus)	Gray or Black Uterine Powder (Pulvis Uterinus griseus or nigricans)	Elixir of Many Virtues (Elixir polychrestum)	Lozenge for Phtisis (Electuarium antiphtisicum)	Saline Mixture (Tinctura salina)	Coral Tincture (Tinctura corallina)	
	Packet at 12 Doses	Lot	Packet at 12 Doses	Packet at 12 Doses	Packet at 12 Doses	Packet at 12 Doses	Lot	16 oz	Lot	Lot	
1791 (Order 1)	30	10	2	10	—	20	20	20	40	40	79
1791 (Order 2)	20	10	1	—	—	10	—	—	—	—	21
1794	40	10	4	—	—	20	10	6	—	—	57
1795	40	10	1	10	30	20	20	6	—	10	62
1796	20	10	4	—	30	20	—	4	—	10	52
1798	—	—	1	—	30	20	—	6	10	10	19
1799 (Order 1)	30	6	1	—	30	—	—	4	—	10	33
1799 (Order 2)	30	—	1	10	30	20	—	—	10	10	45
1801	—	—	1	—	40	40	—	—	10	10	28
Total value, each substance, in Rth	105	11	64	15	48	85	25	46	12	16	426

— No orders.
SOURCE: Missionsarchiv Franckesche Stiftungen (Abteilung 4, Pennsylvanien), 4 D 2, 3, 4, and 5. Monetary values in Reichsthaler, based on Madai, *Brief Account*.
NOTES: Orders shown in original units. Weights are not standardized because of the wide range of unit, packet, and dose sizes. See Table 3.4 for dose sizes and prices, in particular for the various powders, which were usually ordered in multidose packets of doses ranging from 1 grain (*pulvis niger*) and 1/4 grain (*pulvis polychrestus*) to 4 grains (*pulvis solaris*). Package sizes as given in the orders. Reichsthaler at 24 groschen and rounded to the next Thaler. Rounding errors not corrected.

As noted, the *pilulae polychresta* and *contra obstructiones* remained steady after 1794. The *pilulae purgantes*, by contrast, were ordered only four times after an initial large order in 1791. Orders for the *pulvis bezoardicus* continued throughout but decreased substantially after two large orders in 1791 and 1794. Of the items on the B list, the *pulvis solaris*, the Halle stomach and uterine powders, and the expensive and aggressive *pulvis niger* remained in some demand. Orders for the *essentia hypochondriaca*, a botanical emetic and spleen opener both for the sedentary patient and for fury of the womb, dropped off after 1796. It did remain part of Mühlenberg's own armamentarium for his own purposes. Finally, orders for the *essentia dulcis* and the *pulvis stomachicus*, although modest at first, increased after mid-decade and remained stable throughout the next five years. The items Mühlenberg scheduled to prepare by himself thus did not fully replace the *pulvis stomachicus*, the *essentia amara*, and Hoffmann's anodyne liquor (probably with opium). The *essentia amara*, a botanical *arcanum*, remained an item ordered each of the years shown. The *pulvis contra acredinem* was apparently replaced by the suggested mixture with white magnesium (*magnesium album*) prepared locally, or else the public had come to prefer the *tincturae salina* and *corallina*. The *pulvis antispasmodicus*, a Halle chemiatric arcanum, remained a large item on the orders throughout. Bronchial tea from Halle (not shown) and the *electuarium antiphtisicum* also remained popular. (The latter was a heavy item, and the large amounts ordered tend to distort any ranking by weight.) The total monetary value of these orders averaged Rth 165 per year, not counting additional orders placed on behalf of colleagues.

We also have some indication of articles remaining on the shelf because of original overstocking. In 1794, these were *pulvis bezoardicus* and *antispasmodicus*, the polychrest pills, and the *pulvis solaris*. Six years later, the items no longer favored were the *pilulae purgantis* and the *pulvis laxans*. By the end of the century, Mühlenberg himself ranked the Halle items by their popularity and relative price and by their appropriateness for the climate and for patients' needs, in the following order:

1. *Essentia dulcis*
2. *Pilulae contra obstructiones*
3. *Pulvis antispasmodicus*
4. *Pilulae polychrestae*
5. Bronchial tea
6. Stomach powder

7. *Pulvis uterinus*
8. *Essentia antihypochondriaca*
9. *Electuarium antiphtisicum*
10. *Pulvis niger*

In all, this rare set of linked data indicates a continuous North American medical practice that combined local remedies prepared on the premises and the special resource represented by the Richter medications. Increases in shipping and insurance charges and general inflation in 1794 were reflected in increased costs for these medications, the effects of which were offset in Mühlenberg's practice by the economies realized in dispensing mixtures prepared from local herbs. The continued preference for older preparations from the Richter armamentarium is of interest, although this may have reflected difficulties in reproducing complex chemiatric remedies under local conditions.

A Rural Practice in the New Republic: Some Measures of Size

Most of Mühlenberg's orders of Halle medications during the 1790s ran to several hundred ounces troy per year of concentrated extracts, powders, pills, and tinctures,[26] outranking even the generous amounts sent to the Georgia community during the period 1754–64, when the *Medikamentenexpedition* had reached its pinnacle of profitability. Mühlenberg did not order materia medica from Halle.[27] What do these orders mean in terms of relative size for rural American practice at the end of the eighteenth century? A few measures in recently published German work suggest some rough indicators of population size and market penetration for the Halle medicinals. The German numbers are based on pharmaceutical inventories in Braunschweig, a German territory with a well-developed and highly regulated apothecary system and dry goods outlets, many selling Halle Orphanage medications.[28] The population in the Lancaster

26. In this and other orders, I have converted the commercial quantity *Quentchen* usually appearing in the orders to the medical term *drachm*. Both are equal in weight, approximately 4 quentchen making up one lot and eight drachms one ounce; see Table 6.2.
27. Conversely, a substantial order placed by the Brothers Marshall, apothecaries in Philadelphia, in 1785 and reproduced by Edward Kremers, "Historical Fragments, No. 22, Two Invoices of 1785," contains no proprietary or patent medicines.
28. Beisswanger, *Arzneimittelversorgung im 18. Jahrhundert*. The orders she reported are drawn from detailed annual inventories. Individual items were similar to the Pennsylvania orders by Mühlenberg, although there is a considerable range. For comparative data, see 13, 156, 122, 269.

catchment area (3,700 according to the 1790 U.S. Census for the town of Lancaster) was approximately of the same order of magnitude as the 1793 population of two small towns and one village in the Braunschweig duchy. Annual income from total prescriptions of all types for the period 1759–60 sold by the three registered pharmacies in these Braunschweig locations ranged from Rth 310 to Rth 180, excluding any over-the-counter sales of medicinals. All three locations had a full spectrum of Halle medications in stock during 1755–60, and the total inventory value in simples and *composita* of the smallest of these apothecary shops ran to just under Rth 500 per year for the same period.[29]

Thus, the amounts ordered by Mühlenberg over the period 1790–1801 seem to have represented, in quantity, value, and market size, a good-sized semirural practice. Many, but by no means the majority, of the items ordered from Halle were in dispensing sizes (packages or paper boxes holding specific numbers of individual doses; for instance, the *pulvis vitalis* came in boxes of twelve doses each). But orders of fifty lot and above were common, and we know from his journals that Mühlenberg had his own laboratory and made a number of medicinals on his own from local materia medica. He made use of these medications for observed or reported patient complaints in a relatively underserved but economically prosperous semirural area.[30] Not all the population in this area of course was German, nor should we assume that all Germans used Halle medications, or that users used only Halle medications. Also, Mühlenberg's clerical contacts reached well beyond the town of Lancaster into surrounding communities.

In therapeutic terms, his orders embraced, throughout, most of the Halle offering. This included the full range of traditional and modified prescriptions available to the general public, both in the standard medicine chests and on the earlier list dating to the beginning of the eighteenth century, which contained a far greater number of items of chemiatric composition. In other words, based on his personal acquaintance with Orphanage practice during his years in Halle,

29. See Beisswanger, *Arzneimittelversorgung*, tables 1, 6, and 12, for the towns of Schöningen and Schöppenstedt and the village of Vorsfelde in the 1790s. According to the author, this pattern is not representative of the large urban pharmacies in Braunschweig, which had a much larger clientele and sales volume but stocked few if any Halle pharmaceuticals. Quantities held by several dry goods merchants in the smaller town of Wolfenbüttel (appendix table 7) are comparable to merchant orders from the Lancaster area, however. Beisswanger points out that the pharmacy inventory reports may not have corresponded to the commercial reality, because it was not known that the physicians on the *collegium medicum* strongly opposed the Halle medications (154).

30. For the economic significance of the Lancaster region during the latter part of the eighteenth century, see Buel, *In Irons*, 108–9.

the younger Mühlenberg did not feel constrained by the framework implicitly imposed by the standard list, set in stone by the 1740s, but added to these from the chemiatric reservoir of an earlier period.[31] Mühlenberg ordered a good-sized amount (twenty lot in his standing order of 1795) of Hoffmann's famous anodyne liquor, which by that time was available through the Orphanage pharmacy.[32] Although by definition all Richter medications still excluded opium, cinchona bark, and ipecac, the older among them still included antimony and mercury preparations that were part of the regimen of many of the most reputable Pennsylvania physicians, regardless of national background and training. Antimony (both crude and *a. factitia*) in particular remained a respected diaphoretic in a number of expensive proprietary medications throughout the period, James's Fever Powder being one example. A small order placed in 1785 by Justus Heinrich Helmuth of Philadelphia consisted of *pulvis polychrestus* (this was an item rarely ordered by the younger Mühlenberg) containing antimony as a sulfide.[33] Tonics used as female fortifiers abounded, and mercury in small doses remained a familiar laxative.[34]

In Mühlenberg's case, in addition to personal and financial incentives driving these sales,[35] he faced a patient population that, as in Germany, might be tempted to turn to imitations (see Table 7.3 for an example) but who continued to show loyalty to known medicinals with predictable effects and a long-standing reputation for potency in serious cases where all other medicines had failed.[36]

31. Preparations in the standard or A list that were composed entirely or mainly of botanical substances outnumbered mineral and chemiatric preparations two-thirds to one-third. On the B list, this ratio was two to ten. See Tables 3.1 and 3.2.

32. These orders place the sale of some of Hoffmann's arcana by the Orphanage pharmacy earlier than assumed by Lanz based on work by Wolfram Kaiser (*Arzneimittel*, 158, note 293).

33. MAFSt 4 C, Helmuth to Fabricius, 14 April 1785. For sales in North America of James's Fever Powder, see Porter and Porter, "Rise of the English Drugs Industry," 280 passim; and Estes, *Dictionary of Protopharmacology*.

34. For this, see Estes, "Changing Fashions in Therapeutics," and the reply by Crellin, "How Shall I Take My Medicine?"

35. See Chapter 5 for the general fit of German-American orders from Halle with general trading trends observed, for example, by Buel (*In Irons*, in particular 246 and 253ff.) from the 1780s onward. In 1806, during the Continental Blockade, from which American shipping from Hamburg was exempt because of the neutral status of the United States, Mühlenberg in Lancaster ordered medications for Rth 3,238/9. MAFSt 4 G 8, fols. 52–53, 1801–7.

36. For these claims in the original Richter manual, see Chapter 3. They are repeated almost verbatim in a letter from Heinrich Melchior Mühlenberg of 3 March 1759 to Theodor Krome in Einbeck (KM 2: Letter 186): "[E]nough common medications are produced here by chymicis and galenicis. However, the message should be that we will produce ess. dulcis, pulvis vitalis, and essentia antihypochondriaca, etc., *for these can cure where other remedies fail*" (emphasis added).

Table 7.3   Advertisement in German in *Neue Unpartheyische Lancaster Zeitung und Anzeigsnachrichten*, 16 January 1788, for ten medications, imitating the format of the Halle Orphanage medications as advertised in Richter and Madai

I. *Essentia vitalis*, . . . das Unzen Glass kostet 3 schillinge.
II. *Essentia dulcis concentrata*, . . . ein mehreres wozu sie dient zeigt der Unterricht. Das lot 4 schillinge.
III. *Essentia amara*, das Lot 1 schilling.
IV. *Spirito anodino-mineralis*, . . . das Lotglas kostet 1 schilling 6 pence.
V. *Sal minerale*, das Lot kostet 1 schilling 6 pence.
VI. *Pulvis antispasmodicus*, Das Lot Glas 1 schilling.
VII. *Pulvis antiepilepticus niger*, vor allem gegen die grosse Not bei Kindern, jungen und alten Personen . . . 3 schilling.
VIII. *Pulvis laxans*, das Schächtlein ist One schilling 6 pence.
IX. *Pulvis contra aeredinem* [sic], das Schächtlein 1 schilling. Gegen rote und weisse Frieseln, Schärfe und Durchfälle des Leibes, Pocken, Masern.
X. *Pilulae laxantes* . . . befreien Haupt und Brust, den Magen und die Gedärme von ihrer Verschleimung und Schärfe. 2 schilling 6 pence das Schächtlein.

Alle Gläser und Schächtlein sind mit meinem Petschaft versiegelt und werden so unversehret ausgegeben.[a]

[a] The insistence on sealed and unbroken containers was one of the major concerns of the producers of arcana or other proprietary medications and is addressed in the foreword to all Richter and Madai editions.

His orders and reflections show that access to Halle—both in terms of knowledge and of resources—was mitigated by two decades of medical experience that had adapted to and used the resources of the American pharmaceutical environment. His reflections on the wishes and interest of his clientele and his parishioners indicate as well that there remained a German public who both maintained and renewed ties to their culture of origin during a period when the American republic took a neutral stance in the European wars of the period.

The Persistence of a Learned Culture: Books and Medicines

The second commercial pillar of the Francke Foundations was a large Bible press and book trade whose products included not only numerous Bible editions and edification tracts but, as early as 1710, famous grammars from Tamil to Estonian produced by Halle's emissaries to the East.[37] On the North American side of the Atlantic, the audience for this print culture was not only layered vertically, by

37. Lehmann, *Es begann in Tranquebar*; Jeyaraj, *Inkulturation in Tranquebar*.

education, financial means, and interests, but, as we have noted throughout, by language. Orders to Halle for German Bibles of all types, hymnals, and edification literature not only persisted but increased, running to several thousand copies annually during the 1790s, their bindings reflecting the growing prosperity of the German-American middle class. In the medical market, the popularity of Samuel Tissot and of the Richter texts, and of subsequent German imprints of much older works, reflects the complexities of nosological and pharmaceutical nomenclature in multilingual societies and the need to encounter familiar remedies described in the vernacular.[38] But there was in addition an upper end of the German market in North America that also insisted on the learned German book to preserve its access to natural philosophy and the natural sciences.[39] This public found an eager supplier—and competitor with the traditional book dealers in Leipzig and Frankfurt—in the Halle trading mechanisms described in Chapter 5 and discriminating agents in their North American clergy.[40]

Throughout the six decades of substantial book and Bible orders from North American clerics and customers of Halle, first through privileged English channels and later through Holland and Hamburg, we find a wide range of works. Until the 1780s, these included the major authors of the Pietist and evangelical movements of the period: Arndt's *Wahres Christentum*, first printed in 1610–40, Bogatzky's *Paradisgärtlein* and *Güldenes Schatzkästlein*, and the canon of Christian works of contemplation and edification in German editions from Thomas à Kempis and Sontholm to Bunyan's *Pilgrim's Progress*.[41] At the educational end of this wide range of offerings were small educational works and spellers for children and current English-German grammars, a German edition of Bayley's work apparently being a popular choice.[42]

---

38. As argued by Cowen and Wilson, "Traffic in Medical Ideas."

39. Cazden, *Social History of the German Book Trade in America*; Roeber, "German and Dutch Books and Printing."

40. Typical is an order by G. H. E. Mühlenberg, which asked that a book order by Merchant Billmeyer in Lancaster be supplemented by "three small chests, half a dozen packs of stomach powder and polychrest pills each, two dozen Greek testaments, and one dozen *Cornelius nepos* (both bound)."

41. Strangely, and despite a long-standing tradition for the edification literature of the seventeenth century, Halle made no attempt even in Europe to translate the newer evangelical writers such as Whitefield and the Wesleys. For the seventeenth century, see Sträter, *Sontholm, Bayly, Dike, and Hall.*

42. MAFSt 4 G 6, fol. 31, lit. B, 1752, Item 6. These were bound in calf. (*Bailey, Nathan, a compleat English dictionary oder vollständiges . . . englisch-deutsches Wörterbuch . . . anfangs von Nathan Baylie [sic] in einem kurtzen compendio herausgegeben, bey dieser 2. Auflage aber um mehr als die Hälfte verm. von Theodor Arnold, ebd,* 1752, 53). A multivolume German edition was apparently first printed in 1736 in Leipzig, followed by 8 eds.

But as early as the 1750s, there are titles suggesting learned and utilitarian inclinations among a necessarily small but influential group of the reading public, regardless of cost.[43] One example is Johann Jacob Schmidt's *Biblius historicum, geographicum, physicum, metem, et medicum*, a well-known, expensive, and learned five-volume work relating physics, geography, medicine, mathematics, and history to the Scriptures.[44] Standing in the early modern tradition of physico-theology, Schmidt is representative of a Scripture-oriented philosophical and philological approach to the new learning of the eighteenth century. This particular work was not in favor with the Pietist motherhouse, but it is not obvious that this was for reasons of theology. G. A. Francke, for instance, rejected a request from Georgia for the medical part of this work, pointing out that it was useless for daily medical practice.[45] In 1753, H. M. Mühlenberg asked for all five volumes as part of a large book order and requested that it be paid from his inheritance;[46] yet another order for two sets came in 1756,[47] and orders resumed after the Revolutionary War. At the end of the 1750s, Handschuh ordered all parts of Ernstling's *Nucleus Totius Medicinae Quinque partes*, a large pharmaceutical dispensary, requested by "a member of the congregation."[48] Several orders for Mosheim's multivolume, latinate, and costly *History of the Church* also date to this period.

43. One indicator of relative consumer preferences is binding and folio size. The range of bindings provided by Halle over time was extraordinary and indicative of the increasing economic stratification of the German communities by the beginning 1750s. Bindings in many cases equaled and often exceeded the actual value of the printed stock. The last order from Pennsylvania before the Revolution was for close to 500 volumes, including a dozen octavo Bibles in leather cases, eighteen Bibles in sheepskin, and seventy-five copies of the six-volume Arndt (*Wahres Christentum*) with copper engravings and a lengthy foreword. Bindings ordered after the Revolution were often as sumptuous, such as gold-leaf inscriptions and saffian bindings for the seventeen-plus-volume edition of the *Predigernachrichten* (MAFSt 4 D).

44. MAFSt 4 G 6, fol. 79, 28 August 1753. A rare discussion of this work in a medical context is by Dehmel, *Arzneimittel in der Physikotheologie*.

45. Wilson, "Die Halleschen Waisenhausmedikamente." In terms of the link between the Scriptures and the new natural history, however, this work was not really at variance with prevailing Pietist views.

46. MAFSt 4 G 6, fol. 31, Item 3.

47. MAFSt 4 G 6, 1756, fols. 113–14, lit. A.

48. MAFSt 4 G 6, 1744–60, fol. 5, no date: Handschuh listed the work with all part titles and provided the following information: "[P]ars 1 continent lexicon et dispensatorium oder vollkommener und allzeit fertiger Apotheker, etc., darinnen alle und jede Stücke so wirklich in den Apotheken zu finden ihrer Gestalt und Gehalt, Herkunft etc auch was daraus zu machen ist, und wird die Composita auf das beste daraus zu bereiten erklärt worden sind dabey auch nach dem Alphabet die Kunstwörter und viele andere Namen mehr folgen. . . . Helmstedt, 1741," sold at Braunschweig und Leipzig in the Meisser bookstore. (See Wolfgang Schneider, *Arthur Conrad Ernstling, Sachsenburg, 1709–1768, Apotheker und Arzt*.)

These new orders added to the stock of works that Halle clergy—and in Georgia, also the medical mission staff—had brought with them to North America. All came equipped with good-sized libraries in which medical texts were prominent.[49] Usually, when medicine chests were ordered from Halle, they were accompanied by either the original treatise by Richter or the condensed treatise by Madai, but also by surgical works. These texts also came across separately in English, French, and Latin translations and at least in the South seem to have preceded the importation of the writings of Tissot.[50] A 1752 order by Pastor Peter Brunnholz, for instance, included six large Richter texts at Rth 5; thirty copies of the Madai *Kurze Nachricht* at 8 gr; and ten small Latin translations at Rth 1/16 each.[51] We have noted Justus Helmuth's concern for precise printed instructions giving dosages in his pharmaceutical orders during the 1780s (see Chapter 5).

The market for popular and traditional German medical texts reprinted in North America exploded in the 1790s.[52] But the reopening of transatlantic shipping also brought an increase rather than a leveling off of learned titles, indicating a smaller but not trivial public with a continuing and informed interest in German developments in natural philosophy and the new sciences. Among the factors influencing choices from the large European offerings in these fields were the intellectual and scholarly preferences of the second generation of Halle agents. Their training was by now out of line with the new schools of theology at Halle, and several among them tended to be highly conservative in political and philosophical terms. Justus Helmuth rejected Thomas Paine as a "knave" and Priestley as equally out of hand.[53] Other Halle clergy were more relaxed and concentrated on the new branches of natural investigation, above all the immense transatlantic scholarly exchange on post-Linnean classificatory schemes

49. For Georgia in 1737, see Wilson, "Die Halleschen Waisenhausmedikamente," who also describes orders for Juncker's periodicals and Schaarschmidt's *Medizinische Nachrichten*. For Pennsylvania thirty years later, in 1764 (MAFSt 4 G 2, fol. 297), new books ran to Rth 36 for a new incumbent, C. E. Schulze, plus freight for his library dispatched from Saalfeld.

50. Tissot, *Advice to the People*. Some mentions of his work relate to German and French editions; see Cazden, *Social History of the German Book Trade in America*.

51. MAFSt 4 G 2, fol. 230, 1752, Bill for Pastor Brunnholz.

52. Cowen and Wilson, "Traffic in Medical Ideas"; Cowen, "Zum Dienste des Gemeinen Mannes."

53. Roeber, "J. H. C. Helmuth"; idem, "Mosheim Society." As also noted by Roeber, Helmuth's book orders during this period were more heavily oriented to the mid-century Pietist tradition, above all the works of Johann Jacob Rambach, and to Christian education, but also included a recent German geography text, *Büschings Erdbeschreibung, die Theile von Asia, Africa, und America*.

that attempted to integrate American into European botany. The singular contribution of Gotthilf Heinrich Ernst Mühlenberg to the latter enterprise is well recognized.[54] But few scholars of American botany know much if anything about Mühlenberg's medical practice, his trade in pharmaceuticals, and his direct link to the German book trade under the auspices of the Halle Orphanage.

Although G. H. E. Mühlenberg, a compulsive bookworm, continually lamented his own expensive predilection for new European titles, the new traffic in ideas—botanical and pharmaceutical—no longer went only from center to periphery. On 27 October 1796, he sent not only several packages of seeds to Johann Hedwig, professor of botany at Leipzig, but reviewed the new Prussian dispensatories for Professors Adolph Richter and Johann Wilhelm Juncker at Halle. He offered to send seeds and their descriptions to Kurt Sprengel in Halle, in exchange for prints and copper engravings of newly classified plants to be communicated to the American Philosophical Society in Philadelphia as plates for his own work, a study of Lancaster plants. In 1795, shortly before his death, the eminent naturalist Junghans had requested seeds from a range of tree species and dried plant specimens, and similar requests came from Richter in Halle.[55]

Many new book orders of the 1790s were intended for J. H. Helmuth's Philadelphia academy, and a good portion of the botanical works was part of or resulted from G. H. E. Mühlenberg's own interests and those of his extensive network among American botanists, of both German and English extraction.[56] But many titles suggest indigenous and independent demand, such as an 1802 order by Christoph Jacob Hutter in Lancaster for three copies of volume one of "Gren's Pharmacologie, . . . (and his) Chemie, 4 Theile . . . , Junckers Handbuch,

---

54. Maisch, "G. H. E. Mühlenberg als Botaniker," and Müller-Jahnke, "Der Linnaeus Americanus." Note that the Maisch article, appearing in German in the American journal *Pharmazeutische Rundschau*, was published in 1886, when American pharmacy tolerated and even encouraged the incursion of German pharmaceutical standards. Mueller-Jahnke's more recent work relies heavily on the reports of Johann David Schoepf and on little-known German academic correspondence.

55. This and the other correspondence for the years 1795–97 is in MAFSt 4 G 9, 10. The note by Junghans is Item 28, noted as Item 21a, fols. 66 and 67. That by Christian Adolph Richter, a descendant of the Richter family, is from 8 February 1796. For a partial assessment of these exchanges and other botanical correspondence with American, English, and French scholars, see the works by Maisch and Müller Jahnke, cited in note 54 above.

56. For the latter, see Maisch, "G. H. E. Mühlenberg als Botaniker." The old catalogues for the holdings of the German Society Library in Philadelphia list largely educational and theological titles from this period, indicating that the Helmuth school libraries were deposited there. There are no medical titles for our period (to 1820) in the extant catalogue, but holdings are difficult to assess because of the ongoing restructuring of the entire holdings at the time of this study.

3 Theile, und 2 mal Vossens Handbuch der Staatengeschäfte," and serial publications like Buckmann's *Oeconomische Bibliothek*, which Mühlenberg ordered for an unnamed friend.[57]

Thus, during twenty years of resurgent trade with Halle (1790–1810), the network of international exchange by pious and enterprising scholars—begun by August Hermann Francke and Cotton Mather in the early decades of the eighteenth century—was revived by a new generation who exchanged books, observations, copper plates, and botanical and agricultural specimens. These exchanges run counter to the common assumption that until the secular immigrations of the mid-nineteenth century, German philosophy, medicine, and natural history were of little relevance to the development of an early learned culture in North America.

57. MAFSt 4 G 9–10, fol. 195. Friedrich Albrecht Carl Gren, *Handbuch der Pharmacologie oder Lehre von den Arzneimitteln* (Halle: Waisenhausbuchhandlung, part 1, 1790, part 2, 1792, 2 subsequent eds. in 1799/1800 and 1813); idem, *Systematisches Handbuch der gesammten Chemie, zum Gebrauche seiner Vorlesungen entworfen* (Halle: Waisenhausbuchhandlung, 1787–90, and two posthumous eds.). Cited after Seils, *Gren*, 241–42. For the Juncker volume, see Kaiser and Krosch, "Drei Generationen Juncker." These volumes accounted for almost 40 percent of the total Hutter order and ran to Rth 105/6, with a generous discount of 25 percent.

Pietist Medicine and

Pietist Charity

in the New

Republic

8

This study of a transatlantic traffic in medicines and medical ideas has examined Pietist medicine and the pharmaceutical trade of the Francke Foundations as part of the eighteenth-century transatlantic traffic of medical resources and ideas. Both in its origins and its mechanisms, this traffic was an outgrowth of the enterprise of reform and transatlantic mission of a voluntary and independent religious foundation, practicing philanthropy and supporting its work by commerce in books and medicines. On the European side of the Atlantic, we have traced the development of medical charity practice at the Foundations and the closely linked but eventually autonomous manufacture and trade in pharmaceutical products. This trade was conducted on a large scale in a large continental market oriented to domestic German consumption and the territories to the east and southeast that sustained Protestant networks.

The enterprise of reform and mission developed in the early part of the eighteenth century, influenced by similar trends of seventeenth-century European movements, and continued into the English and continental Protestant revival of the first half of the eighteenth century. When this revival reached the shores of colonial North

America in the 1730s, Halle religious and charity reforms were acknowledged by many clergy, from Samuel Mather in Boston to the revivalists George Whitefield and Jonathan Edwards, as a model and inspiration.[1] But when Halle finally gave in to the urgings of German Lutheran congregations in the middle colonies to send out ministers to ensure continued Lutheran observance, education, and church discipline, the ministers went under the auspices of the Bishop of London and the Anglican Society for Promoting Christian Knowledge, with whom Halle had shared the East Indian mission project and the Georgia Plan.[2]

For the Pietist clergy coming to North America between 1740 and 1775 and for their successors, conflict and opportunity in their intended spiritual area of influence arose from many sources. The deeply felt need by many immigrants for a structured congregational life that would preserve Lutheran tenets and the administration of the sacraments in their own language was set off by language differences in this very community and by discord over the validity of calls to arriving and incumbent ministers. Refusal among immigrants newly liberated from European bondage to bow to Pietist church discipline added to the original difficulties of the Pietist ministry in North America, as did the change in the composition of different immigrant cohorts over time and the resulting labor and social stratification in communities. The denominational politics of Halle ministers were encumbered by European relations with an Anglican establishment that banked on the loyalty of their German protégés.[3] In turn, these had to tread carefully in an environment that became increasingly hostile to the Bishop of London and his emissaries, as in the Anglican effort to establish English-language schools and to co-opt the German Lutheran population in the 1750s and 1760s.[4]

1. See Ward, *The Protestant Evangelical Awakening.* This influence ranged from New England (Samuel Mather, *Vita B. Hermanni Augusti Franckii . . . Revisa, et cura Samuelis Mather . . . , cum dedicatione ejus, edita* [Boston, 1733]) to the middle colonies and for a brief moment united the denominations along the eastern seaboard (Lambert, *Inventing the Great Awakening*).

2. For Lutheran North America, the term *mission* may sound like an anachronism. It is generally ceded to the Moravians and their Indian missions, but with few and mainly futile exceptions, the Halle Pietist clergy that started coming over in the 1730s made no attempt to missionize among the Indians, concentrating instead on taking over and asserting the principles of Lutheran church life and church discipline in German congregations. In part, the retention of the older terminology was due to European constraints arising from the conditions of philanthropic bequests supporting missions rather than settlements; with the exception of the Georgia enterprise conducted jointly with the Georgia Trustees and the SPCK in London, Halle had neither the resources nor an agenda that provided for settlement of coherent groups of emigrants.

3. Wilson, "Continental Refugees"; idem, "The Halle Pietists in Georgia."

4. Glatfelter, *Pastors and People,* 2: chap. 6.

The transatlantic migration of medical practice and pharmaceuticals through the agency of Pietist clergy must be seen against the background of these larger transatlantic movements of people and ideas. I have argued that the demographic structure of German immigration over the course of the eighteenth century fostered the development of a distinct medical market and a medical culture in German areas of settlement. In turn, it required the resources and the commercial acumen of the Francke Foundations to secure for their emissaries a corner of this market. The transmission of Pietist medical ideas—a gentler medicine and enlightened therapy—can be documented for some North American practitioners who owed their training to the proponents of this medicine at Halle and who practiced before 1770. More frequent was the adaptation of the therapeutic armamentarium to an environment no longer relying entirely on imports from Europe. This is clear from the eclectic but by no means singular practice of Gotthilf Heinrich Ernst Mühlenberg, who was born in the colonies, was trained at the Halle Foundations, and returned in 1770. In each case, the importance of the remaining cultural and economic ties to Central Europe in the medical domain is well documented in the pattern of orders of pharmaceutical products from Halle to the end of the eighteenth century.

One finding of this study is that the pharmaceutical trade was an indispensable medium through which the Halle Pietists transmitted financial support to their North American diaspora and reinforced its evangelical mission. But in the competitive American market, they could not have succeeded without the close link between the written word and the purchase of proprietary medicines. By the eighteenth century, the growing long-distance trade in such medicines had strengthened this link and made it part of a profitable commodity: The sale of medicines to a large number of unknown buyers required printed manuals of health in the vernacular languages, both by the sellers and users of these medications and by physicians offering domestic manuals that would help the patient find her or his way through both symptoms of illness and cures.[5] As the European reading public and its interests grew and became more selective, print cultures, both secular and oriented to religious lay readers, integrated these writings through the learned book and the nascent journal culture of the new sciences.

That this print culture was of long standing by the eighteenth century and not by any means the singular product of the Enlightenment is well recognized.

---

5. For England, see Smith, "Prescribing the Rules of Help: Self-Help and Advice in the Late 18th Century."

But it played a special role in multicultural colonial North America and opens a window on the social spectrum of German immigrants and the choices of a lay reading public consuming large numbers of printed products. In addition to lay works, imports of learned books from Germany persisted. These may, to some extent, have reflected the persistence of a conservative natural philosophy among readers, for which the public writings and letters of Justus Heinrich Helmuth stand as a representative example among the Pietist clergy.[6] But the scholarly writings and research of Gotthilf Heinrich Ernst Mühlenberg leave little room for arguments of Christian versus secular natural philosophy in botany and medicine. Whether Mühlenberg's lack of an ideological position in the sciences is due to the well-known ability of eighteenth-century clerics to compartmentalize their interests or to a general attitude of tolerance can be established only on examination of the full corpus of his writings and sermons. The same is true for other German representatives of the natural sciences in the new American republic, from Johann Christoph Kunze at Columbia University to Friedrich Melsheimer. Their work and that of others of their cohort remains to be integrated into the history of early American science.

This and other studies indicate a clear need to mine and make accessible generally ignored North American sources to assess the full range of social and economic interests and activities of the German population of the early American republic. In the natural sciences, the only contemporary observer was Johann David Schoepf, who came over with the Hessian troops during the Revolutionary War. His latinate *Materia Medica Americana potissimum regni vegetabilis*, printed in Erlangen in 1787, seems the only work accessible to modern American scholars of the period. This despite the fact that authors like John Maisch in the latter half of the nineteenth century and Wolf Dieter Müller-Jahnke more recently have drawn attention to the indebtedness—largely unknown—not only of Schoepf but of Constantine Samuel Rafinesque and Benjamin Smith Barton to the work of Mühlenberg, with whom they entertained a lively research correspondence.[7]

6. Roeber, "Evangelical Charity."
7. Maisch, "G. H. E. Mühlenberg als Botaniker"; Müller-Jahnke, "Johann David Schoepf"; idem, "Der Linnaeus Americanus." Language and the previous neglect of German sources in this country remain the major barriers to access to the Mühlenberg and Kunze corpus. As a result, the full and valuable overviews of eclectic and physiomedical practice by Haller, *Kindly Medicines*, and of the eclectic materia medica by Flannery, *John Uri Lloyd*, and earlier work by Berman ("Thomsonian Movement") had to skirt the work of early nineteenth-century German-American physicians, leaving us to guess whether they were all allopaths, like John Eberle, or part of a forgotten cohort.

The Practice of Medicine and the Commerce in Pharmaceuticals

One driving force of the medical mission of the Halle clergy in North America was to ensure a market for the Halle Orphanage medications, by both charitable distribution and commercial sales. It is here that the admixture of medical care and ministry that the Francke Foundations had inculcated into their students of theology was put to a test. They passed this test within the niche granted to clergy practicing medicine throughout and beyond the eighteenth century, using the proprietary medicines supplied by their motherhouse in a complex scheme of philanthropic commerce. This commerce survived the colonial period and even grew during the heady days of commercial and medical independence from England, but it does not seem to have survived the growth of homegrown pharmaceutical manufacture in North America.[8]

In Europe, by the early years of the nineteenth century, the link between religion and a Godly medicine and its medicines had been rendered moot by multiple factors—social and economic as much as professional and scientific. Social and health reform in Prussia and other German territories and in most European markets severely curtailed the privileged sales outlets of the *Medikamentenexpedition* and reclassified its medicinals as commercial patent medicines. Sales continued in Germany and the German-speaking enclaves in the east and southeast of Europe, but the medical faculty at Halle had long since ceased collaboration with the Orphanage, maintaining only its bureaucratic rights of visitation. By the 1770s at the latest, the Orphanage hospital and dispensary was strictly a student facility, and the Orphanage educational facilities in turn came under strict Prussian administration and regulation. The eighteenth-century manufacture of pharmaceuticals in apothecary shops and private laboratories and by laying out to pill makers was slowly giving way to commercial and industrial pharmacy, which used the new pharmaceutical chemistry to ensure quality and stability of the materia medica.

Again, North America seems to have offered a much less regulated—some would say entirely unregulated—medical market in terms of drug sales and manufacture. The practice of medicine remained relatively open and fostered market niches and tightly defined customer networks through numerous and competing medical movements, from homeopathy to the various types of eclecticism. The marketing networks and product assurance procedures developed in

8. Haller, *Kindly Medicine*, chap. 5; Flannery, *John Uri Lloyd.*

Halle a good hundred years earlier clearly resembled much in the new and eclectic American market and may well have served as an implicit model. This similarity extended to the much older arguments about the greater safety of medications manufactured by or under the supervision of a knowledgeable physician, and to the religious arguments that buttressed some of the nineteenth-century claims to a kindly and Christian medicine. It would be tempting, therefore, to draw a direct line from Halle pharmaceutical trading practice and its roots in the seventeenth century to nineteenth-century nonallopathic medicinals. But although the channels, market, and mechanisms of commerce may have been similar, little evidence links the composition and indications of the Halle medicinals to the numerous products offered on the American market, the self-declared vitalism of representatives of physiomedicine notwithstanding.[9] Halle medications were not all botanicals but had a strong and lasting chemiatric component. They thus offer a poor fit with the predominant pytho-medicine of many nineteenth-century American medical reformers. In terms of medical philosophy, the fit seems equally poor with the homeopathic scheme of Hahnemann and his followers, despite the obvious similarities of tightly controlled sales and practice networks.

True, the early Halle physicians had proposed a gentler medicine that was opposed to excessive depletion, but any expectational approaches to treatment do not seem to have been carried over into the trends of Halle academic medicine of the second half of the eighteenth century. Stahl's chemical theories were rendered void by Antoine Lavoisier and his contemporaries and by the 1790s had been rejected even by his most explicit supporters, the Halle professor of medicine and materia medica Friedrich Albrecht Carl Gren being among the last.[10] Despite explicit reliance on Stahl's explanatory schemes by many in North America, his medicine seems to have lived on as a symbol rather than a medical reality.

Similar issues remain for the trade in Halle proprietary medicines. Not many historians of medicine and pharmacy deal with questions of the economics of the pharmaceutical trade, although for most of history, the dispensing of drugs in ambulatory practice was and remains the profitable backbone of medicine.[11] Trade on a large scale in any commodity, both domestic and international, in turn affects institutions and the public domain beyond the mechanisms of

9. Haller, *Kindly Medicine*, chap. 5, "Vitalism and the Materia Medica," in particular p. 91.
10. Seils, *Friedrich Carl Gren in seiner Zeit*.
11. Porter and Porter, "Rise of the English Drugs Industry."

finance and commerce. The eighteenth century was on the brink of large-scale commerce that eventually liberated itself and its participants from the tightly defined routes and monopolies of earlier periods. In the case of the Halle Orphanage Foundations, as elsewhere, the commodities of this trade were neither staples nor luxury goods but products consumed by a growing middle-class market. They were books and proprietary medicines consumed in the pursuit of personal spiritual and physical health.

The Halle commerce grew throughout eighteenth-century Europe and flourished in denominational, political, and social constellations that differed in many ways from other trading patterns of the time, but in its essentials exhibited many and probably generic similarities. In France, the trade in proprietary medications benefited from and fed into a growing civil discourse.[12] In England, much of the pharmaceutical trade in the eighteenth century was in the hands of Quakers, who used their network in England and their diaspora abroad to fit this trade into the colonial exchanges formerly reserved to the large merchant companies. In the case of the Halle Orphanage Foundations, which were created by another religious fringe group to reform society, a network of clergy and fellow believers in the nobility and commerce carried the trade first to the east, into Russia and Hungary, in line with Central European migrations of the period. Later, by dint of their English and Danish connections and their evangelical mission, the Foundations gained access to colonial settlements in the East and the West Indies, although they could not count on the protection of German governments and navies.

It is an intriguing question then of historical perspective that this type of trade is seen as liberating in France, whereas in England it is seen as commerce pure and simple, and hardly as one liberating its agents. The Halle people likewise were not French, and many historians would raise their eyebrows at the notion that the Pietist agenda was a precursor of the Enlightenment. But the Halle Pietists sought liberty nonetheless, even if this must be understood in terms of the liberties of an earlier period. In particular, this refers to the God-given assignment, in many of the utopian improvement schemes of the seventeenth century, of specific duties to the three early modern estates, the *Regierstand,* the *Lehrstand,* and the *Hausstand.* As part of the clerisy, the Halle evangelical movement sought freedom from interference by the state with the enterprise of religious reform, and it used the mechanisms of trade and leveraged capital to gain

12. Jones, "The Great Chain of Buying."

it and support its aims. For almost a century, commerce afforded to the Halle Orphanage Foundations these liberties and the freedom to maneuver as a voluntary institution, until the French Revolution and the changed polity of Europe rendered politically independent agencies of religious reform irrelevant.

The New Medical Establishment and the Model of Halle Charity Practice

Replications of the Halle charity model in North America included the Salzburger settlement at Ebenezer and the Savannah Orphanage of George Whitefield. These replications, one fully and publicly sanctioned and supported from Halle and London, the other little known as using Halle precedent, lasted for several decades but did not in themselves inspire renewed replication in turn. Both Georgia orphanages remained poor replicas of the German motherhouse, being severely limited by the shortage of white labor and local demand for potential orphans as house servants.[13]

By contrast, there were potential charity populations in the middle urbanized colonies, but the motherhouse withheld its full support when it could have laid the basis for a strong German presence linking charity to medical care on the Halle dispensary model. Heinrich Melchior Mühlenberg's attempt in the 1770s at partial replication of at least the money-making components of the Halle institutions never took off. Although the orphanage movement of the early American republic seems to have been influenced by Francke's writings,[14] Heinrich Melchior Mühlenberg's earlier use of the term *orphanage* for North America was largely emblematic; in his plans, the orphanage was intended to support not so much orphans as the aging and disabled American pastorate who had come from Halle. Although funds that could have been be used in its support seem to have been available from a large earlier legacy, the Halle fathers were unable or unwilling to grant this request.

During the colonial period, there was indeed much planning for German schools and even colleges, but the split among the Quaker factions and the general suspicion of Anglican schemes in Philadelphia, the Congregational tradition in Boston, and above all the prudent policy of mutual religious tolerance in running community affairs seem to have mitigated against a Lutheran

13. Wilson, "Land, Population, and Labor." Both Bremner (*American Philanthropy*, 21) and Lambert (*Pedlar in Divinity*, 18) refer to the Francke institutions as a precedent for George Whitefield, without noting that a direct replication was in operation twenty-five miles down the Savannah River.
14. Porter, "Francke's Transatlantic Legacy."

institution openly subservient to metropolitan English interests. But what the ministers from Halle did achieve—whether as conscious agents or as a byproduct of their number and their labors—was to create a congregational network stretching across social classes and recreating, mutatis mutandis on foreign soil, the conditions in which voluntary charity on the Halle model could be practiced. The Halle mission clergy slowly turned into North American clergy of German origin forced to compete for the loyalty of the God-fearing public with Methodists and Baptists during the Second Great Awakening of the 1820s. It is only fair then to ask what remained of the specifically Pietist agenda in the new forms of American medical charity that was on its way to being fully launched.

Although German immigration had slowed to a trickle in the late eighteenth and early nineteenth centuries, the leaders of the Lutheran clergy and their descendants had become full participants in the American educational and scholarly culture, passing along German educational models, if not always the German language, at various academic institutions and theological seminaries of the new republic. They took their place among the members of the new learned societies and as trustees of numerous institutions. Justus Helmuth pioneered German charity and Christian education in Philadelphia beginning in the 1780s.[15] After the earlier failure of his Philadelphia seminary,[16] we can trace Johann Christopher Kunze, for instance, to an endowed professorship at King's College in New York and to a decade of faithful attendance at the meetings of the Board of Governors of New York Hospital. Until his death in 1807, he served ex officio as senior pastor of the united Lutheran congregations and actively participated in hospital administration and oversight, his often-stated aversion to English apparently not constituting a hindrance.[17]

It is doubtful whether the apparent reluctance of the German clerical leaders in North America to explicitly perpetuate the Halle traditions was due to their inability to stand their ground—linguistically or otherwise—among their American peers. Rather, we seem to be faced in this early national period with a general unwillingness to acknowledge any European roots for American

15. Roeber, "J. H. C. Helmuth"; idem, "Mosheim Society."
16. For a full account of this often-ventured plan, see letter of 13 and 14 June 1773 (quoted from the *Mühlenberg Journals*, 1772–74), reprinted in Haussmann, *Kunze's Seminarium and the Society for the Propagation of Christianity and Useful Knowledge Among the Germans in America*, 25–28.
17. *Minutes of the New York Hospital, 1795–1810.* The only language problem arising was the spelling of his name, which ranged from "Cuncie" to "Kunzie." I thank Adele Lerner, archivist of New York Hospital—Cornell Medical School, for guiding me to these sources.

charity institutions, a phenomenon that, as noted above, found its match in the not entirely successful insistence on an American medicine that would take full account of a unique disease environment and less costly native materia medica.[18] Although the exchange of medical ideas and medical education with Europe continued, the makers of public charity and public health at the municipal level seem to have had little inclination to model themselves consciously on either England or Germany or, for that matter, France. Although the beloved Quaker mentor of many American physicians in London, Dr. John Fothergill, sat on the founding board of New York Hospital in 1771, its minutes for the period 1795–1810 show little reference to English precedent. What we do see by the turn of the century is increasing deference to the medical profession as charity policymakers. In an address celebrating the opening of the New York Dispensary in 1830, the speaker, a man clearly of German extraction but by now an Episcopal minister, invoked the emblematic names of physicians from Sydenham to Stahl, but had little to say of the institutional antecedents of the American dispensary for the poor, whether in England or in Central Europe.[19]

Continuing a colonial tradition, the municipal and state institutions under civil government and the numerous voluntary hospitals and dispensaries were multiconfessional to reflect local constituencies and to permit mixed voluntary and public financing.[20] In New York, where the senior ministers of all confessions were ex officio members of the New York Hospital board, the state government was expected to and did cover the annual deficits. In 1813, commemorating the seventeenth anniversary of the Boston dispensary, John Coffin did not lose a word on English or other models that may be presumed to have influenced the structure of this institution.[21] It took another sixty years for a lengthy record of English practices to be introduced into the discussion. The wars with England had been forgotten, and renewed and continuing debates about financing this

18. That this was a futile endeavor in antebellum pharmacy is noted by Higby, In Service to American Pharmacy, introduction. The native physician movement among a section of full-time physicians of some standing is discussed in the work of Warner, The Therapeutic Perspective, chap. 6.

19. Schroeder, "Plea for the Industrious Poor."

20. An early example of an apparently tolerant multiconfessionalism under Protestant leadership is the Charleston orphanage, founded in 1790, which had both Jewish and Catholic representatives on its board. It goes almost without saying that it did not admit black children. (King, ed., History and Records of the Charleston Orphan House, 1790–1860; Bellows, Benevolence of Slaveholders).

21. Coffin, "An Address Delivered Before the Contributors of the Boston Dispensary at Their Seventeenth Anniversary, October 21, 1813."

by now venerable dispensary and preventing the abuse of its services looked back to historical parallels.[22]

There is little recent work on charity dispensaries in North America, and what there is has adopted the English paradigm without much question. A classic 1918 study of urban dispensaries was not written from a historical but a public health perspective. Its authors confined their discussion of the origins of the dispensary for the poor to ten pages, focusing on the London institution opened in 1696 by the College of Physicians and their eighteenth-century successors from Burwell to Lettsom. They did add a modest disclaimer to these historical observations, to the effect that "[n]o reference is made here to the Dispensaries on the Continent. They do not appear to have affected the early development of dispensaries in the United States."[23] The early nineteenth-century orphanage movement did generate some reference to the Halle Orphanage as a model, particularly in New York and Philadelphia. Here, the influence of the Pietist clergy and the tradition of edification literature apparently remained visible, despite the many, and probably unarticulated, differences in the populations covered and the educational goals.[24]

Thus, we may owe to a historical artifact—partly arising from a historiography focusing on national European traditions to the detriment of a framework oriented to larger religious and secular trends—the poverty of information on whether and how continental philanthropy and medical charity care were received and incorporated into American charity care. The early nineteenth-century agenda of American patrons of the poor and of physicians seeking opportunities for patient-oriented teaching in urban charitable dispensaries are too similar to those proposed by the Protestant reformers a century earlier to have been entirely coincidental. However, in the multicultural and multi-

22. I base these observations on the valuable collection of printed sources by Charles Rosenberg, *Caring for the Working Man*, introduction, 17ff. and 63ff.

23. Davis and Warner, *Dispensaries, Their Management and Development*, 4.

24. A biography of August Hermann Francke (*Memoirs of Augustus Hermann Francke*, prepared for the American Sunday School Union, Philadelphia, 1831) was published by the American Sunday School Union in 1831. I thank Dr. Markus Mathias at Halle for this reference. Porter ("Francke's Transatlantic Legacy") stresses the conceptual and practical differences between the Halle and the North American models, although her insistence on rational and utilitarian versus religious and Christian goals is one that, as I have tried to show, does not hold for the Halle Orphanage if we strip Francke's writings of their eighteenth-century rhetoric. That populations and educational goals differed between settings that were two continents and one hundred years apart goes without saying. Porter's work does stress the emergence of female agency in voluntary orphanage construction and management and their emphasis on female orphans and half-orphans.

confessional urban settings of the Jeffersonian period, European precedents may well have been implicit and taken for granted unless they were specifically rejected.

A Legacy of Voluntarism

Although his legacy as one of the forgotten pioneers of eighteenth-century charity receded into a hazy myth and was resurrected only occasionally, August Hermann Francke and his Foundations became part of the generic model for the nineteenth century and beyond of the private, voluntary, and nonprofit organization. Even today, institutions and organizations that make up this sector are mainly dedicated to charity—relief of dependent men, women, and children ravaged by natural and manmade catastrophes, and education and medical care in unprovided areas or for marginalized populations. To a large extent, these organizations are drawn from religious groupings and are well connected and well supported by definable and well-regarded social groups. They have considerable international connections and areas of expertise and work and enjoy considerable autarchy. Thus, they occupy a recognized societal place that is to my mind strikingly reminiscent of the position sought and for almost a century held by the Francke Foundations: They are legitimized by but not dependent on the state and their own churches. They seek and are assigned tasks outside the state social sector and budget and rely on voluntary labor and contributions, but they use rather than represent both the state and the for-profit sector and its mechanisms. To paraphrase Karl Gabriel,[25] in both the domestic and the international fields, they can claim their place and gather support because of the failure of governments in periods of political and social transition.

In Germany as in much of Europe, this applies above all to the Catholic *Caritas* agencies and the Protestant voluntary bodies.[26] In North America, their role at all levels of need and services has been recognized since the early nineteenth century, when they owed their influence specifically to their ability to speak for immigrant populations defined by ethnicity—mainly language and religion.[27]

25. Gabriel, "Caritas angesichts fortschreitender Säkularisierung."
26. For the development of *Caritas* and *Diakonie* in the field of social services, see Gatz, *Caritas und soziale Dienste*.
27. August Hermann Francke's *Pietas Halensis*, first translated into English in 1705 by the London printer of the SPCK, was published in an American translation in 1867 by William L. Gage (*Faith's Work Perfected, or Francke's Orphan House at Halle*, New York: Anson D. F. Randolph).

The traffic in Halle medical traditions and pharmaceutical products was part of colonial charity practice and fed these larger developments.

The social history of North American medicine at the end of our period of study has increasingly turned to the poverty of rural medical practice, the preponderance of domestic medicine, and the rejection of traditional and often heroic medicine in favor of eclectic practices and medical sectarianism. But except for American work on nineteenth-century care for the mentally ill, which specifically invokes European models,[28] we remain largely ignorant of antecedents of community and medical charity in rural and small urban settlements, which encompassed much of the American population in the old colonies and the northwestern territories settled during the first decades of the new republic. We know that there were a number of German orphanages and old age homes founded on a voluntary basis during the first decades of the nineteenth century. The community institutions of sects like the Schwenkfelders and the Moravians in areas with large German populations are preserved in their institutional histories. But we do not know which, if any, was the modal experience. There is continuing and unresolved contemporary debate on whether the financial mechanisms of charity care should be in the public domain, should be commercial, or should rely on voluntary and religious institutions for funding and labor, and whether they should or even can follow European models, both secular and religious. If a historical perspective has any use, it is surely worth asking not whether but how European traditions of religiously driven social reform, of which *Francke's Anstalten* were an early and spectacular example, created attitudes and expectations that influenced practices of American medical charity.

28. For example, Rothman, *The Discovery of the Asylum: Social Order, and Disorder in the New Republic*.

In citing works in the footnotes, shortened titles are generally used. Primary sources and frequently cited works are identified by abbreviations in the text and footnotes.

The major primary sources for this book are in the archives of the Francke Foundations in Halle, Germany. The following abbreviations denote these archival materials:

AFSt—Archiv der Franckeschen Stiftungen (Hauptarchiv), followed by folder and item number.

MAFSt—Missionsarchiv der Franckeschen Stiftungen, Series 1–5.

 Series 1–3 refer to the East Indian Missions, Series 4 to Pennsylvania, and Series 5 to Georgia. This study relies mainly on the American mission records, although some materials, particularly those regarding donations and bequests, are cross-filed.

  MAFSt 4 (Pennsylvania): Series (A–G): Stück were available: fol(s).
  MAFSt 5 (Georgia): Series (A–E): Stück were available: fol(s).

VAFSt—Wirtschafts- und Verwaltungsarchiv der Franckeschen Stiftungen.

 Accessible through three volumes of indexes (*Repertorien*) compiled in 1866. This study relies mainly on Repertorium ii, which contains the ledgers of the various accounting departments of the Foundations (*Rechnungen der verschiedenen Kassen*). At the time of my research, these were indexed in the original *Repertorien* by file drawer, with additional identification by item in some folders. These references are used here as:

  (W) VAFSt/Repertorium/Title (i–xx)/*Fach* (Roman numerals): fol. (if available).

Frequently cited works are identified by the following abbreviations:

Brief Account—David Samuel von Madai, *A Brief Account of the Effects and Use of Some Approved Medicines Which are Dispensed in the Orphanhouse at Halle* (1784).

Detailed Reports—George F. Jones et al., eds., *Detailed Reports of the Salzburger Emigrants Who Settled in America.*

Höchst-nöthige Erkenntnis—Christian Friedrich Richter, *Seeligen Hn. D. Christian Friedrich Richters Höchst-nöthige Erkenntnis des Menschen* . . . (1710, and subsequent editions).

KM—Kurt Aland, ed., *Die Korrespondenz Heinrich Melchior Mühlenbergs*, 4 vols.

Kurzer und deutlicher Unterricht—Christian F. Richter, *Kurzer und deutlicher Unterricht von dem Leibe und natürlichen Leben des Menschen* (1705).

Dates are stated as given throughout, without attempting to reconcile the differences between the Julian and Gregorian calendars. Direct quotations are my translations.

Abelove, Henry. *The Evangelist of Desire: John Wesley and the Methodists.* (Stanford, Calif.: Stanford University Press, 1990).

Adams, Willi Paul. "The Colonial German Language Press and the American Revolution." In *The Press and the American Revolution*, ed. Bernard Bailyn and John B. Hench. (Worcester, Mass.: American Antiquarian Society, 1980).

Aland, Kurt. "Pietismus und soziale Frage." In *Pietismus und moderne Welt*, ed. Kurt Aland, Erhard Peschke, and Manfred Schmidt. Arbeiten zur Geschichte des Pietismus. (Witten: Luther Verlag, 1974), 12:99–137.

Aland, Kurt, ed. *Die Korrespondenz Heinrich Melchior Mühlenbergs: Aus der Anfangszeit des Deutschen Luthertums in Nordamerika, vol. 1, 1740–1752, vol. 2, 1753–1762, vol. 3, 1763–1768, vol. 4, 1768–1780.* (Berlin and New York: de Gruyter, 1986–93).

Aland, Kurt, Erhard Peschke, and Manfred Schmidt, eds. *Pietismus und moderne Welt*. (Witten: Luther Verlag, 1974).

Alberti, Michael. *Specimen Medicinae Theologicae*. (Halle: Joannis Christiani Hendelii, 1726).

Altmann, Eckhard. *Christian Friedrich Richter (1676–1711): Arzt, Apotheker, und Liederdichter der Halleschen Pietisten*. (Witten: Luther Verlag, 1972).

Altmann, Ida, and James Horn, eds. *To Make America: European Emigration in the Early Modern Period*. (Berkeley and Los Angeles: University of California Press, 1991).

Amburger, Erik. *Geschichte des Protestantismus in Russland*. (Stuttgart: Evangelisches Verlagswerk, 1961).

American Sunday School Union. *Memoirs of Augustus Hermann Francke*. (Philadelphia, 1831).

Andersson, Bo. "Die Autorität der Prophetin: Eva Margaretha Frölich und der prophetische Diskurs." *Pietismus und Neuzeit* 17 (1991): 9–35.

Arndt, Johann. *Garden of Paradise, or Holy Prayers and Exercises; Pursuing the Design of the Famous Treatise on True Christianity . . . now done into English from the German original*. (London: Downing, 1716).

———. *Johann Arndts . . . Sechs Bücher vom Wahren Christenthum nebst desselben Paradiesgärtlein*. (1605, and many subsequent editions).

Arndt, K. J. R., and May E. Olson, eds. *The German Language Press of the Americas*, vol. 1, 3d rev. ed. (1976).

Arndt, K. J. R., and Reimer C. Eck, eds. *The First Century of German Language Printing in the United States of America: A Bibliography Based on the Studies of Oswald Seidensticker and Wilbur H. Oda*. (Göttingen: Niedersächsische Staats- und Universitätsbibliothek, 1989).

Bailyn, Bernard. *The Peopling of British North America: An Introduction*. (New York: Knopf, distributed by Random House, 1986).

———. *Voyagers to the West: A Passage in the Peopling of North America on the Eve of the American Revolution*. (New York: Knopf, 1988).

Bailyn, Bernard, and Philip D. Morgan, eds. *Strangers in the Realm: Cultural Margins of the First British Empire*. (Chapel Hill: University of North Carolina Press, 1991).

Ball, Dr. John. *The Modern Practice of Physic or a method of judiciously treating several disorders incident to the human body, together with a recital of their causes, symptoms, diagnostics, and prognostics, and the regimen necessary to be observed in regard of them, etc.*, 3d ed. (London: A. Millar, 1768).

Barr Rothenberg, Winifred. *From Marketplaces to a Market Economy: The Transformation of Rural Massachusetts, 1750–1850*. (Chicago: University of Chicago Press, 1992).

Barry, Jonathan. "Piety and the Patient: Medicine and Religion in Eighteenth-Century Bristol." In *Patients and Practitioners: Lay Perceptions of Medicine in Pre-Industrial Society*, ed. Roy Porter. Cambridge History of Medicine. (Cambridge: Cambridge University Press, 1985), 145–75.

Barry, Jonathan, and Colin Jones, eds. *Medicine and Charity Before the Welfare State*. (London: Routledge, 1991).

Barton, William. *Vegetable Materia Medica of the United States*. (Philadelphia: Carey and Son, 1817–19).

Bartz, Ernst. *Die Wirtschaftsethik August Hermann Franckes*. (Hamburg, 1934).

Bauer, Rudolph. "Spener Francke & Co.: Pietismus und Wohltätigkeit des städtischen Bürgertums und der adeligen Damen im 17./18. Jahrhundert." In *Die liebe Not: Zur historischen Kontinuität der freien Wohlfahrtspflege*, ed. Rudolph Bauer. (Weinheim and Basel: Beltz, 1984).

———. "Voluntary Welfare Associations in Germany and the United States: Theses on the Historical Development of Intermediary Systems." *Voluntas* 1.1 (1990): 97–111.

Beck, John B. *An Historical Sketch of the State of Medicine in the American Colonies, from Their First Settlement to the Period of the Revolution*. (Albany: C. Van Benthuysen, 1850).

Becker-Cantarino, Barbara. *Der lange Weg zur Mündigkeit: Frauen und Literatur in Deutschland von 1500 bis 1800*. (Munich: Deutscher Taschenbuch Verlag, 1989).

Beiler, Rosalind J. "From the Rhine to the Delaware Valley: The Eighteenth-Century Transatlantic Trade and Communication Channels of Caspar Wistar." In Hartmut Lehmann et al., eds., *In Search of Peace and Prosperity: New Settlements in Eighteenth-Century Europe and America*. (University Park: The Pennsylvania State University Press, 2000), 172–88.

Beisswanger, Gabriele. *Arzneimittelversorgung im 18. Jahrhundert: Die Stadt Braunschweig und die ländlichen Distrikte im Herzogthum Braunschweig-Wolfenbüttel*. Braunschweiger Veröffentlichungen zur Geschichte der Pharmazie und Naturwissenschaften 36. (Braunschweig: Deutscher Apothekerverlag, 1996).

Bell, Albert Dehner. *The Life and Times of Dr. George de Benneville, 1703–1793*. (Boston: Department of Publications of the Universalist Church of America, 1953).

Bell, Whitfield J., Jr. *John Morgan, Continental Doctor*. (Philadelphia: University of Pennsylvania Press, 1965).

———. "A Portrait of the Colonial Physician." *Bulletin of the History of Medicine* 44 (1970): 497–517.

———. *The Colonial Physician and Other Essays*. (New York: Science History Publications, 1975).

———. "Medicine in Boston and Philadelphia, 1750–1820: Comparisons and Contrasts." In *Medicine in Colonial Massachusetts, 1620–1820: A Conference Held 25 and 26 May 1978 by the Colonial Society of Massachusetts*. (Boston: Colonial Society, distributed by University Press of Virginia, 1980).

———. *The College of Physicians of Philadelphia, A Bicentennial History*. (Canton Mass.: Science History Publications, 1987).

Bellers, John. *The First Workers Co-operators: Proposals for Raising a College of Industry*. (Reprint Nottingham, 1980).

Benassi, Enrico, ed. *The Clinical Consultations of Giambattista Morgagni.* (Boston, 1984).

Benneville, George de. *Medicina Pennsylvania; or, The Pennsylvania Physician.* (Manuscript, College of Physicians, Philadelphia, c. 1770).

Berky, Andrew S. *Practitioner in Physick: A Biography of Abraham Wagner, 1717–1763.* (Pennsburg, Pa.: Schwenkfelder Library, 1954).

Berman, Alex. "Thomsonian Movement." *Bulletin of the History of Medicine* 225 (1951): 405–28, 519–38.

———. "The Heroic Approach in Nineteenth-Century Therapeutics." *Bulletin of the American Society of Hospital Pharmacists* 11 (1954): 320–27.

———. "Neo-Thomsonianism." *Journal of the History of Medicine and the Allied Sciences* 11 (1956): 133–55.

Berns, Jörg Jochen. "Utopie und Medizin: Der Staat der Gesunden und der gesunde Staat: Utopische Entwürfe des 16. und 17. Jahrhunderts." In *Heilkunde und Krankheitserfahrung in der frühen Neuzeit,* ed. Udo Benzendörfer and Wilhelm Kühlmann. (Tübingen: Max Niemeyer, 1992), 55–93.

Beyerlein, Berthold. *Die Entwicklung der Pharmazie zur Hochschuldisziplin (1750–1875): Ein Beitrag zur Universitäts- und Sozialgeschichte.* (Stuttgart: Wissenschaftliche Verlagsgesellschaft, 1991).

Bigelow, Jacob. *American Medical Botany.* (Boston: Cummings and Hilliard, 1817–20).

Bone, K. "Dosage Considerations in Herbal Medicine." *British Journal of Phytotherapy* 3 (1993–94): 128–37.

Bonner, Thomas Neville. *Becoming a Physician: Medical Education in Britain, France, Germany, and the United States.* (New York and Oxford: Oxford University Press, 1995).

Bonomi, Patricia U. *Under the Cope of Heaven: Religion, Society, and Politics in Colonial America.* (Oxford: Oxford University Press, 1986).

Brecht, Martin. "Der Hallesche Pietismus in der Mitte des 18. Jahrhunderts: Seine Ausstrahlung und sein Niedergang." In *Geschichte des Pietismus,* ed. M. Brecht, K. Deppermann, U. Gäbler, and H. Lehmann. (Göttingen: Vandenhoeck and Ruprecht, 1995), 2:319–57.

Brecht, Martin, ed. *Der Pietismus vom siebzehnten bis zum frühen achtzehnten Jahrhundert.* Vol. 1 of *Geschichte des Pietismus,* ed. M. Brecht, K. Deppermann, U. Gäbler, and H. Lehmann. (Göttingen: Vandenhoeck und Ruprecht, 1993).

Brecht, Martin, and Klaus Deppermann, eds. *Der Pietismus im achtzehnten Jahrhundert.* Vol. 2 of *Geschichte des Pietismus,* ed. M. Brecht, K. Deppermann, U. Gäbler, and H. Lehmann. (Göttingen: Vandenhoeck and Ruprecht, 1995).

Brecht, Martin, K. Deppermann, U. Gäbler, and H. Lehmann, eds. *Geschichte des Pietismus,* 2 vols. (Göttingen: Vandenhoeck und Ruprecht, 1993 and 1995).

Breen, Timothy H. "An Empire of Goods: The Anglicanization of Colonial America, 1690–1776." *Journal of British Studies* (1986) 25: 467–99.

Bremner, Robert H. *American Philanthropy,* 2d ed. (Chicago: University of Chicago Press, 1988).

Brendle, Thomas R., and Claude W. Unger. *Folk Medicine of the Pennsylvania Germans: The Non-Occult Cures.* (New York: A. M. Kelley, 1935; reprint 1970).

Brewer, John. *The Sinews of Power: War, Money, and the English State, 1688–1783.* (Cambridge, Mass.: Harvard University Press, 1990).

Bridenbaugh, Carl, and Jessica Bridenbaugh. *Rebels and Gentlemen: Philadelphia in the Age of Franklin*. (New York: Reynal and Hitchcock, 1942).

Brink, Andreas. *Die deutsche Auswanderungswelle in die britischen Kolonien Nordamerikas um die Mitte des 18. Jahrhunderts*. (Stuttgart: Steiner, 1993).

Brock, Helen C. "The Influence of Europe on Colonial Massachusetts Medicine." In *Medicine in Colonial Massachusetts, 1620–1820: A Conference Held 25 and 26 May 1978 by the Colonial Society of Massachusetts*. (Boston: Colonial Society, distributed by University Press of Virginia, 1980).

———. "North America, A Western Outpost of European Medicine." In *The Medical Enlightenment of the Eighteenth Century*, ed. Andrew Cunningham and Roger French. (Cambridge: Cambridge University Press, 1990).

Brockliss, Laurence, and Colin Jones. *The Medical World of Early Modern France*. (Oxford: Oxford University Press, 1997).

Brown, Marion E. "Adam Kuhn, Eighteenth-Century Physician and Teacher." *Journal of Medicine and Allied Sciences* (1950): 163–77.

Brunner, Daniel L. *Halle Pietists in England: Anthony William Boehm and the Society for Promoting Christian Knowledge*. (Göttingen: Vandenhoeck und Ruprecht, 1993).

Buchan, William. *Domestic Medicine; or, The Family Physician*. (Philadelphia: Crukshank, 1774).

———. *Domestic Medicine, or a Treatise on the Prevention and Cure of Diseases by Regimen and Simple Medicines, with an Appendix Containing a Dispensatory for the Use of Private Practitioners*, 5th, 7th, 20th eds., with improvements ed. (London: Publisher varies with edition, 1776, 1781, 1797).

Buel, Richard, Jr. *In Irons: Britain's Naval Supremacy and the American Revolutionary Economy*. (New Haven: Yale University Press, 1998).

Bureau of the Census. *Historical Statistics of the United States: Colonial Times to 1970*, Part 2, Series Z (Colonial and Prefederal Statistics). (Washington, D.C.: U.S. Government Printing Office, 1974).

Butler, Jon. *Awash in a Sea of Faith: Christianizing the American People*. (Cambridge, Mass.: Harvard University Press, 1990).

Butterfield, H., ed. *A Letter by Dr. Benjamin Rush Describing the Consecration of the German College at Lancaster in June 1787*. (Lancaster, Pa., 1945).

Bylebyl, Jerome J. "Teaching Methodus Medendi in the Renaissance." In *Galen's Method of Healing: Proceedings of the 1982 Galen Symposium*, ed. Fridolf Kudlien and Richard J. Durling. (Leiden: E. J. Brill, 1991), 157–89.

Cabot, Richard C. "Suggestions for the Reorganization of Hospital Out-Patient Departments, with Special Reference to the Improvement of Treatment." In *Caring for the Working Man: The Rise and Fall of the Dispensary, An Anthology of Sources*, ed. Charles E. Rosenberg. (New York: Garland, 1989), 273–85.

Canny, Nicholas P., ed. *Europeans on the Move: Studies on European Migration, 1500–1800*. (Oxford: Oxford University Press and Clarendon Press, 1994).

Cappon, Lester, ed. *Atlas of Early American History, Revolutionary Era, 1760–1790*. (Princeton: Princeton University Press, 1976).

Carl, Johann Samuel. *Medicina pauperum oder Armen-Apothek*. (Büdingen: n.p., 1719).

Cassedy, James. "Meteorology and Medicine in Colonial America." *Journal of the History of Medicine and Allied Sciences* (1969): 193–204.

————. "Church Record Keeping and Public Health in Early New England." In *Medicine in Colonial Massachusetts, 1620–1820: A Conference Held 25 and 26 May 1978 by the Colonial Society of Massachusetts*. (Boston: Colonial Society, distributed by the University Press of Virginia, 1980), 57, 249–63.

Cavallo, Sandra. "Conceptions of Poverty and Poor Relief in Turin in the Second Half of the Eighteenth Century." In *Domestic Strategies: Work and Family in France and Italy, 1600–1800*, ed. Stuart Woolf. (Cambridge: Cambridge University Press, 1991), 199.

————. "The Motivations of Benefactors: An Overview of Approaches to the Study of Charity." In *Medicine and Charity before the Welfare State*. (London: Routledge, 1991), 46–62.

Cazden, Robert E. *A Social History of the German Book Trade in America to the Civil War.* (Columbia, S.C.: Camden House, 1984).

Cipolla, Carlo M., and K. Borchardt, eds. *Europäische Wirtschaftsgeschichte, vol. 2: Sechzehntes und siebzehntes Jahrhundert.* (Stuttgart: Gustav Fischer, 1979).

Coffin, John G. "An Address Delivered Before the Contributors of the Boston Dispensary at Their Seventeenth Anniversary, October 21, 1813." In *Caring for the Working Man: The Rise and Fall of the Dispensary, An Anthology of Sources*, ed. Charles E. Rosenberg. (New York: Garland, 1989), 17–34.

Cook, Harold J. *The Decline of the Old Medical Regime in Stuart London.* (Ithaca: Cornell University Press, 1986).

————. "Henry Stubbe and the Virtuosi-Physicians." In *The Medical Revolution of the Seventeenth Century*, ed. Roger K. French and Andrew Wear. (Cambridge: Cambridge University Press, 1989), 256–65.

————. *Trials of an Ordinary Doctor: Joannes Groenevelt in Seventeenth Century London.* (Baltimore: Johns Hopkins University Press, 1994).

————. "Natural History and 17th Century English and Dutch Medicine." In *The Task of Healing: Medicine, Religion, and Gender in England and the Netherlands, 1450–1800*, ed. Hilary Marland and Margaret Pelling. (Rotterdam: Erasmus, 1996).

Cowen, David L. "The Edinburgh Pharmacopoeia." *Medical History* 1 (1957): 125–39, 340–51.

————. *Medicine and Health in New Jersey: A History.* (Princeton: Van Nostrand, 1964).

————. "The British North American Colonies as a Source of Drugs." *Veröffentlichungen der internationalen Gesellschaft für Geschichte der Pharmazie* 28 (1966): 47–59.

————. *A Bibliography on the History of Colonial and Revolutionary Medicine and Pharmacy.* (Madison, Wis.: American Institute of the History of Pharmacy, 1975).

————. *Medicine in Revolutionary New Jersey.* (Trenton: New Jersey Historical Commission, 1975).

————. *Colonial and Revolutionary Heritage of Pharmacy in America.* (Trenton: New Jersey Pharmaceutical Association, 1976).

————. "The Impact of the Materia Medica of the North American Indians on Professional Practice." In *Botanical Drugs of the Americas in the Old and New Worlds*, ed. Wolfgang-Hagen Hein. (Stuttgart: Wissenschaftliche Verlagsgesellschaft, 1984).

————. "'Zum Dienst des Gemeinen Mannes insonderheit für die Landleute': The Domestic and Veterinary Medical Books Printed in Colonial North America and the United

States in the German Language." In *Orbis Pictus: Kultur- und pharmaziehistorische Studien: Festschrift für Wolfgang-Hagen Hain zum 65. Geburtstag*, ed. Werner Dressendörfer and Wolf-Dieter Müller-Jahncke. (Frankfurt am Main: Govi-Verlag, 1985), 60–66.

———. "The Folk Medicine of the Pennsylvania Dutch." In *Folklore and Folk Medicines*, ed. John Scarborough. (Madison, Wisc.: American Institute of the History of Pharmacy, 1987).

———. "The Letters of Dr. William Brown to Andrew Craigie." *Pharmacy in History* 39 (1997): 140–47.

Cowen, David L., ed. *The Spread and Influence of British Pharmacopoeial and Related Literature: An Historical and Bibliographical Study*. (Stuttgart: Wissenschaftliche Verlagsgesellschaft, 1974).

Cowen, David L., and Renate Wilson. "The Traffic in Medical Ideas: Popular Medical Texts as German Imports and American Imprints." *Caduceus* 13.1 (1997): 67–80.

Coxe, John Redman. *The American Dispensatory*. (Philadelphia: Dobson, 1806).

Crellin, John K. "How Shall I Take My Medicine? Dosages and Other Matters in Eighteenth-Century Medicine." *Caduceus* 13.1 (1997): 39–50.

Crellin, John K., and J. R. Scott. "Pharmaceutical History and Its Sources in the Wellcome Collections, II: Drug Weighing in Britain, 1700–1900." *Medical History* 13 (1969): 51–67.

———. "Pharmaceutical History and Its Sources in the Wellcome Collections, III: Fluid Medicines, Prescription Reform, and Posology, 1700–1900." *Medical History* 14 (1970): 132–53.

Cressy, David. *Coming Over: Migration and Communication Between England and New England in the Seventeenth Century*. (Cambridge and New York: Cambridge University Press, 1987).

Culpepper, Nicholas, Gent. Student in Physick and Astrology. *The English Physician Enlarged, with 369 Medicines Made of English Herbs, that were not in any impression until this, being an astrolog-physical discourse of the vulgar herbs of this nation; containing a compleat method of physick, wherein a man may preserve his body in health or cure himself, being sick, for threepence charge, with such things only as grow in England, they being most fit for English bodies, etc. etc.* (London: Bettesworth and C. Hitch, 1733), 386 and index.

Cunningham, Andrew, and Roger French, eds. *The Medical Enlightenment of the Eighteenth Century*. (Cambridge: Cambridge University Press, 1990).

Curtin, Philip D. *Cross-Cultural Trade in World History*. (Cambridge: Cambridge University Press, 1984).

Davis, Michael M., Jr. "The Functions of a Dispensary or Out-Patient Department." In *Caring for the Working Man: The Rise and Fall of the Dispensary, An Anthology of Sources*, ed. Charles E. Rosenberg. (New York: Garland, 1989), 285–99.

Davis, Michael M., Jr., and Robert A. Warner. *Dispensaries, Their Management and Development: A Book for Administrators, Public Health Workers, and All Interested in Better Medical Service for the People*. (New York: Macmillan, 1918).

de Boor, Friedrich. "Pietismus, Enthusiasmus, und Separatismus an der Wende des 17./18. Jahrhunderts." *Nachrichten der Lutherakademie* (1968–69): 37–41.

———. "Die Franckeschen Stiftungen als 'Fundament' und 'Exempel' lokaler, territorialer, und universaler Reformziele des Hallischen Pietismus." *Pietismus und Neuzeit: Jahrbuch zur Geschichte des Neueren Protestantismus* 10 (1984): 215–26.

Debus, Allen G. *The English Paracelsians.* (London: Oldbourne, 1965).

———. "History with a Purpose: The Fate of Paracelsus." *Pharmacy in History* 26 (1984): 83–96.

———. *The French Paracelsians: The Chemical Challenge to Medical and Scientific Tradition in Early Modern France.* (Cambridge: Cambridge University Press, 1991).

Debus, Allen G., ed. *Science, Medicine, and Society in the Renaissance: Essays to Honor Walter Pagel.* (New York: Science History Publications, 1972).

Debus, Allen G., and Michael Walton, eds. *Reading the Book of Nature: The Other Side of the Scientific Revolution.* (16th Century Journal Publishers, 1998).

Dehmel, Gisela. *Arzneimittel in der Physikotheologie.* (Münster: Lit Verlag, 1996).

Denzel, Markus A. "Der Aufstieg und die Einbindung der Vereinigten Staaten von Amerika in die Weltwirtschaft." In *Währungen der Welt, I: Europäische und nordamerikanische Devisenkurse, 1777–1914,* ed. Jürgen Schneider, Oskar Schwarzer, and Friedrich Zellfelder. Beiträge zur Wirtschafts- und Sozialgeschichte 49. (Stuttgart, Franz Steiner Verlag, 1991), 146–77, 157ff.

Denzel, Markus A., ed. *Geld- und Wechselkurse der deutschen Messeplätze Leipzig und Braunschweig (18. Jahrhundert bis 1823).* Beiträge zur Wirtschafts- und Sozialgeschichte 61. (Stuttgart: Franz Steiner Verlag, 1996).

Depperman, Klaus. *Der hallesche Pietismus und der preussische Staat unter Friedrich III.* (Göttingen: Vandenhoeck and Rupprecht, 1961).

———. "Pietismus und moderner Staat." In *Pietismus und moderne Welt,* ed. Kurt Aland, E. Peschke, and M. Schmidt. Arbeiten zur Geschichte des Pietismus. (Witten: Luther-Verlag, 1974), vol. 12.

De Vorsey, Louis, Jr., ed. *De Brahm's Report of the General Survey in the Southern District of North America.* (Columbia: University of South Carolina Press, 1967).

Dinges, Martin. "Frühneuzeitliche Armenfürsorge als Sozialdisziplinierung? Probleme mit einem Konzept." *Geschichte und Gesellschaft* 17.1 (1991): 5–29.

Dinges, Martin, ed. *History of Homeopathy.* (Stuttgart: Steiner, 1997).

Doerflinger, Thomas M. *A Vigorous Spirit of Enterprise: Merchants and Economic Development in Revolutionary Philadelphia.* (Chapel Hill: Institute for Early American History and Culture, University of North Carolina Press, 1986).

Dr. Robert James's Powder for Fevers and all Inflammatory Disorders. Published by Virtue of His Majesty's Royal Letters Patent (n.p., n.d.).

Dreyhaupt, Johannes Friedrich. *Ausführlich diplomatisch historische Beschreibung . . . des Saalkreises,* 2 vols. (1780).

Duden, Barbara. *Geschichte unter der Haut: Ein Eisenacher Arzt und seine Patientinnen um 1730.* (Stuttgart, 1978).

Düffer, Johann C. F. *Dr. David Samuel von Madais . . . Kurze Beschreibung der Wirkungen und Anwendungsart der bekannten Hallischen Waisenhaus-Arzneyen.* (Halle: Verlag der Medicamentenexpedition und in Commission der Buchhandlung des Waisenhauses, 1808).

Duffy, Eamon. "Correspondence Fraternelle: The SPCK, the SPG, and the Churches of Switzerland in the War of the Spanish Succession." In *Reform and Reformation: England and the Continent*, ed. Derek Baker. (Oxford: Blackwell, 1979).

———. "The Society of [*sic*] Promoting Christian Knowledge and Europe: The Background to the Founding of the Christentumsgesellschaft." *Pietismus und Neuzeit* 7 (1981): 728–42.

Duffy, John. *Epidemics in Colonial America*. (Baton Rouge: Louisiana State University Press, 1953).

———. *The Healers: The Rise of the Medical Establishment*. (New York: McGraw-Hill, 1976).

———. *From Humors to Medical Science: A History of American Medicine*, 2d ed. (Urbana and Chicago: University of Illinois Press, 1993).

Duffy, John, ed. *The Rudolf Matas History of Medicine in Louisiana*. (Baton Rouge: Louisiana State University Press, 1957).

Dumschat, Sabine. "Deutsche Ärzte im Moskauer Russland." *Hamburger Beiträge zur Geschichte der Deutschen im europäischen Osten*, no. 5.

Eamon, William. *Science and the Secrets of Nature: Books of Secrets in Medieval and Early Modern Culture*. (Princeton: Princeton University Press, 1994).

Die Egenolff-Lutherische Schriftgiesserei in Frankfurt am Main und ihre geschäftlichen Verbindungen mit den Vereinigten Staaten von Nord Amerika. (Frankfurt am Main: D. Stempel AG, 1926).

Elmer, Peter. "Medicine, Religion, and the Puritan Revolution." In *The Medical Revolution of the Seventeenth Century*, ed. Roger K. French and Andrew Wear. (Cambridge: Cambridge University Press, 1989), 10–45.

Estes, J. Worth. "Therapeutic Practice in Colonial New England." In *Medicine in Colonial Massachusetts, 1620–1820: A Conference Held 25 and 26 May 1978 by the Colonial Society of Massachusetts*. (Boston: Colonial Society, distributed by University Press of Virginia, 1980).

———. "Patterns of Drug Usage in Colonial America." *New York State Journal of Medicine* 87.1 (1987): 37–45.

———. "The Pharmacology of Nineteenth-Century Patent Medicines." *Pharmacy in History* 30.1 (1988): 3–18.

———. *Dictionary of Protopharmacology: Therapeutic Practices, 1700–1850*. (Canton, Mass.: Science History Publications, 1990).

———. "The European Reception of the First Drugs from the New World." *Pharmacy in History* 37 (1995): 3–23.

Estes, J. Worth, ed. "Changing Fashions in Therapeutics." *Caduceus* 11.3 (1995): 65–72.

Fertig, Georg. "German Migration." In *Europeans on the Move: Studies on European Migration, 1500–1800*, ed. Nicholas P. Canny. (Oxford: Oxford University Press and Clarendon Press, 1994), 200–220.

Finzsch, Norbert, and Robert Jütte, eds. *Institutions of Confinement: Hospitals, Asylums, and Prisons in Western Europe and North America, 1500–1950*. (Cambridge: Cambridge University Press, 1996).

Fissell, Mary E. "Charity Universal? Institutions and Moral Reform in Eighteenth-Century Bristol." In *Stilling the Grumbling Hive: Debates on Social and Economic*

Problems in England, 1698–1740, ed. Lee Davison et al. (Stroud, England: Allan Sutton, 1992).

———. "Readers, Texts, and Context: Vernacular Medical Works in Early Modern England." *The Popularization of Medicine*, ed. Roy Porter. (London: Routledge, 1992), 72–96.

———. *Patients, Power, and the Poor in Eighteenth-Century Bristol*. (Cambridge: Cambridge University Press, 1991).

Fogleman, Aaron Spencer. "Migration to the Thirteen British North American Colonies, New Estimates." *Journal of Interdisciplinary History* 22 (1992): 691–709.

———. *Hopeful Journeys: German Immigration, Settlement, and Political Culture in Colonial America, 1717–1775*. (Philadelphia: University of Pennsylvania Press, 1995).

Forman Craine, Elaine, ed. *The Diary of Elizabeth Drinker*. (Boston: Northeastern University Press, 1991).

Foust, Clifford M. *Rhubarb: The Wondrous Drug*. (Princeton: Princeton University Press, 1992).

Francke, August Hermann. *Project von der Verpflegung der Krancken*. (Halle: Wirtschaftsarchiv der Franckeschen Stiftungen XIX/II/1: Acta der beym Waisenhause eingerichteten Kranckenpflege, generalia, vol. I, 1718, fols. 1–14, 1708).

———. *Segens-volle Fusstapfen des noch lebenden und waltenden liebreichen und getreuen Gottes . . .*, 3d ed. (Halle: Verlag des Waisenhauses, 1709).

———. *Nicodemus, or, A Treatise Against the Fear of Man . . . Rendered into English from the High-Dutch and Dedicated to the Honorable Society for Reformation of Manners*. (Boston: Rogers and Fowle, 1744).

———. "Project: Zu einem Seminario Universali oder Anlegung eines Pflantzgartens, von welchem man eine reale Verbesserung in allen Ständen in und auserhalb Teutschlandes, ja in Europa und allen übrigen Theilen der Welt zugewarten." In *August Hermann Francke: Werke in Auswahl*, ed. Erhard Peschke. (Witten: Luther-Verlag, 1969), 108–15.

French, Roger. "Sickness and the Soul: Stahl, Hoffmann, and Sauvages on Medical Pathology." In *The Medical Enlightenment of the Eighteenth Century*, ed. Andrew Cunningham and Roger French. (Cambridge: Cambridge University Press, 1990).

French, Roger K., and Andrew Wear, eds. *The Medical Revolution of the Seventeenth Century*. (Cambridge: Cambridge University Press, 1989).

Fritschi, Alfred. *Schwesterntum: Zur Sozialgeschichte der weiblichen Berufskrankenpflege in der Schweiz 1850–1930*. (Zurich: Chronos, 1990).

Gabriel, Karl. "Caritas angesichts fortschreitender Säkularisierung." In *Caritas und soziale Dienste*, ed. E. Gatz: *Geschichte des kirchlichen Lebens in den deutsch-sprachigen Ländern seit dem Ende des 18.* Jahrhunderts, vol. 5. (Freiburg and Basel: Herder, 1997), 438–55.

Gage, William. *Faith's Work Perfected, or Francke's Orphan House at Halle*. (New York: Anson D. F. Randolph, 1867).

Gartrell, Elizabeth G. "Women Healers and Domestic Remedies in Eighteenth-Century America: The Recipe Book of Elizabeth Coates Paschall." In *Early American Medicine*, ed. Robert Goler and Pascal J. Imperato. (New York: Fraunces Tavern Museum, 1987).

Gatz, Erwin, ed. *Caritas und soziale Dienste*, vol. 5: *Geschichte des kirchlichen Lebens in den deutsch-sprachigen Ländern seit dem Ende des 18. Jahrhunderts*. (Freiburg and Basel: Herder, 1997).

Gay, George W. "Abuse of Medical Charity: Discussion by Drs. Hasket Derby, J. W. Elliot, Alfred Worcester, Farrar Cobb, John C. Munro, Frederic A. Washburn, Jr., E. W. Cushing, Samuel Crowell, and Charles Cook, Boston Medical and Surgical Journal, March 16, 1905." In *Caring for the Working Man: The Rise and Fall of the Dispensary, An Anthology of Sources*, ed. Charles E. Rosenberg. (New York: Garland, 1989), 179–248.

Gelfand, Toby. "The Origins of a Modern Concept of Medical Specialization: John Morgan's Discourse of 1765." *Bulletin of the History of Medicine* 50 (1976): 511–35.

———. "Medicine in New France." In *Medicine in the New World*, ed. Ronald L. Numbers. (Knoxville: University of Tennessee Press, 1987).

Getz, Faye Marie. "Charity, Translation, and the Language of Medical Learning in Medieval England." *Bulletin for the History of Medicine* 64 (1990): 1–17.

Gevitz, Norman. *Other Healers: Unorthodox Medicine in America.* (Baltimore: Johns Hopkins University Press, 1988).

———. "But All Those Authors Are Foreigners: American Literary Nationalism and Domestic Medical Guides." In *The Popularization of Medicine, 1650–1850*, ed. Roy Porter. (London: Routledge, 1992).

Gevitz, Norman, and Micaela Sullivan-Fowler. "Making Sense of Therapeutics in Seventeenth-Century New England." *Caduceus* 11.2 (1995): 87–102.

Geyer-Kordesch, Johanna. "Fevers and Other Fundamentals: Dutch and German Medical Explanations, ca. 1680 to 1730." *Medical History* Supplement no. 1 (1981): 99–120.

———. "The Enlightened and the Pious in Eighteenth-Century Germany." In *Patients and Practitioners: Lay Perceptions of Medicine in Pre-Industrial Society*, ed. Roy Porter. (Cambridge: Cambridge University Press, 1985), 67–86.

———. "Georg Ernst Stahl: Pietismus, Medizin, und Aufklärung in Preussen im 18. Jahrhundert. " Unpublished *Habilitationsschrift*, University of Münster, 1987.

———. "Die Medizin im Spannungsfeld zwischen Aufklärung und Pietismus: Das unbequeme Werk Georg Ernst Stahls und dessen kulturelle Bedeutung." In *Zentren der Aufklärung, 1, Halle: Aufklärung und Pietismus*, ed. Norbert Hinske. Wolfenbütteler Studien zur Aufklärung 15. (Heidelberg: Lambert Schneider, 1989), 255–73.

———. "Court Physicians and State Regulation in Eighteenth-Century Prussia: The Emergence of Medical Science and the Demystification of the Body." In *Medicine at the Courts of Europe, 1500–1837*. (London: Routledge, 1990).

———. "Georg Ernst Stahl's Radical Pietist Medicine and Its Influence on the German Enlightenment." In *The Medical Enlightenment of the Eighteenth Century*, ed. Andrew Cunningham and Roger French. (Cambridge: Cambridge University Press, 1990), 67–87.

Gibson, James E. *Bodo Otto and the Medical Background of the American Revolution.* (Baltimore: Charles C. Thomas, 1937).

Glatfelter, Charles Henry. *Pastors and People: German Lutheran and Reformed Churches in the Pennsylvania Field, 1717–1793*, 2 vols. (Kutztown, Pa.: Kutztown Publishers, 1980, 1981).

Goldwater, S. S. "Dispensary Ideals: With a Plan for Dispensary Reform Based upon the Adoption of the Principle of Restricted Numbers." In *Caring for the Working Man: The Rise and Fall of the Dispensary, An Anthology of Sources*, ed. Charles E. Rosenberg. (New York: Garland, 1989), 249–73.

Golz, Hermann. "Repertorium Epistolarum Sibiriacum I, aus Curt Friedrich von Wreechs 'Wahrhafter und umständlicher Historie von denen Schwedischen Gefangenen in Russland und Siberien . . .' (Sorau 1725) zusammengestellt." In *Halle und Osteuropa*, ed. J. Wallmann and U. Sträter. (Halle: Niemeyer; Tübingen: Verlag der Franckeschen Stiftungen, 1997), 19–48.

Gottsched, Louise Adelgunde Victorie. *Die Pietisterey im Fischbein-Rocke*. (Reprint Stuttgart: Wolfgang Martens, 1986).

Grabbe, Hans-Jürgen. "Besonderheiten der europäischen Einwanderung in die USA während der frühen nationalen Periode, 1783–1820." *American Studies* 33 (1988): 271–90.

Granshaw, Lindsay, and Roy Porter, eds. *The Hospital in History*. (New York: Routledge, 1989).

Grell, Ole Peter. "Plague in Elizabethan and Stuart London: The Dutch Response." *Medical History* 34 (1990): 424–39.

Grell, Ole Peter, and Andrew Cunningham, eds. "German Immigration." *Journal of Interdisciplinary History* 20 (1990).

———. *Religio Medici: Medicine and Religion in Seventeenth-Century England*. (Aldershot, England: Scholar Press, 1996).

———. *Health Care and Poor Relief in Protestant Europe, 1500–1700*. (London: Routledge, 1997).

Guerra, Francisco. "Drugs from the Indies and the Political Economy of the Sixteenth Century." *Analecta Medico Historica* 1 (1966): 29–54.

Habrich, Christa. "Therapeutische Grundsätze pietistischer Ärzte des 18. Jahrhunderts." *Beiträge zur Geschichte der Pharmazie* 31.16 (1982): 121–23.

———. "Untersuchungen zur pietistischen Medizin und ihrer Ausprägung bei Johann Samuel Carl und seinem Kreis." Unpublished *Habilitationsschrift*, Ludwig-Maximilians-Universität, 1982.

———. "Zur Ethik des pietistischen Arztes im 18. Jahrhundert." In *Ethik in der Geschichte der Medizin und Naturwissenschaften*, ed. Wolfram Kaiser and Arina Völker. (Halle and Wittenberg: Martin-Luther Universität Halle-Wittenberg, 1985), 55, E77.

———. "Characteristic Features of Eighteenth-Century Therapeutics in Germany." *Clio Medica* 22 (1991): 39–49.

Haller, John S. *Medical Protestants, the Eclectics in American Medicine, 1825–1939*. (Carbondale: Southern Illinois University Press, 1994).

———. *Kindly Medicines: Physio-Medicalism in America, 1836–1911*. (Kent: Kent State University Press, 1997).

Hart, Simon, and Harry J. Kreider, eds. *Evangelisch Luthersche Kerk (Netherlands): Protocols of the Lutheran Church in New York City, 1702–1750, Correspondence with Lutheran Bodies in Amsterdam, Hamburg, London, and Skara*. (Excerpts published New York: New York Public Library, 1958).

———. *Lutheran Church in New York and New Jersey, 1722–1760: Lutheran Records in the Ministerial Archives of the Staatsarchiv, Hamburg, Germany*. (Ann Arbor: University of Michigan Press, 1962).

Hatfield, M. P., and Clark Roswell. "Report of the Special Committee of the Medical Association of the District of Columbia, on the 'Hospital and Dispensary Abuse in the City of Washington.'" In *Caring for the Working Man: The Rise and Fall of the*

Dispensary, An Anthology of Sources, ed. Charles E. Rosenberg. (New York: Garland, 1989).

Haussmann, Carl Frederick. "Kunze's Seminarium, and the Society for the Propagation of Christianity and Useful Knowledge among the Germans in America." *Americana Germanica (Philadelphia)* 27 (1917): 25–28.

Helm, Jürgen. "Der Umgang mit dem kranken Menschen im halleschen Pietismus des frühen 18. Jahrhunderts." *Medizinhistorisches Journal* 31 (1996): 67–87.

———. "Kinder und Lehrkrankenhaus im frühen 18. Jahrhundert? Die Einrichtungen zur Krankenfürsorge in den Franckeschen Stiftungen." *Medizinhistorisches Journal* 3.33 (1998): 107–41.

Helmuth, Justus Heinrich Christian. *Kurze Nachricht von dem sogenannten gelben Fieber in Philadelphia, für den nachdenkenden Christen.* (Philadelphia: Stein and Kämmerer, 1793–94).

Henderson, John. "The Hospitals of Late-Medieval and Renaissance Florence: A Preliminary Survey." In *The Hospital in History*, ed. Lindsey Granshaw and Roy Porter. (London: Routledge, 1989), 63–92.

Hickel, Erika. "Britische Pharmakopieliteratur des 17.–19. Jahrhunderts." In *The Spread and Influence of British Pharmacopoeial and Related Literature: An Historical and Bibliographical Study*, ed. D. L. Cowen. (Stuttgart: Wissenschaftliche Verlagsgesellschaft, 1974).

Higby, Gregory J. *In Search of American Pharmacy: The Professional Life of William Procter, Jr.* (Tuscaloosa: University of Alabama Press, 1992).

Hinrichs, Carl. *Friedrich Wilhelm I, König in Preussen.* (Hamburg: Hanseatische Verlagsanstalt, 1941).

———. *Preussentum und Pietismus: Der Pietismus in Brandenburg-Preussen als religiös-soziale Reformbewegung.* (Göttingen: Vandenhoeck und Ruprecht, 1971).

Hitchcock, Tim. "The English Workhouse: A Study in Institutional Poor Relief in Selected Counties, 1696–1750." Doctoral dissertation, Oxford University, 1985.

———. "Paupers and Preachers: The SPCK and the Parochial Workhouse Movement." In *Stilling the Grumbling Hive: The Response to Social and Economic Problems in England, 1689–1750*, ed. Lee Davison et al. (New York: St. Martin's Press, 1992), 145–66.

Hoffmann, Friedrich. *Fundamenta Medicinae ex principiis naturae mechanicis in usum Philiatrorum succinte proposita . . .* (Halle: Impens. Simon Joh. Hubneri, literis viduae Salfeldianae, 1695).

———. *Medicinae rationalis systematicae tomus primus quo philosophia corporis humani vivi et sani ex solidis physico-mechanicis et anatomicis principiis methodo plane demonstrativa per certa theoremata ac scholia traditur . . .*, 2d ed. (Halle: Officina Rengeriana, 1729 [first publication 1707]).

Hoffmann, Friedrich, comp. *Popular German Names of Domestic Drugs and Medicines* (Volksthümliche Deutsche Arzneimittel-Namen), 3d. ed. (1901).

Holmes, Geoffrey. *Augustan England: Professions, State, and Society, 1680–1730.* (London: Allen and Unwin, 1982).

Hubatsch, Walther. *Geschichte der evangelischen Kirche in Ostpreussen.* (Göttingen: Vandenhoeck und Ruprecht, 1968).

Hunter, Michael. "The Reluctant Philanthropist: Robert Boyle and the 'Communication of Secrets and Receits in Physick.'" In *Religio Medici: Medicine and Religion in Seventeenth-Century England*, ed. Ole Peter Grell and Andrew Cunningham. (Aldershot, England: Scholar Press, 1996).

Imbert, Jean. *Le Droit hospitalier de l'Ancien Regime*. (Paris: Presses Universitaires de France, 1993).

Imhof, Arthur. *Lebenserwartungen in Deutschland vom 17. bis 19. Jahrhundert*. (Weinheim, 1990).

Jarcho, Saul. *Quinine's Predecessor: Francesco Torti and the Early History of Cinchona*. (Baltimore: Johns Hopkins University Press, 1993).

Jewson, N. D. "Medical Knowledge and the Patronage System in Eighteenth-Century England." *Sociology* 8 (1974): 369–85.

Jeyaraj, Daniel. *Inkulturation in Tranquebar: Der Beitrag der frühen dänischen-halleschen Mission zum Werden einer indisch-einheimischen Kirche, 1706–1730*. (Erlangen: Verlag der evangelisch Lutherischen Mission, 1996).

Jones, Colin. *Charity and Bienfaisance: The Treatment of the Poor in the Montpellier Region, 1740–1815*. (Cambridge: Cambridge University Press, 1982).

———. "The Constitution of the Modern Hospital Patient." In *Institutions of Confinement: Hospitals, Asylums, and Prisons in Western Europe and North America, 1500–1950*, ed. Norbert Finzsch and Robert Jütte. (New York: Cambridge University Press, 1996), 55–74.

———. "The Great Chain of Buying." *American Historical Review* 101 (1996): 13–40.

Jones, George F. "German-Speaking Settlers in Georgia, 1733–1741." *The Report: A Journal of German-American History* 38 (1982): 35–51.

———. *Salzburger Saga*. (Athens: University of Georgia Press, 1983).

———. "Report of Mr. Ettwein's Journey to Georgia and South Carolina." *South Carolina Historical Journal* 91 (1991): 147–60.

———. *The Georgia Dutch*. (Athens: University of Georgia Press, 1992).

———. "German-Speaking Settlers in Georgia, 1733–1741." *The Report: A Journal of German-American History* 38 (1982): 35–51.

Jones, George F., Renate Wilson et al., eds. *Detailed Reports of the Salzburger Emigrants Who Settled in America . . .* (Vols. 1–17, Athens: University of Georgia Press; vol. 18, Rockland, Me.: Picton Press, 1966–95).

Jones, Gordon W., ed. *Cotton Mather: The Angel of Bethesda*. (Barre, Mass.: American Antiquarian Society and Barre Publishers, 1972).

Juncker, Johann. "Vom schädlichen Fieber-Vertreiben." *Wöchentliche Hallische Anzeigen* 25 (1737): 432–37.

———. *Entwurf zu einer Instruction eines Medici ordinarii*. (Halle: Wirtschaftsarchiv der Franckeschen Stiftungen XIX/II/1: Acta der beym Waisenhause eingerichteten Kranckenpflege, generalia, vol. I, 1718, fols. 78–89).

Jütte, Robert. *Obrigkeitliche Armenfürsorge in deutschen Reichsstädten der frühen Neuzeit: Städtische Armenwesen in Frankfurt am Main und Köln*. (Cologne: Böhlau, 1984).

———. "Disziplinierungsmechanismen in der städtischen Armenfürsorge der Frühneuzeit." In *Soziale Sicherheit und soziale Disziplinierung: Beiträge zu einer historischen Theorie der Sozialpolitik*, ed. Florian Tennstedt and Christoph Sachse. (Frankfurt am Main: Suhrkamp, 1986).

———. "Die medizinische Versorgung einer Stadtbevölkerung im 16. und 17. Jahrhundert am Beispiel der Reichsstadt Köln." *Medizinhistorisches Journal* 22.1 (1987): 173–84.

———. Die Persistenz des Verhütungswissens in der Volkskultur: Sozial- und medizinhistorische Anmerkungern zur These von der 'Vernichtung der weisen Frauen.'" *Medizinhistorisches Journal* 24 (1989): 214–31.

———. *Ärzte, Heiler, und Patienten: Medizinischer Alltag in der frühen Neuzeit.* (Munich and Zurich: Artemis and Winkler, 1991).

Jütte, Robert, and Wolfgang Eckart, eds. *Das europäische Gesundheitssystem: Gemeinsamkeiten und Unterschiede in historischer Perspektive.* (Stuttgart: Franz Steiner Verlag, 1994).

Kaiser, Wolfram. "Der Lehrkörper der Medizinischen Fakultät in der halleschen Amtszeit von Georg Ernst Stahl." In *Georg Ernst Stahl, 1659–1734: Hallesches Symposium, 1984,* ed. Wolfram Kaiser and Arina Völker. Wissenschaftliche Beiträge der Martin-Luther-Universität Halle-Wittenberg. (Halle and Wittenberg: Martin-Luther-Universität Halle-Wittenberg, 1985).

Kaiser, Wolfram, ed. *Johann Juncker und seine Zeit.* (Halle and Wittenberg: Martin-Luther-Universität Halle-Wittenberg, 1979).

Kaiser, Wolfram, and Arina Völker. *Michael Alberti 1682–1757.* (Halle and Wittenberg: Martin-Luther-Universität Halle-Wittenberg, 1982).

———. "Repräsentanten der Ars medica halensis in der russischen Medizingeschichte des 18. Jahrhunderts." *Forschungen zur osteuropäischen Geschichte: Osteuropa Institut der Freien Universität Berlin: Historische Veröffentlichungen* 44 (1990): 61–95.

Kaiser, Wolfram, and Arina Völker, eds. *Georg Ernst Stahl (1659–1734): Hallesches Symposium, 1984.* (Halle and Wittenberg: Martin-Luther-Universität Halle-Wittenberg, 1985).

Kaiser, Wolfram, and Heinz Krosch. "Drei Generationen Juncker." *Wissenschaftliche Zeitschrift der Martin-Luther-Universität Halle-Wittenberg: Mathematisch-naturwissenschaftliche Reihe* 14 (1965): 397–432.

———. "Zur Geschichte der medizinischen Fakultät der Universität Halle im 18. Jahrhundert (VIII): Zum 250. Geburtstag von Dorothea Christiane Erxleben." *Wissenschaftliche Zeitschrift der Martin-Luther-Universität Halle-Wittenberg: Mathematisch-Naturwissenschaftliche Reihe* 14.4 (1965): 269–302.

———. "Die Statuten der Medizinischen Fakultät im 18. Jahrhundert." *Wissenschaftliche Beiträge Universität Halle* 3 (1967): 77–104.

———. "Zur Geschichte der medizinischen Fakultät der Universität Halle im 18. Jahrhundert (XX): Hallesche Doktoranden als Mitglieder der Academie Imperialis Leopoldina-Carolina Naturae Curiosorum." *Wissenschaftliche Zeitschrift der Martin-Luther-Universität Halle-Wittenberg: Mathematisch-naturwissenschaftliche Reihe* 16 (1967): 603–44.

———. "Die Statuten der Medizinischen Fakultät im 18. Jahrhundert." *250 Jahre Collegium Clinicum Halense, 1717–1767: Beiträge zur Geschichte der Medizinischen Fakultät der Universität Halle. Wissenschaftliche Beiträge der Martin-Luther-Universität Halle-Wittenberg* 673 (R2). (Halle: Martin-Luther-Universität Halle-Wittenberg, 1967).

Katz, Michael B., ed. *In the Shadow of the Poorhouse: A Social History of Welfare in America.* (New York: Basic Books, 1986).

Keeny, Elisabeth Barnaby. "Unless Powerful Sick: Domestic Medicine in the Old South." In *Science and Medicine in the Old South,* ed. Ronald L. Numbers and Todd L. Savitt. (Baton Rouge: Louisiana State University Press, 1989), 276–94.

King, Lester S. "Stahl and Hoffman: A Study in Eighteenth-Century Animism." *Journal of the History of Medicine and Allied Sciences* 19 (1964): 118–30.

———. *The Road to Medical Enlightenment, 1650–1695.* (London: Macdonald, 1970).

King, Susan, ed. *History and Records of the Charleston Orphan House, 1790–1860.* (Easley, S.C.: Southern Historical Press).

King, William Harvey. *History of Homeopathy and Its Institutions in America*, 4 vols. (New York: Lewis Publishing, 1905).

Kinzelbach, Annemarie. *Gesundbleiben, Krankwerden, Armsein in der frühneuzeitlichen Gesellschaft: Gesunde und Kranke in den Reichsstädten Überlingen und Ulm, 1500–1700.* (Stuttgart: Franz Steiner Verlag, 1995).

Klingebiehl, Thomas. "Huguenot Settlements in Central Europe." In Hartmut Lehmann et al., eds., *In Search of Peace and Prosperity: New Settlements in Eighteenth-Century Europe and America.* (University Park: The Pennsylvania State University Press, 2000), 39–67.

Konert, Jürgen. "Caritas est viva: Gedanken zu einem Forschungsprojekt über den Einfluss des Pietismus auf die Entwicklung von Medizin und Pharmazie." *Das achtzehnte Jahrhundert: Mitteilungen der deutschen Gesellschaft für die Erforschung des 18. Jahrhunderts* 16 (1992): 137–52.

———. "Friedrich Hoffmann (1660–1742)." *Zeitschrift für ärztliche Fortbildung* 17 (1993): 413–17.

———. "Academic and Practical Medicine in Halle During the Era of Stahl, Hoffmann, and Juncker." *Caduceus* 13.1 (1997): 23–38.

Krafka, Joseph. "An Account of the Attempt of the Society of Apothecaries to Establish the Drug Trade in Colonial America." *Journal of the American Pharmaceutical Association* 28 (1939): 616–19.

———. "Medicine in Colonial Georgia." *Georgia Historical Quarterly* 31 (1947): 326–44.

Kramer, Gustav. *August Hermann Francke: Ein Lebensbild.* (Halle, 1880–82).

Kramer, Gustav, ed. *August H. Franckes pädagogische Schriften, nebst der Darstellung seines Lebens und seiner Stiftungen.* (Langensalza: H. Beyer & Söhne, 1885; reprint Osnabrück, 1966).

Kredel, F. E., and J. H. Hoch. "Early Relations of Pharmacy and Medicine in the United States." *Journal of the American Pharmaceutical Association* 28 (1939): 702–7.

Kreider, Harry J. "The Lutheran Church in New York, 1649–1772." *Bulletin of the New York Public Library* (1954): 48–50.

Kremers, Edward. "Historical Fragments, No. 22, Two Invoices of 1785." *Journal of the American Pharmaceutical Association* 20 (7) 1931: 682–95

Kuppermann, Karen O. *Providence Island, 1630–1641: The Other Puritan Colony.* (Cambridge: Cambridge University Press, 1993).

Labisch, Alfons. *Homo Hygienicus: Gesundheit und Medizin in der Neuzeit.* (Frankfurt am Main: Campus, 1992).

Lachmund, Jens, and Gunnar Stolberg. *Patientenwelten, Krankheit, und Medizin vom späten 18. bis zum frühen 20. Jahrhundert im Spiegel von Autobiographien.* (Opladen: Leske and Budrich, 1995).

Lambert, Frank. *"Pedlar in Divinity": George Whitefield and the Transatlantic Revivals, 1737–1770.* (Princeton: Princeton University Press, 1994).

———. *Inventing the Great Awakening.* (Princeton: Princeton University Press, 1999).

Lane, Joan. "'The Doctor Scolds Me': The Diaries and Correspondence of Patients in Eighteenth-Century England." In *Patients and Practitioners: Lay Perceptions of Medicine in Pre-Industrial Society,* ed. Roy Porter. (Cambridge: Cambridge University Press, 1985), 205–48.

Lanz, Almut. *Arzneimittel in der Therapie Friedrich Hoffmanns (1660–1742): Unter besonderer Berücksichtigung der Medicina consultatoria (1721–1723).* (Braunschweig: Deutscher Apotheker-Verlag, 1995).

La Vopa, Anthony J. *Grace, Talent, and Merit: Poor Students, Clerical Careers, and Professional Ideology in Eighteenth-Century Germany.* (Cambridge: Cambridge University Press, 1988).

Lawrence, William. "Medical Relief to the Poor, September, 1877." In *Caring for the Working Man: The Rise and Fall of the Dispensary: An Anthology of Sources,* ed. Charles E. Rosenberg. (New York: Garland, 1989), 63–116.

Leavitt, Judith Walzer. *Brought to Bed: Childbearing in America, 1750 to 1950.* (New York: Oxford University Press, 1986).

Lehmann, Arno. *Es begann in Tranquebar: Die Geschichte der ersten evangelischen Kirche in Indien.* (Berlin: Evangelische Verlagsanstalt, 1956).

———. *Hallesche Mediziner und Medizinen am Anfang deutsch-indischer Beziehungen.* (Halle: Verlag des Waisenhauses, 1956).

Lehmann, Hartmut. *Pietismus und weltliche Ordnung in Württemberg vom 17. bis zum 20. Jahrhundert.* (Stuttgart: Kohlhammer, 1969).

———. *Das Zeitalter des Absolutismus.* (Stuttgart: Kohlhammer, 1980).

———. "Pietismus und soziale Reform in Brandenburg-Preussen." In *Preussen, Europa, und das Reich,* ed. Oswald Hauser. (Cologne and Vienna: Böhlau, 1987).

Lehmann, Hartmut, Hermann Wellenreuther, and Renate Wilson, in cooperation with John B. Frantz and Carola Wessel, eds. *In Search of Peace and Prosperity: New Settlements in Eighteenth-Century Europe and North America.* (University Park: The Pennsylvania State University Press, 2000).

Leibrock-Plehn, Larissa. *Hexenkräuter oder Arznei: Die Abtreibungsmittel im 16. und 17. Jahrhundert.* (Stuttgart: Wissenschaftliche Verlagsgesellschaft, 1992).

Lempa, Heikki. *Bildung der Triebe: der deutsche Philanthropismus, 1768–1788.* (Turku: Turun yliopisto, 1993).

Lesky, Erna. *Österreichisches Gesundheitswesen im Zeitalter des aufgeklärten Absolutismus.* (Vienna, 1959).

Lesky, Erna, ed. *A System of Complete Medical Police: Selections from Johann Peter Frank.* (Baltimore, 1976).

Lettsom, John Coakley. "Hints Designed to Promote the Establishment of a Dispensary, for Extending Medical Relief to the Poor at Their Own Habitations." In *Caring for the Working Man: The Rise and Fall of the Dispensary, An Anthology of Sources,* ed. Charles E. Rosenberg. (New York: Garland, 1989), 1–16.

Lewis, William. *The Edinburgh New Dispensatory.* (Philadelphia: Dobson, 1791).

Lieburg, Mart van. "Religion and Medical Practice in the Netherlands in the 17th Century." In *The Task of Healing: Medicine, Religion, and Gender in England and the Netherlands, 1450–1800,* ed. Hilary Marland and Margaret Pelling. (Rotterdam: Erasmus, 1996), 135–44.

Lindberg, Carter. "The Lutheran Tradition." In *Caring and Curing: Health and Medicine in the Western Religious Traditions*, ed. Ronald L. Numbers and Darrel W. Amundsen. (New York: Macmillan, 1986).

Lindemann, Mary. *Patriots and Paupers: Hamburg, 1712–1830*. (New York: Oxford University Press, 1990).

———. *Health and Healing in Eighteenth-Century Germany*. (Baltimore: Johns Hopkins University Press, 1996).

Loetz, Franziska. "Medikalisierung in Frankreich, Grossbritannien, und Deutschland, 1750–1850: Ansätze, Ergebnisse, und Perspektiven der Forschung." In *Das europäische Gesundheitssystem: Gemeinsamkeiten und Unterschiede in historischer Perspektive*, ed. Robert Jütte and Wolfgang Eckart. (Stuttgart: Franz Steiner Verlag, 1994), 123–62.

Lovelace, Richard L. *The American Pietism of Cotton Mather: Origins of American Evangelicalism*. (Grand Rapids: Christian University Press/Bermans, 1979).

Madai, David Samuel von. *Kurtze Nachricht von dem Nutzen und Gebrauch einiger bewährten Medicamente: Welche zu Halle im Magdeburgischen in dem Waisenhaus dispensiret werden*. (Halle: Waisenhaus, 1746).

———. *Abhandlung von den sogenannten kalten Fiebern*. (Halle: Verlag des Waisenhauses, 1747).

———. *Kort bericht van de nuttigheid en 't gebruik van eenige beproefde geneesmiddelen*. (Amsterdam: n.p., 1760).

———. *A Brief Account of the Effects and Use of Some Approved Medicines Which Are Dispensed in the Orphanhouse at Halle*. (Halle: Orphanhouse, 1784).

Mair, John. *Book-Keeping Modernized, or Merchant Accounts by Double Entry, According to the Italian Form*, 8th ed. (Edinburgh, 1800).

Maisch, John M. "G. H. E. Mühlenberg als Botaniker." *Pharmaceutische Rundschau* 4.6 (1886): 119–29.

Marland, Hilary, and Margaret Pelling, eds. *The Task of Healing: Medicine, Religion, and Gender in England and the Netherlands, 1450–1800*. (Rotterdam: Erasmus, 1996).

Mather, Samuel. *Vita B. Hermanni Augusti Franckii . . . Revisa, et cura Samuelis Mather . . . , cum dedicatione ejus, edita*. (Boston, 1733).

Matthias, Markus. "Enthusiastische Hermeneutik des Pietismus, dargestellt an Johanna Eleonora Petersens Gespräche des Herzens mit Gott." *Pietismus und Neuzeit* 17 (1991): 36–61.

McCusker, John J. *Money and Exchange in Europe and America, 1600–1775*. (Chapel Hill: University of North Carolina Press, 1978).

McCusker, John L., and Russell R. Menard. *The Economy of British America, 1607–1789*. (Chapel Hill: University of North Carolina Press, 1985).

Meier, Louis A. *Early Pennsylvania Medicine: A Representative Early American Medical History, Montgomery County, Pennsylvania, 1682–1799*. (Boyertown, Pa.: Gilbert Printing Co., 1976).

Mols, Roger, S. J. "Die Bevölkerung Europas 1500–1700." In *Europäische Wirtschaftsgeschichte: Sechzehntes und siebzehntes Jahrhundert*, ed. C. M. Cipolla and K. Borchardt. (Stuttgart: Gustav Fischer, 1979).

Müller, Thomas. *Kirche zwischen zwei Welten: Die evangelische Obrigkeitsproblematik bei Heinrich Melchior Mühlenberg*. (Stuttgart: Franz Steiner, 1994).

Müller-Jahncke, Wolf-Dieter. "Der 'Linnaeus Americanus' und seine Beziehungen zu deutschen Botanikern: G. H. E Mühlenberg: Beiträge zu amerikanisch-deutschen Beziehungen in den Naturwissenschaften des 18. und 19. Jahrhunderts." *Deutsche Apothekerzeitung* 117 (1977): 1323–30.

———. "Johann David Schoepf, 1752–1800: A German Physician as a Botanist and Zoologist in North America." *Pharmacy in History* 20 (1978): 43–64.

———. "Astrologisch-magische Theorie und Praxis in der Heilkunde der frühen Neuzeit." *Sudhoffs Archiv: Zeitschrift für Wissenschaftsgeschichte* 25 (1985): 121–33.

———. "Die Medicina Pennsylvania des George de Benneville." In *Dixhuitieme: Zur Geschichte von Medizin und Naturwissenschaften im 18. Jahrhundert*, ed. Arina Völker. (Halle and Wittenberg: Martin-Luther-Universität Halle-Wittenberg, 1988), 25, 121–33.

Müller-Jahncke, Wolf-Dieter, and Christoph Friedrich. *Geschichte der Arzneimitteltherapie*. (Stuttgart: Deutscher Apotheker Verlag, 1996).

Murphy, Lamar Riley. *Enter the Physician: The Transformation of Domestic Medicine, 1760–1860*. (Tuscaloosa: University of Alabama Press, 1991).

Newman, William R. "Alchemical and Baconian Views on the Art-Nature Division." In *Reading the Book of Nature: The Other Side of the Scientific Revolution*, ed. Allen G. Debus and Michael T. Walton. (Kirksville, Mo.: Sixteenth-Century Journal Publishers, 1998), 81–90.

Numbers, Ronald L. "'Do-It-Yourself the Sectarian Way.'" In *Medicine Without Doctors*, ed. G. B. Risse, R. L. Numbers, and J. W. Leavitt. (New York: Science History Publications, 1977), 49–72.

Numbers, Ronald L., ed. *Medicine in the New World*. (Knoxville: University of Tennessee Press, 1987).

Numbers, Ronald L., and Darrel W. Amundsen, eds. *Caring and Curing: Health and Medicine in the Western Religious Traditions*. (New York: Macmillan, 1986).

Numbers, Ronald L., and Todd L. Savitt, eds. *Science and Medicine in the Old South*. (Baton Rouge: Louisiana State University Press, 1989).

Oschlies, Wolf. *Die Arbeits- und Berufspädagogik A. H. Franckes*. Arbeiten zur Geschichte des Pietismus 6. (Witten, 1969).

Owen, David. *English Philanthropy, 1660–1960*. (Cambridge, Mass.: Harvard University Press, 1964).

Pagel, Walter. "Helmont-Leibniz-Stahl." *Sudhoffs Archiv für Geschichte der Medizin* (1931) 24: 19–59.

———. *Paracelsus: An Introduction to Philosophical Medicine in the Era of the Renaissance*. (New York: S. Karger, 1958).

Paletschek, Sylvia. "Adelige und bürgerliche Frauen, 1770–1870." In *Adel und Bürgertum in Deutschland, 1770–1848*, ed. Elisabeth Fehrenbach. Schriften des Historischen Kollegs 31. (Munich: Oldenbourg, 1994).

Palmer, Michael A. *John Uri Lloyd, the Great Eclectic*. (Carbondale: Southern Illinois University Press, 1998).

Palmer, Richard. "Thomas Corbyn, Quaker Merchant." *Medical History* 33 (1989): 371–76.

Parker, Geoffrey. "Die Entstehung des modernen Geld-und Finanzwesens in Europa, 1500–1730." In *Europäische Wirtschaftsgeschichte, vol. 2: Sechzehntes und siebzehntes*

Jahrhundert, ed. Carlo M. Cipolla and K. Borchardt. (Stuttgart: Gustav Fischer, 1979).

Parrish, Edward. "Eclectic Pharmacy." *American Journal of Pharmacy* 23 (1851): 329–25.

———. "Pharmacy in Philadelphia." *American Journal of Pharmacy* 14 (1869): 97–108.

Partington, James Reddick. *A History of Chemistry*. (London: Macmillan and St. Martin's Press, 1960, vol 1; 1961, vol 2; 1962, vol. 3).

Peickert, Heinz. *Geheimmittel im deutschen Arzneiverkehr: Ein Beitrag zur Wirtschaftsgeschichte der Pharmazie und zur Arzneispezialitätenfrage*. (Leipzig: Edelmann, 1932).

Pele, Ortwin, and Gertrud Pickhan. *Zwischen Lübeck und Novgorod: Wirtschaft, Politik, und Kultur im Ostseeraum vom frühen Mittelater bis ins 20. Jahrhundert*. (Lüneburg: Institut Nordostdeutsches Kulturwerk, 1998).

Pelling, Margaret. "Healing the Sick Poor: Social Policy and Disability in Norwich, 1550–1640." *Medical History* 29 (1985): 115–37.

Pelling, Margaret, and Charles Webster. "Medical Practitioners." *Health, Medicine, and Mortality in Sixteenth-Century England*, ed. Charles Webster. (Cambridge: Cambridge University Press, 1979), 165–236.

Peschke, Erhard. *Francke Werke in Auswahl*. (Berlin: Evangelische Verlagsanstalt, 1969).

Piechocki, Werner. "Gesundheitsfürsorge und Krankenpflege in den Franckeschen Stiftungen in Halle/Saale." *Acta Historica Leopoldina* 2 (1965): 29–66.

———. "Das Testament des Halleschen Klinikers Friedrich Hoffmann d. J." *Acta Historica Leopoldina* 2 (1965): 112–14.

Podczeck, Ottto, ed. *Der grosse Aufsatz: August Hermann Franckes Schrift über eine Reform des Erziehungs-und Bildungswesens als Ausgangspunkt einer geistlichen und sozialen Neuordung der Evangelischen Kirche des 18. Jahrhunderts*. (Leipzig: Abhandlungen der Sächsischen Akademie der Wissenschaften zu Leipzig, Philologisch-historische Klasse, 1962).

Poeckern, Hans Joachim. *Die Halleschen Waisenhausarzeneyen*. (Leipzig: Edition Leipzig, 1984).

———. "300 Jahre Waisenhausapotheke." Unpublished manuscript (Halle: Hallesche Waisenhausapotheke, 1998).

Porter, Roy. "The Gift Relation: Philanthropy and Provincial Hospitals in 18th-Century England." In *The Hospital in History*, ed. Lindsay Granshaw and Roy Porter. (New York: Routledge, 1989), 149–78.

Porter, Roy, ed. *Patients and Practitioners: Lay Perceptions of Medicine in Pre-Industrial Society*. (Cambridge and New York: Cambridge University Press, 1985).

———. *The Popularization of Medicine*. (London: Routledge, 1992).

Porter, Roy, and Andrew Wear, eds. *Problems and Methods in the History of Medicine*. (London: Croom Helm, 1987).

Porter, Roy, and Dorothy Porter. "The Rise of the English Drugs Industry: The Role of Thomas Corbyn." *Medical History* 33 (1989): 277–95.

Porter, Susan. "Francke's Transatlantic Legacy." In *Waisenhäuser vor und nach August Hermann Franckes Gründing 1698. Hallesche Forschungen*. (Tübingen: Max Niemeyer Verlag, 2000).

Rappaport, George David. *Stability and Change in Revolutionary Pennsylvania: Banking, Politics, and Social Structure*. (University Park: The Pennsylvania State University Press, 1996).

Richter, Christian F. *Kurzer und deutlicher Unterricht von dem Leibe und natürlichen Leben des Menschen.* (Halle: Im Waisenhause, 1705).

———. *Ausführlicher Bericht von der Essentia Dulci.* (Halle: Waisenhaus, 1708).

———. *Seeligen Hn. D. Christian Friedrich Richters Höchst-nöthige Erkenntnis des Menschen, sonderlich nach dem Leibe und natürlichen Leben, oder ein deutlicher Unterricht, von der Gesundheit und deren Erhaltung; auch von deren Ursachen, Kennzeichen, und Namen der Krankheiten, damit ein jeder, auch ungelehrter bei Ermangelung eines Medici, sonderlich durch XI hierzu hinlänglich erfundene, und Gebrauch dieses Traktats, vermöge bisheriger reicher Erfahrung die gewöhnlichen, auch schweren Krankheiten sicher und mit gutem Success kurieren Könne, nun zum viertenmale gedruckt und herausgegeben von D. Christian Sigismund Richter und D. Johann Wolfgang Künstlin, Med. Pract. in Halle.* (Leipzig: Johann Friedrich Gleditsch and Son, 1712; other eds. are Halle: Waisenhaus, 1708, 1710, 1715, et seq.).

Riddle, John M. *Contraception and Abortion from the Ancient World to the Renaissance.* (Cambridge, Mass.: Harvard University Press, 1992).

———. *Eve's Herbs: A History of Contraception and Abortion in the West.* (Cambridge, Mass.: Harvard University Press, 1997).

Riley, James C. "Disease Without Death: New Sources for a History of Sickness." *Journal of Interdisciplinary History* 17.3 (1987): 537–63.

———. *The Eighteenth-Century Campaign to Avoid Disease.* (New York: Macmillan, 1987).

Risse, Guenter B. *Hospital Life in Enlightenment Scotland: Care and Teaching at the Royal Infirmary of Edinburgh.* (Cambridge: Cambridge University Press, 1986).

———. "Hospital History: New Sources and Methods." In *Problems and Methods in the History of Medicine*, ed. Roy Porter and Andrew Wear. (London: Croom Helm, 1987), 175–204.

———. "Medicine in New Spain." In *Medicine in the New World*, ed. Ronald L. Numbers. (Knoxville: University of Tennessee Press, 1987).

———. "Before the Clinic Was 'Born': Methodological Perspectives in Hospital History." In *Institutions of Confinement: Hospitals, Asylums, and Prisons in Western Europe and North America, 1500–1950*, ed. Norbert Jütte and Robert Finzsch. (Washington, D.C.: Cambridge University Press, 1996), 75–96.

Risse, Guenter B., Ronald L. Numbers, and Judith Walzer Leavitt, eds. *Medicine Without Doctors.* (New York: Science History Publications, 1977).

Ritschl, Albrecht. *Geschichte des Pietismus*, 3 vols. (1880–86; reprint Berlin: de Gruyter, 1966).

Roeber, A. Gregory. "In German Ways." In *Strangers in the Realm: Cultural Margins of the First British Empire*, ed. Bernard Bailyn and Philip D. Morgan. (Chapel Hill: University of North Carolina Press, 1991).

———. *Palatines, Liberty, and Property: German Lutherans in Colonial British America.* (Baltimore: Johns Hopkins University Press, 1993).

———. "The Mosheim Society and the Preservation of German Education and Culture in the New Republic, 1789–1813." In *Mutual Influence on Education in Germany and the United States*, ed. Hartmut Lehmann, and Kenneth F. Ledford. (Cambridge: Cambridge University Press, 1995).

———. "J. H. C. Helmuth, Evangelical Charity, and the Public Sphere in Pennsylvania, 1793–1800." *Pennsylvania History* 121.1–2 (1997): 77–100.

———. "German and Dutch Books and Printing. In *A History of the Book in America: The Colonial Book in the Atlantic World*, ed. Hugh Amory and David D. Hall. (Cambridge and New York: Cambridge University Press, 1999), 298–313.

Rose, Craig, "Politics and the London Royal Hospitals, 1683–1692." In *The Hospital in History*, ed. Lindsay Granshaw and Roy Porter. (New York: Routledge, 1989).

Rosen, George. *A History of Public Health*. (New York, 1958).

———. "Cameralism and the Concept of Medical Police." In *From Medical Police to Social Medicine: Essays on the History of Health Care*. (New York: Science History Publications, 1974).

Rosenberg, Charles E. "Medical Text and Social Context: Explaining William Buchan's Domestic Medicine." *Bulletin of the History of Medicine* 23 (1983): 22–42.

Rosenberg, Charles E., ed. *Caring for the Working Man: The Rise and Fall of the Dispensary, An Anthology of Sources*. (New York: Garland, 1989).

Rothermund, Dietmar. *The Layman's Progress: Religious and Political Experience in Colonial Pennsylvania, 1740–1770*. (Philadelphia: University of Pennsylvania Press, 1961).

Rothman, David J. *The Discovery of the Asylum: Social Order, and Disorder in the New Republic*. (Boston: Little Brown, 1971).

Rush, Benjamin. "Account of the Manners of the German Inhabitants of Pennsylvania." In *Proceedings of the Pennsylvania German Society*, ed. T. E. Schmauk. (1910).

———. *A Letter by Dr. Benjamin Rush Describing the Consecration of the German College at Lancaster in June 1787*. (With an introduction and notes by H. Butterfield; Lancaster, Pa., 1945).

Rutten, A. M. G. "Slavenhandel, ziekten en mortaliteit in de Curacaose medisch-farmaceutische geschiedenis." *Farmaceutisch Weekblad* 27.15 (1992): 389–406.

———. "Drinkbaar goud voor zwarte slaven; de geneesmiddel farbriktie op Curaçao in 1707 en de Hallese piëtisten." *GEWINA* 21 (1998): 127–30.

Sachse, Julius Friedrich. *History of the German Role in the Discovery, Exploration, and Settlement of the New World*. (Bowie, Md.: Heritage Books, 1991).

Sachsse, Christoph, and Florian Tennstedt. *Geschichte der Armenfürsorge in Deutschland: Vom Spätmittelalter zum 1. Weltkrieg*. (Stuttgart: Kohlhammer, 1980).

Sames, Arnold. *Anton Wilhelm Böhme, 1673–1722: Studien zum ökumenischen Denken und Handeln eines halleschen Pietisten*. Arbeiten zur Geschichte des Pietismus 26. (Göttingen: Vandenhoeck and Ruprecht, 1990).

Savacool, Jacob Woodrow. "Illness and Therapy in Two Eighteenth-Century Physician Texts." *Caduceus* 13.1 (1997): 51–66.

Savitt, Todd L., and J. Harvey Young, eds. *Disease and Distinctiveness in the American South*. (Knoxville: University of Tennessee Press, 1988).

Scarborough, John, ed. *Folklore and Folk Medicines*. (Madison, Wisc.: American Institute of the History of Pharmacy, 1987).

Schicketanz, Peter. *Carl Hildebrand von Cansteins Beziehungen zu Philipp Jacob Spener*. Arbeiten zur Geschichte des Pietismus 1. (Witten, 1963).

Schicketanz, Peter, ed. *Der Briefwechsel Carl Hildebrand von Cansteins mit August Hermann Francke*. (Berlin and New York: De Gruyter, 1972).

Schlenther, Boyd Stanley. "'To Convert the Poor People in America': The Bethesda Orphanage and the Thwarted Zeal of the Countess of Huntingdon." *Georgia Historical Quarterly* 77.2 (1994): 225–56.

Schneider, Jürgen, Oskar Schwarzer, Friedrich Zellfelder, and Markus Denzel, eds. *Geld und Währungen in Europa im 18. Jahrhundert*. Beiträge zur Wirtschafts-und Sozialgeschichte 49. (Stuttgart: Franz Steiner Verlag, 1992).

———. *Europäische Wechselkurse im 17. Jahrhundert*. Beiträge zur Wirtschafts-und Sozialgeschichte 46. (Stuttgart: Franz Steiner Verlag, 1993).

Schneider, Wolfgang. "Geheimmittel und Spezialitäten." In *Lexikon zur Arzneimittelgeschichte*, Band iv. (Frankfurt: Govi-Verlag, 1969).

Schoultz, Martin Weyer von der. *Stadt und Gesundheit im Ruhrgebiet, 1850–1929: Verstädterung und kommunale Gesundheitspolitik dargestellt am Beispiel der jungen Industriestadt Gelsenkirchen*. (Essen: Klartexte, 1994).

Schrader, Hans-Jürgen. *Literaturproduktion und Büchermarkt des radikalen Pietismus: Johann Heinrich Reitz: "Historie Der Wiedergebohrnen" und ihr geschichtlicher Kontext*. (Göttingen: Vandenhoeck und Ruprecht, 1989).

Schroeder, John Frederick. "Plea for the Industrious Poor and Strangers, in Sickness: An Address Delivered at the Opening of and Edifice Erected by the Trustees of the New York Dispensary, January 11, 1830." In *Caring for the Working Man: The Rise and Fall of the Dispensary, An Anthology of Sources*, ed. Charles E. Rosenberg. (New York: Garland, 1989), 35–62.

Schwartz, Sally. *A Mixed Multitude*. (New York and London: New York University Press, 1987).

Schweinitz, Edmund de. "The Financial History of the Province and Its Sustentation Fund." Unpublished typescript. (Bethlehem, Pa.: Moravian Archives, 1877).

Scofield, Roger, and John Walter, eds. *Famine, Disease, and the Social Order in Early Modern Society*. (Cambridge: Cambridge University Press, 1989).

Seils, Markus. "Friedrich Albrecht Carl Gren in seiner Zeit, 1760–1798." *Heidelberger Schriften zur Pharmazie und Naturwissenschaftsgeschichte*, ed. Wolf-Dieter Müller-Jahncke. (Stuttgart: Wissenschaftliche Verlagsgesellschaft, 1995).

Shackelford, Jole. "Rosicrucianism, Lutheran Orthodoxy, and the Rejection of Paracelsianism in Early Seventeenth-Century Denmark." *Bulletin of the History of Medicine* 70 (1996): 181–204.

Shoemaker, Robert. "Reforming the City: The Reformation of Manners Campaign in London, 1690–1738." In *Stilling the Grumbling Hive: The Response to Social and Economic Problems in England, 1689–1750*, ed. Robert B. Shoemaker et al. (New York: St. Martin's Press, 1992), 99–120.

Shoemaker, Robert B., et al., eds. *Stilling the Grumbling Hive: The Response to Social and Economic Problems in England, 1689–1750*. (New York: St. Martin's Press, 1992).

Shryock, Richard H. *Medicine and Society in America, 1650–1860*. (New York: New York University Press, 1960).

———. *Medical Licensing in America, 1650–1965*. (Baltimore, 1967).

Silverman, Kenneth. *The Life and Times of Cotton Mather*. (New York, 1984).

Smaby, Beverly P. *The Transformation of Moravian Bethlehem: From Communal Mission to Family Economy*. (Philadelphia, 1988).

Smith, C. Earle. "Henry Mühlenberg, Botanical Pioneer." *Proceedings of the American Philosophical Society* 106 (1962): 443–60.

Smith, Ginnie. "Prescribing the Rules of Health: Self-Help and Advice in the Late 18th Century." In *Patients and Practitioners*, ed. Roy Porter. (Cambridge: Cambridge University Press, 1985), 249–82.

Sonnedecker, Glenn. "The Rise of Drug Manufacture in America." *Emory University Quarterly* 21 (1965): 73–87.

Sonnedecker, Glenn, ed. *Kremers and Urdang's History of Pharmacy.* 4th ed. (Philadelphia: J. D. Lippincott, 1976).

Sonnedecker, Glenn, and Gregory J. Higby. *Pharmacy in the Individual States.* (Madison, Wisc.: American Institute for the History of Pharmacy, 1984).

Spierenburg, Pieter. *The Prison Experience, Disciplinary Institutions, and Their Inmates in Early Modern Europe.* (New Brunswick: Rutgers University Press, 1982).

Splitter, Wolfgang M. "A Free People in the American Air: The Evolution of German Lutherans from British Subjects to Pennsylvania Citizens, 1740–1790." Doctoral dissertation, Johns Hopkins University, 1993.

Stahl, Georg Ernst. *Observationes clinico-practicae: Worinnen gezeigt wird, wie ein Praktikus die menschlichen Kranckheiten nach den verschiedenen Eigenschaften . . . gründlich heilen solle.* (Leipzig: Caspar Jacob Eyssel, 1718).

———. *Über den mannigfaltigen Einfluss von Gemütsbewegungen auf den menschlichen Körper (neben drei weiteren Arbeiten von Stahl).* (Leipzig: Barth, 1961).

Steele, Ian Kenneth. *Atlantic Merchant-Apothecary: Letters of Joseph Cruttenden, 1710–1717.* (Toronto and Buffalo: University of Toronto Press, 1977).

Stoeffler, F. Ernest. *The Rise of Evangelical Pietism.* (Leiden: E. J. Brill, 1965).

———. *German Pietism During the 18th Century.* (Leiden: E. J. Brill, 1973).

Stoeffler, F. Ernest, ed. *Continental Pietism and Early American Christianity.* (Grand Rapids: Bermans, 1976).

Stolleis, Michael. "Veit Ludwig von Seckendorff." In *Staatsdenker im 17. und 18. Jahrhundert, Reichspublizistik, Politik, Naturrecht,* ed. Richard Stolleis. (Frankfurt am Main, 1977), 148–73.

Sträter, Udo. "Pietismus und Sozialtätigkeit." *Pietismus und Neuzeit: Jahrbuch zur Geschichte des Neueren Protestantismus* 8 (1982): 201–30.

———. "Soziales Engagement bei Spener." *Pietismus und Neuzeit: Jahrbuch zur Geschichte des Neueren Protestantismus* 12 (1986): 70–83.

———. *Sonthom, Bayly, Dike, und Hall: Studien zur Rezeption der englischen Erbauungsliteratur in Deutschland im 17. Jahrhundert.* (Tübingen, 1987).

Sudhoff, Carl, ed. *Johann Christian Reil, Von der Lebenskraft.* (Leipzig, 1910).

Sykes, Norman. *Church and State in England in the 18th Century.* (Cambridge: Cambridge University Press, 1934).

Szindely, E. *Krankheit und Heilung im älteren Pietismus.* (Stuttgart, 1962).

Tappert, Theodore G., and John W. Doberstein, eds. *The Journals of Henry Melchior Mühlenberg, vol. 1, 1742–1763, vol. 2, 1764–1776, vol. 3, 1777–1787.* (Philadelphia: Mühlenberg Press, 1942–58; reprint Picton Press, 1982).

Telle, Joachim. "Arzneikunst und der 'gemeine Mann': Zum deutsch-lateinischen Sprachenstreit in der frühneuzeitlichen Medizin." In *Ausstellungskatalog der Herzog August Bibliothek.* (Wolfenbüttel, 1982), 36, 43–50.

Tennent, John. *Every Man His Own Doctor: or, The Poor Planter's Physician.* (Philadelphia: Benjamin Franklin, 1736).

Thomas, Keith. *Religion and the Decline of Magic: Studies in Popular Beliefs in 16th and 17th Century England.* (London: Weidenfeld and Nicolson, 1971).

Tischner, Rudolf. *Geschichte der Homeopathie*. (Leipzig: Wilmar Schwabe, 1939).

Tissot, Samuel Auguste. *Advice to the People in General, with Regard to Their Health* . . . (Philadelphia: Sparhawk, 1771).

Trokhatchev, Sergey, and Renate Wilson. "Laurentius Blumentrost, Scion of a Russian-German Medical Family." In *Mezhdunarodnye medicinskie obzory*. (1993).

Ulrich, Laurel. *A Midwife's Tale*. (Cambridge, Mass.: Harvard University Press, 1990).

Urlsperger, Johann August, ed. *Americanisches Ackerwerk Gottes, der zuverlässigen Nachrichten, den Zustand der americanischen erbauten Pflanzstadt Ebenezer in Georgien betreffend*. (Augsburg: vol. 4, 1766).

Urlsperger, Samuel, ed. *Americanisches Ackerwerk Gottes, der zuverlässigen Nachrichten, den Zustand der americanischen erbauten Pflanzstadt Ebenezer in Georgien betreffend*. (Augsburg: vol. 1, 1753; vol. 2, 1755; vol. 3, 1759).

———. *Ausführliche Nachricht(en) von den Sal(t)zburgischen Emigranten, die sich in America niedergelassen haben* . . . *18 Continuationen*. (Halle: in Verlegung des Waisenhauses, 1735–52).

Van Horne, John, ed. *Religious Philanthropy and Colonial Slavery: The American Correspondence of the Associates of Dr. Bray, 1717–1777*. (Urbana: University of Illinois Press, 1985).

Vanja, Christina. "Aufwärterinnen, Narrenmägde, und Siechenmütter—Frauen in der Krankenpflege der frühen Neuzeit." *Medizin, Gesellschaft, und Geschichte* 11 (1992): 9–24.

Völker, Arina. "Die medizinischen und pharmazeutischen Einrichtungen der Franckeschen Stiftungen während der halleschen Amtsphase von Georg Ernst Stahl." In *Georg Ernst Stahl (1659–1734): Hallesches Symposiumm 1984*, ed. Wolfram Kaiser and Arina Völker. (Halle and Wittenberg: Martin-Luther-Universität Halle-Wittenberg, 1985), 66 (E 73).

———. "Die Medizin der Aufklärungsepoche und die heilkundliche Konzeption des Pietismus hallescher Prägung." In *Dixhuitieme: Zur Geschichte von Medizin und Naturwissenschaften im 18. Jahrhundert*, ed. Arina Völker. Wissenschaftliche Beiträge der Martin-Luther-Universität Halle-Wittenberg. (Halle and Wittenberg, 1988), 20 (T. 67).

Völker, Arina, and Burchhard Thaler, eds. *Die Entwicklung des medizinhistorischen Unterrichts: Wolfram Kaiser zum 60. Geburtstag*. (Wittenberg: Martin-Luther-Universität Halle-Wittenberg, 1982).

von Wreech, Curt Friedrich. *Wahrhafte und umständliche Historie von denen schwedischen Gefangenen* . . . (Rothe: Sorau, 1728).

Vorsey De, Louis, Jr., ed. *De Brahm's Report of the General Survey in the Southern District of North America*. (Columbia: University of South Carolina Press, 1967).

Walker, Mack. *The Salzburg Transaction: Expulsion and Redemption in Eighteenth-Century Germany*. (Ithaca: Cornell University Press, 1992).

Wallace, Paul A. W. *The Mühlenbergs of Pennsylvania*. (Philadelphia: University of Pennsylvania Press, 1950).

Wallmann, Johannes. *Philipp Jakob Spener und die Anfänge des Pietismus*, 2d ed. (Tübingen: Mohr, 1986).

———. "Beziehungen des frühen Pietismus zum Baltikum und zu Finnland." In *Der Pietismus in seiner europäischen und aussereuropäischen Ausstrahlung: Suomenkieliset tiivistelmat*, ed. Johannes Wallmann and Pentti Laasonen. (Helsinki: Suomen Kirkkohistori-allinen Seura, 1992), 50–53.

Ward, William Reginald. *The Protestant Evangelical Awakening.* (Cambridge: Cambridge University Press, 1992).

Waring, John I. *Medicine in South Carolina.* (Charleston: South Carolina Medical Association, 1964).

Warner, John H. *The Therapeutic Perspective, Medical Practice, Knowledge, and Identity in America, 1820–1885.* (Cambridge, Mass.: Harvard University Press, 1986).

Watson, Patricia A. *The Angelical Conjunction: The Preacher-Physicians of Colonial New England.* (Knoxville: University of Tennessee Press, 1991).

Wear, Andrew. "Medical Practice in Late 17th and Early 18th Century England: Continuity and Union." In *The Medical Revolution of the Seventeenth Century*, ed. Roger K. French and Andrew Wear. (Cambridge: Cambridge University Press, 1989).

———. "The Popularization of Medicine in Early Modern England." In *The Popularization of Medicine, 1650–1850*, ed. Roy Porter. (London: Routledge, 1992), 17–41.

———. "Religious Beliefs in Early Modern England." In *The Task of Healing: Medicine, Religion, and Gender in England and the Netherlands, 1450–1800*, ed. Hilary Marland and Margaret Pelling. (Rotterdam: Erasmus, 1996), 145–70.

———. *Health and Healing in Early Modern England: Studies in Social and Intellectual History.* (Aldershot, England: Ashgate, 1998).

Webster, Charles. *The Great Instauration: Science, Medicine, and Reform, 1626–1660.* (London: Duckworth, 1975).

———. "Alchemical and Paracelsian Medicine." In *Health, Medicine, and Mortality in the Sixteenth Century*, ed. Charles Webster. (Cambridge: Cambridge University Press, 1979), 312–15.

———. "Paracelsus: Medicine as Popular Protest." In *Medicine and the Reformation*, ed. Ole Peter Grell and Andrew Cunningham. (London: Routledge, 1993), 57–77.

Weiser, Frederick, Paulette Weiser, and Edward Weiser, eds. *The Weiser Families in North America*, vol. 1. (Re-edit of 1924 and 1960 eds.; Rockport, Me.: Picton Press, 1996).

Welsch, Heinz. "Die Franckeschen Stiftungen als wirtschaftliches Grossunternehmen." In *August Hermann Francke: Das humanistische Erbe des grossen Erziehers.* (Halle: Francke Komittee, 1965), 28–44.

Wesley, John. *Primitive Physick: or, An Easy and Natural Method of Curing Most Diseases.* (Philadelphia: Crukshank, 1770).

———. *Primitive Physick: or, An Easy and Natural Method of Curing Most Diseases*, 15th ed. (London: Hawes, 1772).

Wessel, Carola. "'We Do Not Want to Introduce Anything New . . .': Transplanting the Communal Life from Herrnhut to the Upper Ohio Valley." In Hartmut Lehmann et al., eds., *In Search of Peace and Prosperity: New Settlements in Eighteenth-Century Europe and America.* (University Park: The Pennsylvania State University Press, 2000), 246–62.

Wiggin, Frederick Holme. "The Abuse of Medical Charity, Medical News Oct. 23, 1897." In *Caring for the Working Man: The Rise and Fall of the Dispensary, An Anthology of Sources*, ed. Charles E. Rosenberg. (New York: Garland, 1989), 157–78.

Wilson, Adrian. "Participant or Patient: Seventeenth-Century Childbirth from the Mother's Point of View." In *Patients and Practitioners: Lay Perceptions of Medicine in Pre-Industrial Society*, ed. Roy Porter. (Cambridge: Cambridge University Press, 1985), 133–37.

Wilson, Renate. "Die Halleschen Waisenhausmedikamente und die 'Höchst-nöthige Erkenntnis' im Kolonialstaat Georgien, 1733–1765." *Schriftenreihe für Technik, Naturwissenschaften, und Medizin* 28 (1991): 108–28.

———. "Public Works and Piety: The Missing Salzburger Diaries for 1744–1745." *Georgia Historical Quarterly* 77 (Summer 1993): 336–66.

———. "Continental Protestant Refugees and Their Protectors in Germany and London: Commercial and Charitable Networks." *Pietismus und Neuzeit* 20 (1994): 107–24.

———. "Pietist Universal Reform and Care of the Sick and the Poor: The Medical Institutions of the Francke Foundations and Their Social Context." In *Institutions of Confinement: Hospitals, Asylums, and Prisons in Western Europe and North America, 1500–1950*, ed. Norbert Finzsch and Robert Jütte. (New York: Cambridge University Press, 1996), 133–54.

———. "Heinrich Wilhelm Ludolf, August Hermann Francke, und der Eingang nach Russland." In *Halle und Osteuropa*, ed. J. Wallmann and U. Sträter. (Halle: Niemeyer; Tübingen: Verlag der Franckeschen Stiftungen, 1997), 83–108.

———. "The Traffic in Halle Orphanage Medications: Medicinals, Philanthropy, and Colonial Mission." *Caduceus* 13.1 (Spring 1997): 6–22.

———. "The Development of Eighteenth-Century Voluntary Institutions: Medical Care and Social Reform." *Voluntas* 9 (Spring 1998): 81–101.

———. "The Halle Pietists in Georgia." *Lutheran Quarterly* 12 (Summer 1998): 271–301.

———. "Land, Population, and Labor: Lutheran Immigrants in Colonial Georgia." In Hartmut Lehmann et al., eds., *In Search of Peace and Prosperity: New German Settlements in Eighteenth-Century Europe and North America*. (University Park: The Pennsylvania State University Press, 2000), 217–45.

Wilson, Renate, and Hans Joachim Poeckern. "A Continental System of Medical Care in Colonial Georgia." *Medizin, Gesellschaft, und Geschichte: Jahrbuch des Instituts für Geschichte der Medizin der Robert Bosch Stiftung* 9 (1992): 99–126.

Wilson, Renate, and Peter Nolte. "The Diary of a Country Parson in Colonial Georgia." In *The German Language in America, 1683–1991*, ed. J. Salmons. (Madison: University of Wisconsin Press, 1993), 13–29.

Winter, Eduard. *Halle als Ausgangspunkt der deutschen Russlandkunde im 18. Jahrhundert.* (Berlin: Akademie-Verlag, 1953).

Witt, Ulrike. *Bekehrung, Bildung, und Biographie: Frauen im Umkreis des Halleschen Pietismus.* (Halle, Franckesche Stiftungen-Thieme, 1996).

Wokeck, Marianne S. "The Flow and Composition of German Immigration to Philadelphia, 1727–1755." *Pennsylvania Magazine of History and Biography* 105 (1981): 244–78.

———. "Harnessing the Lure of the 'Best Poor Man's Country': The Dynamics of German-Speaking Immigration to British North America, 1683–1783." In *To Make America: European Emigration in the Early Modern Period*, ed. I Altman and J. Horn. (Berkeley and Los Angeles: University of California Press, 1991).

———. "Charting Courses Between Assimilation and Persistence: German Settlements in the American Colonies." In Hartmut Lehmann et al., eds., *In Search of Peace and Prosperity: New German Settlements in Eighteenth-Century Europe and North America* (University Park: The Pennsylvania State University Press, 2000), 191–216.

———. *Trade in Strangers: The Beginnings of Mass Migration to North America*. (University Park: The Pennsylvania State University Press, 1999).

Wolf, Evemarie. *Über die Anfänge der Pharmaziegeschichtschreibung, Von Johannes Ruellius (1529) bis David Peter Hermann Schmidt (1835)*. (Stuttgart: Wissenschaftliche Verlagsgesellschaft, 1996).

Woods, Jean W., and Fürstenwald, Maria A. *Schriftstellerinnen, Künstlerinnen, und gelehrte Frauen des deutschen Barock: Ein Lexikon*. (Stuttgart: Metzler, 1984).

Woodward, Josiah. *Francke's Pietas Halensis*. Bound with other Francke tracts. (London, 1708).

Woolf, Stuart, ed. *Domestic Strategies: Work and Family in France and Italy, 1600–1800*. (Cambridge: Cambridge University Press, 1991).

Wunder, Heide. *Er ist die Sonn, sie ist der Mond: Frauen in der Frühen Neuzeit*. (Munich: Beck, 1992).

Wunder, Heide, and Christina Vanja. *Wandel der Geschlechterbeziehungen zu Beginn der Neuzeit*. (Frankfurt am Main: Suhrkamp, 1991).

Young, J. Harvey. "Patent Medicines: Early Example of Competitive Marketing." *Journal of Economic History* 20 (1960): 649.

Young, James Harvey. *Toadstool Millionaires: A Social History of Patent Medicines in America Before Federal Regulation*. (Princeton: Princeton University Press, 1962).

Zaunick, Rudolph. *Beiträge zur Geschichte des Gesundheitswesens der Stadt Halle und der medizinischen Fakultät der Universität Halle: Acht Abhandlungen*. (Leipzig: Joh. Ambrosius Barth, 1965).

Zäpernick, Gertraud. "Johann Georg Gichtels und seiner Nachfolger Briefwechsel mit den hallischen Pietisten, besonders mit A. M. Francke." *Pietismus und Neuzeit* 8 (1982): 74–118.

Zimmermann, Heinz. *Arzneimittelwerbung in Deutschland vom Beginn des 16. bis zu Ende des 18. Jahrhunderts*. (Würzburg: Jal-Verlag, 1974).

Index

Page numbers in *italics* refer to tables and figures.